Shahid M. Hussain

Liver MRI

Correlation with Other Imaging Modalities
and Histopathology

Forewords by
John L. Gollan, MD, PhD and Richard C. Semelka, MD

With 114 Figures in 1.865 Parts

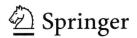 Springer

Shahid M. Hussain, MD, PhD
Professor of Radiology
Director of Body MRI
Chief Abdominal Imaging
Department of Radiology
University of Nebraska Medical Center
981045 Nebraska Medical Center
Omaha, NE 68198
USA
Email: smhussain@unmc.edu

ISBN 3-540-25552-4   Springer-Verlag Berlin Heidelberg New York

Library of Congress Control Number: 2006929204

Springer is a part of Springer Science+Business Media
http://www.springer.com

© Springer-Verlag Berlin Heidelberg 2007

Printed in Germany

Editor: Dr. Ute Heilmann
Desk Editor: Wilma McHugh
Copy-editing: WS Editorial Ltd, Shrewsbury, UK
Production Editor: Joachim W. Schmidt
Cover design: eStudio Calamar, Spain

Typesetting: FotoSatz Pfeifer GmbH, D-82166 Gräfelfing
Printed on acid-free paper – 21/3151 – 5 4 3 2 1 0

To Ellen, Emma, and Charlotte

Foreword I

In March 1973, a short paper was published in *Nature*, entitled „Image formation by induced local interaction; examples employing nuclear magnetic resonance." The author was Paul C. Lauterbur, a Professor of Chemistry at the State University of New York at Stony Brook. In this seminal manuscript the author described a new imaging technique which moved the single dimension of NMR spectroscopy to the dual dimension of spatial orientation, thereby resulting in the foundation of modern magnetic resonance (MR) imaging. Over the ensuing years, MR imaging has assumed an increasingly important role in clinical imaging. It distinguishes itself from other imaging modalities, such as ultrasound (US) or computed tomography (CT), by the unique ability to visualize specific tissue components in a non-invasive manner.

In the earlier days, diagnostic MR imaging was limited to cerebral and musculoskeletal diseases. Imaging of other areas which are more prone to movement through breathing (abdominal) or pulsation motions (cardiac) became available more recently, with the introduction of faster sequences and the development of more dedicated MR imaging coils. Currently, liver MRI is considered the cornerstone of abdominal imaging. In most centers, however, liver MRI is still employed largely as a problem solving modality, when US and CT have provided an unsatisfactory outcome. This truly is an unfortunate misconception, which should be abandoned in favor of MR imaging as the primary modality for detection and characterization of liver abnormalities. If applied in the form of state-of-the-art technology, MR imaging has the potential of providing an accurate diagnosis of focal liver lesions in the majority of cases, frequently obviating the need for more invasive strategies.

We are standing on the verge of a new breakthrough in MR imaging, with the introduction of clinical high field MRI systems, such as 3.0T, multiple coil elements, parallel imaging capabilities, stronger gradients, and faster computers. Collectively, these developments will undoubtedly initiate a new era in MR imaging of the liver. The author of this impressive text, Dr. Shahid Hussain, and our institution are on the forefront of these important developments. This textbook with its numerous high quality illustrations, including computer-generated drawings, state-of-the-art MR images and radiology-pathology correlations, provides an accurate and up-to-date overview of imaging findings of a wide spectrum of liver lesions. The manner in which the contents of this book are presented provides an intuitive, easy to read approach, albeit on the topic of liver nodules or the analysis of parenchymal disorders. This textbook will be of particular benefit for clinicians and radiologists involved in the diagnosis and management of hepatic diseases.

MRI imaging will most certainly continue to emerge as a key, primary imaging modality for a broad spectrum of liver diseases. Likewise, it is essential that MRI becomes increasingly familiar to those who provide care for patients with liver abnormalities. Hence, I highly recommend this book as a routine companion for radiologists whilst reviewing MR examinations in the clinical setting, as study book for professionals in-training, such as radiology and gastroenterology fellows, and as reference for more experienced hepatologists, gastroenterologists, surgeons and pathologists. This is an easy way to acquire new knowledge on the topic of MR imaging.

John L. Gollan, MD, PhD, FRACP, FRCP, FACP
Dean, College of Medicine,
University of Nebraska Medical Center,
Omaha, Nebraska, USA

Foreword II

Annually, many thousands of patients worldwide undergo imaging for the workup of a suspected or known abnormality of the liver. Cross-sectional imaging modalities, such as ultrasound (US), computed tomography (CT), and magnetic resonance imaging (MRI), are utilized in most centers to assess liver abnormalities. These modalities, often used in various combinations, have fundamental differences in data acquisition and hence differences in the type of physical characteristics of tissues that they interrogate.

The major focus of this book is to describe that MR imaging is an accurate technique for the evaluation of focal liver lesions. MR imaging can also be used to evaluate diffuse hepatic diseases, hepatic vascular abnormalities (MR angiography), and biliary diseases (MR cholangiography). In the near future, it will be feasible to evaluate functional aspects of the liver through the use of one or more combinations of current fast breath hold MR imaging sequences, and MR spectroscopy, diffusion-weighted imaging, perfusion imaging and non-proton imaging. MR imaging may soon play a unique role in molecular imaging of the liver, including the specific targeting of diseased tissues, as well as providing imaging guidance for future smart drugs or cell delivery systems.

The introduction of multiple coil elements, parallel imaging, stronger gradients, and faster computers will undoubtedly increase the cranio-caudal (z-) coverage substantially. High resolution MR imaging of the abdomen and pelvis in a single exam (like CT) without the use of ionizing radiation and nephrotoxic iodine contrast media will become a reality. Liver MRI, however, will remain a crucial part of such a strategy that is important for staging malignancies in the abdomen.

By nature MR imaging is considered a complex modality by many radiologists and clinicians. This book succeeds in making liver MRI more accessible to the experienced as well as novice users who intend to use MR imaging for evaluation of liver abnormalities. MR imaging findings and concepts are presented and explained in simple-to-interpret computer-generated drawings. Additional explanation is provided by the radiology-pathology correlation and comparison to other imaging modalities. A particular strength of Dr. Hussain's book is the extensive correlation with other imaging modalities, to allow the reader to have a fuller understanding of how the imaging modalities interrelate.

Shahid Hussain is one of the world's recognized authorities on imaging of diseases of the liver. This book reveals his breadth of knowledge on this subject. Therefore, I can highly recommend this book to radiologists, clinicians, residents, radiology technicians, and students. Radiologists and radiology residents may particularly find this book useful during the reporting process of liver MR imaging exams.

Richard C. Semelka, MD
Professor and Vice-Chair of Research,
Director of MRI Services,
Department of Radiology,
University of North Carolina at Chapel Hill,
Chapel Hill, North Carolina, USA

Preface

This book provides a practical approach for MR imaging of the focal and diffuse liver lesions based on the state-of-the-art MR imaging sequences, computer-generated drawings, concise figure captions, relevant and systematic (differential) diagnostic information, recent literature references, and patient management possibilities. MR imaging findings are correlated to ultrasound, computed tomography, and pathology when appropriate. This book will greatly benefit all professionals interested and involved in imaging, diagnosis, and treatment of focal and diffuse liver lesions, including radiologists, gastroenterologists, surgeons, pathologists, MR physicists, MRI clinical scientists, radiology and other residents, MR technicians, and students.

This manuscript has especially benefited from the critical review by the following Body MR imaging experts and colleagues: Franz Sulzer, MD and Indra C. van den Bos, MD.

In addition, I am grateful to the following colleagues and friends for their continuous support during the past several years: Richard C. Semelka, MD, Donald G. Mitchell, MD, Eric K. Outwater, MD, Caroline Reinhold, MD, Michèle A. Brown, MD, Masayuki Kanematsu, MD, Nikolaos L. Kelekis, MD, Susan M. Ascher, MD, Sat Somers, MD, N. Cem Balci, MD, Diego R. Martin, MD, Till R. Bader, MD, PhD, Kees van Kuijk, MD, PhD, Peter M.T. Pattynama, MD, PhD, Abida Z. Ginai, MD, PhD, Jan C. den Hollander, MD, Robert A. de Man, MD, PhD, Pieter E. Zondervan, MD, Türkan Terkivatan, MD, PhD, Jan N.M. IJzermans, MD, PhD, Kees Verhoef, MD, Gabriel P. Krestin, MD, PhD, Johannes L. Bloem, MD, PhD, Reginald Goei, MD, PhD, Roy S. Dwarkasing, MD, Remy W.F. Geenen, MD, Jayant R. Kichari, MD, and Steven D. Wexner, MD, FACS, FRCS.

Finally, I am thankful to John L. Gollan, MD, PhD, Dean of the College of Medicine, and Craig W. Walker, MD, Professor and Chairman of the Department of Radiology at the University of Nebraska Medical Center, for their incessant support and for providing a positive and a stimulating academic environment.

Shahid M Hussain, MD, PhD
Professor of Radiology
Director of Body MRI
Chief Abdominal Imaging
Department of Radiology
University of Nebraska Medical Center
981045 Nebraska Medical Center
Omaha, NE 68198
USA
Email: smhussain@unmc.edu

How To Use This Book

MR imaging is a unique imaging modality which allows a comprehensive evaluation of the liver and includes the visualization of the soft tissue components based on various T1- and T2-weighted sequences, the vascularity based on routine dynamic gadolinium-enhanced imaging and MR angiography, and the biliary tree based on MR cholangiography. The versatility of MR imaging and the amount of the diagnostic information obtained from a single liver MRI examination may intimidate the reader. This book provides a unique approach to simplifying liver MRI.

To diagnose most liver diseases, four sequences are most important to evaluate. These include: (1) a fat-suppressed T2-weighted sequence (or an equivalent sequence); (2) a T1 in-phase gradient-echo sequence; (3) arterial-phase dynamic gadolinium-enhanced images; and (4) delayed-phase gadolinium-enhanced images. This book provides computer-generated drawings of these or four similar MRI sequences to highlight and explain the most important diagnostic findings. The direct MRI drawing comparison facilitates the interpretation of the important imaging findings. In addition, background information and up-to-date available literature is provided, with correlation to other imaging modalities (US, CT) and pathology.

Liver abnormalities are divided into five major categories. Within each category, subcategories are provided and more specific diagnoses are listed alphabetically. Based on this book, liver MRI can be approached as follows:

- Step I: Categorize the liver abnormality into one of the five groups:
    1. High-fluid content liver lesions (high signal on T2 which persists on longer T2)
    2. Solid liver lesions (moderately high signal on T2; similar to the spleen or lower)
    3. Diffuse liver lesions (expressed by the diffuse or segmental abnormal signal or enhancement)
    4. Vascular liver lesions (visible mainly in the arterial phase)
    5. Biliary tree abnormalities (visible on T2-weighted and MRCP sequences)
- Step II: Evaluate the signal intensity on fat-suppressed T2- and T1-weighted sequences as well as gadolinium-enhanced images and attempt a more specific diagnosis.
- Step III: Compare your working diagnosis to the specific examples within each category systematically and confirm your finding into a more definitive (differential) diagnosis.

This approach is consistently applied throughout the book, which shows that most liver lesions can be detected and characterized based on this method. At the end of the book, several examples of differential diagnostic comparisons have been provided of the most common liver lesions. The reader is encouraged to develop a similar approach during reading liver MRI exams in daily clinical practice. In addition, two appendices have been provided to explain a typical liver MR imaging protocol and the normal segmental anatomy of the liver.

Contents

High-Fluid Content Liver Lesions

I

1 Abscesses – Pyogenic Type

Hepatic abscesses result from an infectious process of bacterial origin associated with destruction of the hepatic parenchyma and stroma in 0.006–2.2% of hospital admissions. Gram-negative bacteria of colonic origin (*E. coli, Klebsiella,* and *Enterobacter*) can often be isolated from such abscesses. Pyogenic liver abscesses may result from obstruction of the biliary tract with stasis of bile and bacterial overgrowth, or as a complication of direct biliary tract infection. Hematogenous spread and bacterial seeding of the liver may occur via the portal vein secondary to abdominal infection. Other less common routes are hematogenous and direct perihepatic spread.

MR Imaging Findings

Hepatic abscess presents as a relatively complicated fluid collection, which is composed of central areas with low signal intensity on T1-weighted images and high signal intensity on T2-weighted images. Particularly, on T2-weighted images the central cavity may show septa and debris. A central fluid-containing cavity is often surrounded by a few millimeters (in most cases: 1–5 mm; in some cases: >5 mm) of thick inflamed liver parenchyma (wall of the abscess), which most likely contains microabscesses. Perilesional (wedge-shaped) edema may be present. Most abscesses show early persistent enhancement of the wall (Figs. 1.1–1.3A, B). Although in most patients the diagnosis and follow-up is carried out on computed tomography (CT), magnetic resonance (MR) imaging is increasingly being performed on acutely ill patients; therefore, it is important for radiologists to understand the appearance of hepatic abscesses at MR imaging.

Differential Diagnosis

In ambiguous cases, the differential diagnosis may include: (1) metastases (the ring enhancement progresses in a centripetal fashion with a decrease in intensity on delayed images); (2) infected metastases (difficult to differentiate; thicker and more irregular wall; clinical history important); (3) hepatosplenic candidiasis (multiple lesions <10 mm in diameter); (4) hydatid cysts (internal septa); (5) echinococcus abscesses (thicker septa and daughter cysts) (Fig. 1.3C, D).

Management

Management options include: (1) percutaneous drainage; (2) open surgical drainage; and (3) antibiotic therapy. Single dominant hepatic abscess with a large fluid cavity can be treated with percutaneous drainage. Treatment should be tailored to each patient.

Literature

1. Mendez RJ, Schiebler ML, Outwater EK, Kressel HY (1994) Hepatic abscesses: MR imaging findings. Radiology 190:431–436
2. Balci CN, Semelka RC, Noone TC, et al. (1999) Pyogenic hepatic abscesses: MRI findings on T1- and T2-weighted and serial gadolinium-enhanced gradient-echo images. J Magn Reson Imaging 9:285–290
3. Perez JAA, Gonzalez JJ, Baldonedo RF, et al. (2001) Clinical course, treatment, and multivariate analysis of risk factors for pyogenic liver abscess. Am J Surg 181:177–186

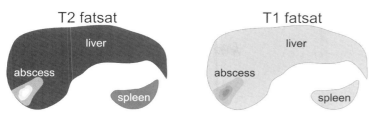 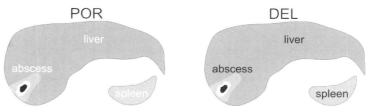

Fig. 1.1. Abscess, pyogenic type, drawings. T2 fatsat: in the right liver, a small fluid collection (high signal) is surrounded by a wedge-shaped area of edema; **T1 fatsat:** the fluid is slightly hypointense to the liver with faintly visible edema; **POR:** an evenly thick layer of liver tissue surrounding the fluid collection shows enhancement; **DEL:** the thick wall of the abscess remains enhanced in the delayed phase

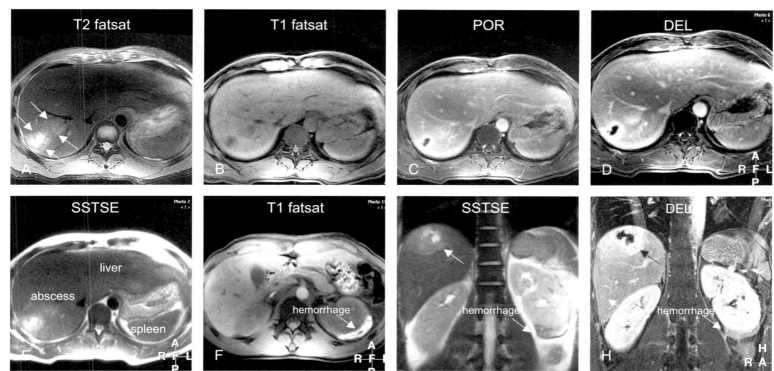

Fig. 1.2. Abscess, pyogenic type, MR imaging findings at 3.0T. A Axial fat-suppressed T2-weighted turbo spin echo (TSE) image (T2 fatsat): In the right liver, a small fluid collection is surrounded by a wedge-shaped area of edema (*arrows*). **B** Axial fat-suppressed T1-weighted gradient recalled echo (GRE) (T1 fatsat): The fluid collection is hypointense to the liver with faintly visible edema. **C** Axial portal phase gadolinium (Gd)-enhanced three-dimensional (3D) T1-w GRE image (POR): The fluid collection has a thick wall. **D** Axial delayed phase GRE image (DEL): The wall of the abscess shows persistent enhancement (no washout). **E** Axial T2-weighted single-shot TSE image (SSTSE): The central part of the abscess contains fluid due to necrosis. **F** Axial fat-suppressed GRE image through the kidneys (T1 fatsat): Perinephric hemorrhage (an incidental finding) shows high signal (*arrow*). **G** Coronal SSTSE image (SSTSE): The abscess is subcapsular to the liver (*arrow*). **H** Coronal delayed phase image (DEL): The wall of the abscess has a ragged appearance (*arrow*)

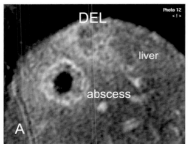 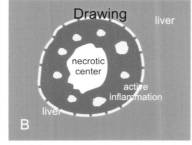 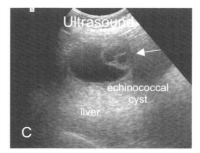 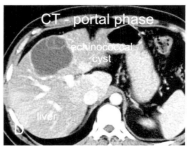

Fig. 1.3. Abscess anatomy. A A detailed view of the coronal high resolution delayed phase image (from the patient above) shows small cavities within the wall of the abscess. **B** Drawing of the abscess: the central cavity is filled with fluid that is surrounded by a wall of inflammation with (most likely) micro-abscesses and edema. **C** Ultrasound (US) (another patient) shows a typical echinococcal cyst with daughter cysts (*arrow*). **D** CT in portal phase confirms the US findings

2 Biliary Hamartomas (von Meyenberg Complexes)

Biliary hamartomas are benign biliary malformations, which are currently considered as part of the spectrum of fibropolycystic diseases of the liver due to ductal plate malformation. This entity is common and estimated to be present in approximately 3% of patients. These lesions are often discovered as incidental findings during cross-sectional imaging or during palpation of the surface of the liver during laparotomy, usually in the setting of colorectal malignancy. Biliary hamartomas may be solitary or multiple, and multiple tumors can be extensive.

MR Imaging

On MR images, tumors are small (usually < 1 cm), often multiple, and well defined. The high fluid content renders these lesions low signal on T1, high signal on T2, and negligible enhancement on early and late post-gadolinium images. Although this appearance resembles simple cysts, biliary hamartomas demonstrate a thin rim of enhancement on early and late post-contrast images (Figs. 2.1, 2.2).

Differential Diagnosis

The major potential diagnostic error is to misclassify these lesions as metastases due to the presence of ring enhancement. The thin enhancing rim of biliary hamartomas, visualized on imaging, may be correlated histopathologically with the presence of compressed hepatic parenchyma bordering the lesion. In contrast, the pattern of ring enhancement displayed by metastases relates histopathologically to the outermost vascularized portion of the tumor. Peritumoral enhancement is also observed in some metastases. MR imaging further corroborates the different histologic profiles of the two processes through the observation that enhancement in biliary hamartoma does not progress centrally, while enhancement in metastases most often progresses centrally.

Pathology

Histopathologically biliary hamartomas consist of a collection of small, sometimes dilated, irregular and branching bile ducts embedded in a fibrous stroma. A few of the ducts may contain inspissated bile. In general, biliary hamartomas contain no or few vascular channels (Fig. 2.3).

Management

No treatment or follow-up with imaging is required for typical biliary hamartomas.

Literature

1. Semelka RC, Hussain SM, Marcos HB, Woosley JT (1999) Biliary hamartomas: solitary and multiple lesions shown on current MR techniques including gadolinium enhancement. JMRI 10:196–201
2. Semelka RC, Hussain SM, Marcos HB, Woosley JT (2000) Perilesional enhancement of hepatic metastases: correlation between MR imaging and histopathologic findings – initial observations. Radiology 215:89–94
3. McLoughlin MJ, Phillips MJ (1975) Angiographic findings in multiple bile-duct hamartomas of the liver. Radiology 116:41–43

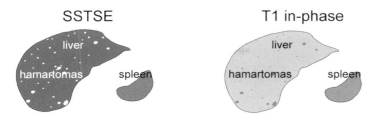
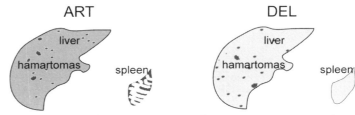

Fig. 2.1. Biliary hamartomas, drawings. SSTSE: hamartomas appear as multiple bright (cyst-like) lesions within a darker liver; **T1 in-phase**: hamartomas are predominantly hypointense compared to the liver; **ART**: hamartomas often show a faint rim of enhancement; **DEL**: hamartomas remain unenhanced like cysts in the liver but may have some residual rim of enhancement

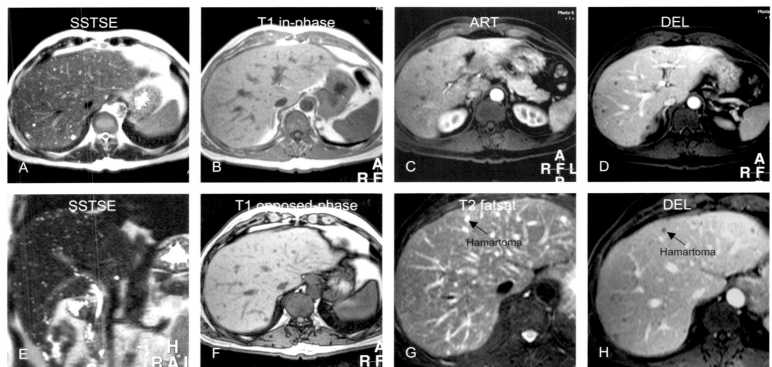

Fig. 2.2. Biliary hamartomas, multiple, typical MRI findings. A Axial SSTSE image (SSTSE): Biliary hamartomas are hyperintense (cyst-like) to the liver. **B** Axial in-phase image (T1 in-phase): Biliary hamartomas are hypointense and less obvious than on the T2-w images. **C** Axial arterial phase image (ART): Biliary hamartomas show a faint rim of enhancement. **D** Axial delayed phase image (DEL): Biliary hamartomas remain unenhanced like cysts in the liver but may have a faint persistent rim of enhancement. **E** Coronal SSTSE image (SSTSE): Biliary hamartomas are very bright and scattered throughout the liver, including the subcapsular region. **F** Axial opposed-phase image (T1 opposed-phase): No fatty infiltration is present. **G** Detailed view of axial fat-suppressed T2-w TSE image (T2 fatsat): Biliary hamartomas may be difficult to distinguish from surrounding vessels. **H** Detailed view of axial delayed phase image (DEL): Biliary hamartomas are predominantly non-enhancing lesions with a faint persistent rim of enhancement

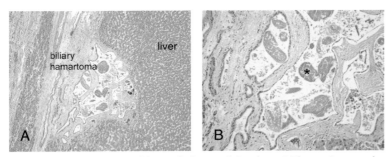
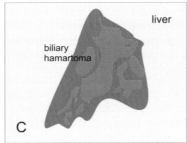
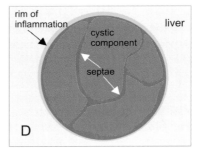

Fig. 2.3. Biliary hamartoma, histopathology and drawings. A Photomicrograph shows a biliary hamartoma that consists of a group of several small cysts filled with bile. Note the normal liver that surrounds the hamartoma. H&E, ×100. **B** Photomicrograph shows in detail the cystic components of the hamartoma filled with bile (*), which explains the high signal on T2-weighted images. H&E, ×200. **C** Drawing shows the collapsed biliary hamartoma in vitro. **D** Drawing shows the distended biliary hamartoma in vivo

3 Cyst I – Typical Small

Hepatic cysts are common lesions (they may occur in up to 20% of the general population). These lesions are usually divided into unilocular (95%) and multilocular varieties. Although the pathogenesis of these cysts is not clear, most hepatic cysts are considered to be developmental in origin. Currently, most hepatic cysts are discovered as incidental findings on cross-sectional imaging. Smaller cysts (<10 mm) at US and CT may be difficult to distinguish from solid lesions, and may cause diagnostic problems especially in patients with an underlying (colorectal) malignancy.

MR Imaging

At MR imaging, cysts are low in signal intensity on T1-weighted images, high in signal intensity on T2-weighted images, and retain signal intensity on longer echo time (e.g., >120 ms) T2-weighted images. After injection of contrast, cysts do not show any enhancement. On delayed post-gadolinium images (up to 5 min), cysts remain unenhanced. The latter findings may be useful to ensure that lesions are cysts and not poorly vascularized metastases that show gradual enhancement. T2-weighted sequences with a long echo time (TE) in combination with delayed phase images are especially effective at showing small (≤5 mm) cysts. MRI is particularly valuable when lesions are small and the patient has a known primary malignancy (Figs. 3.1, 3.2). Typical and relatively larger cysts can be characterized at CT as well as US (Figs. 3.3A, B).

Differential Diagnosis

Typical simple cysts at MR imaging do not cause any diagnostic problems and can be distinguished from other cystic lesions with confidence. Atypical cysts or cysts with septa may show overlapping features with other entities such as: (1) mucinous or cystic metastases (look for multiple septa and perilesional enhancement); and (2) ciliated foregut cysts (congenital lesions, frequently located at the anterior margin of the liver with mucinous content and a slightly bulging liver contour). The presence of a cystic lesion with an enhancing wall and extension beyond the contour of the liver may also be observed in some forms of metastatic disease such as hepatic metastasis from ovarian malignancies. For this reason, a diagnosis of foregut cyst on imaging studies should only be made in the absence of peritoneal disease and a clinical history of malignancy.

Pathology

Pathologically, the lining of the cyst shows a single layer of cuboidal to columnar epithelial cells. Lining epithelium rests on an underlying fibrous stroma (Fig. 3.3C, D).

Management

No treatment or follow-up with imaging is required for typical small hepatic cysts.

Literature

1. Rossai J (1995) Ackerman's surgical pathology, vol 1, 8th edn. Mosby, St. Louis, p 898
2. Mortele KJ, Ros PR (2001) Cystic focal liver lesions in the adult: differential CT and MR imaging features. Radiographics 21:895–910
3. Shoenut JP, Semelka RC, Levi C, Greenberg H (1994) Ciliated hepatic foregut cysts: US, CT, and contrast-enhanced MR imaging. Abdom Imaging 19:150–152

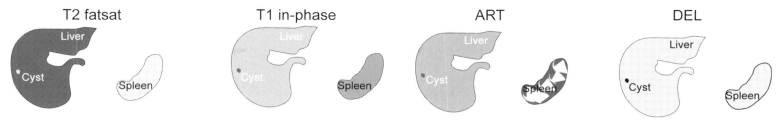

Fig. 3.1. Cyst, drawings. T2 fatsat: cyst is very bright (fluid-like) compared to the liver with smooth and sharp margins; T1 in-phase: cyst is hypointense to the liver; ART: cyst shows no enhancement; DEL: cyst remains unenhanced

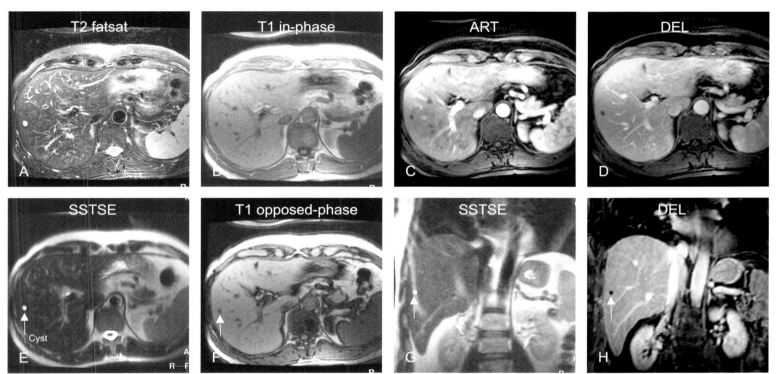

Fig. 3.2. Cyst, typical MRI findings. A Axial fat-suppressed T2-w TSE image (T2 fatsat) shows a small sharply marginated bright cyst. B Axial in-phase image (T1 in-phase): The cyst has low signal intensity. C Axial gadolinium-enhanced 3D GRE image in the arterial phase (ART): The cyst shows no enhancement. D Axial delayed phase (DEL): The cyst remains unenhanced. E Axial T2-w SSTSE image with longer TE of 120 ms (SSTSE): The cyst (arrow) retains its high signal intensity due to high fluid content (typical sign of non-solid liver lesions). F Axial opposed-phase image (T1 opposed-phase): The cyst (arrow) has low signal intensity. G Coronal SSTSE image (SSTSE): The bright cyst is well recognizable (arrow). H Coronal delayed phase image (DEL): The cyst is clearly visible as a small non-enhancing lesion with excellent correlation and confirmation of the T2 information (arrow). The ability of MRI to combine the information on various T1, T2, gadolinium-enhanced sequences is unparalleled and allows a highly confident and reliable diagnosis for sound medical and surgical decision making

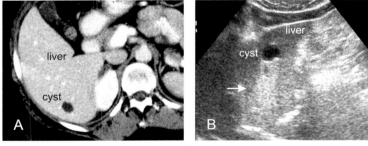
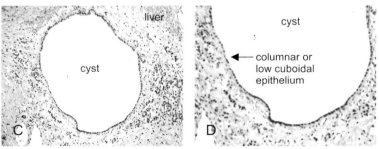

Fig. 3.3. Cyst, CT, US, and histology. A CT (another patient) shows a small un-enhanced cyst. B Ultrasound (another patient) shows a typical cyst with sharp margins and increased sound transmission (arrow). C Photomicro-graph shows a typical cyst that is surrounded by the liver tissue with inflammatory infiltrates. H&E, ×100. D A detailed view of the previous photomicrograph shows the epithelial lining more closely (arrow)

4 Cyst II – Typical Large with MR-CT Correlation

Large hepatic cysts are less common than the smaller or multiple cystic lesions in the liver. Such lesions may be detected incidentally but patients are more likely to present with symptoms such as upper abdominal discomfort, pain, or even obstructive jaundice due to the biliary compression by the cyst. Intracystic hemorrhage may also occur and cause symptoms.

MR Imaging

Very large liver cysts have a similar MR imaging appearance to smaller cysts. Cysts are low in signal intensity on T1-weighted images, high in signal intensity on T2-weighted images, and retain signal intensity on longer echo time (e.g., > 120 ms) T2-weighted images. Cysts, as non-solid liver lesions, share this T2 characteristic with hemangiomas in the liver. Because cysts do not enhance with gadolinium on MR images, delayed post-gadolinium images (up to 5 min) may be useful to ensure that lesions are simple cysts without any solid nodules or thickened septa. In addition, MR imaging can reliably exclude hemorrhage on T1-weighted GRE with fat suppression as well as any biliary dilatation (Figs. 4.1, 4.2). CT is also well able to visualize these lesions (Fig. 4.3). CT may be less accurate for small amounts of hemorrhage or solid components.

Differential Diagnosis

Differential diagnosis of a large cystic liver lesion includes: (1) infectious cystic lesions, such as abscess (clinical history and enhancing wall at imaging), intrahepatic hydatid cyst (clinical history and daughter cysts in 75% at MRI and CT and calcifications in 50% at CT); and (2) neoplastic lesions, such as undifferentiated embryonal sarcoma, biliary cystadenoma or cystadenocarcinoma, and cystic metastases. Hallmarks of neoplastic lesions are solid components with intralesional or perilesional enhancement. Such findings should not be present in large simple developmental liver cysts.

Management

Several types of treatment have been advocated for large (symptomatic) hepatic cysts, including: (1) percutaneous drainage and sclerosis using alcohol, tetracycline, doxycycline, or a combination (this method is associated with recurrence of cysts and symptoms); (2) drainage in combination with various types of surgery; and (3) drainage in combination with minocycline injection (a more recent type of treatment). Percutaneous treatments may be contraindicated in patients with bleeding tendency, echinococcal cysts, and cysts communicating with the biliary tree.

Literature

1. vanSonnenberg E, et al. (1994) Symptomatic hepatic cysts: percutaneous drainage and sclerosis. Radiology 190:387–392
2. Cellier C, Cuenod CA, Deslandes P, et al. (1998) Symptomatic hepatic cysts: treatment with single-shot injection of minocycline hydrochloride. Radiology 206:205–209
3. Regev A, Reddy KR, Bercho M, et al. (2001) Large cystic lesions of the liver in adults: a 15-year experience in a tertiary center. J Am Coll Surg 193:36–45

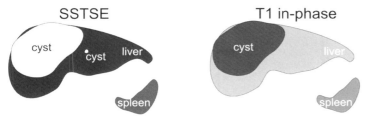
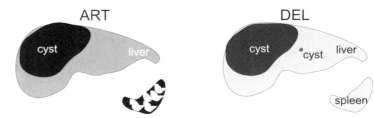

Fig. 4.1. Cyst, drawings. T2 long TE: a large cyst with smaller cysts is much brighter with sharp demarcation to the liver; **T1 in-phase:** the large cyst is hypointense to the liver; the smaller cyst is less well visible; **ART:** the large cyst shows no enhancement in the arterial phase after contrast; **DEL:** the large cyst shows no enhancement in the delayed phase after contrast; the smaller cyst is also visible

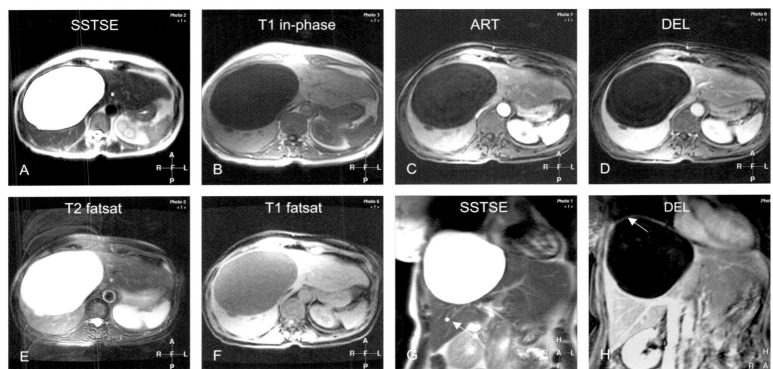

Fig. 4.2. Cyst, large and small. A Axial T2-w SSTSE image (SSTSE) shows a very large and a smaller cyst with sharp margins and high signal to the liver. **B** Axial in-phase image (T1 in-phase): Cysts are hypointense to the liver. **C** Axial arterial phase GRE image (ART): Cysts show no enhancement. **D** Axial delayed phase image (DEL): Cysts remain unenhanced. **E** Axial fat-suppressed TSE image (T2 fatsat): Bright signal of the larger cyst causes ghosting on this respiratory-triggered image. **F** Axial fat suppressed GRE image (T1 fatsat): Cysts show signal that is comparable to fluid (simple cysts). Note the perilesional liver tissue with a rim of higher signal due to compression. **G** Coronal SSTSE image (SSTSE): The larger cyst is in a subphrenic location with the smaller cyst adjacent to it (*arrow*). **H** Coronal delayed phase post-Gd 2D T1-w GRE image (DEL): The larger cyst shows a thin wall (*arrow*)

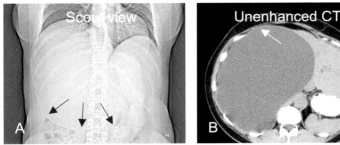
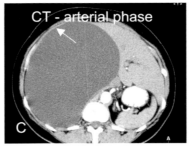
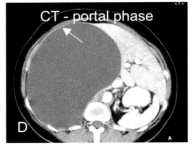

Fig. 4.3. Cyst, large, CT findings (another patient). A Scout view shows the space-occupying effect of the large hepatic cyst with displacement of the bowel loops (*arrows*). **B** Unenhanced CT of a large cyst in the right liver with thin wall. **C** CT in the arterial phase shows no enhancement of the cyst with the thin wall (*arrow*). **D** CT in the portal phase shows no enhancement of any other structures within the cyst with the thin wall (*arrow*)

5 Cyst III – Multiple Small Lesions with MR-CT-US Comparison

Recent studies suggest that small (<15 mm) liver lesions seen at computed tomography (CT) are benign in more than 80% of patients with known malignancy. With the application of multi-row detector CT and thinner collimation, it is likely that more liver lesions will be detected that will need additional imaging for characterization, most likely with MR imaging. It is particularly important to distinguish benign from metastatic and primary malignant lesions.

MR Imaging Versus Computed Tomography and Ultrasound

The appearance and the ability to characterize small hepatic cysts differ considerably between MR imaging, CT, and US (Figs. 5.1–5.3). At MR imaging, hepatic cysts can be characterized based on a unique combination of findings including very bright signal on T2-weighted sequences with sharp margins and absence of enhancement on all phases of dynamic gadolinium-enhanced as well as on delayed phase images. Due to large intrinsic tissue differences between the background liver (dark) and cysts (very bright), even very small cysts of only a few millimeters in diameter can be detected and characterized on images with much larger slice thickness. CT and ultrasound lack these properties, and hence the characterization of small hepatic lesions (mainly distinction between solid and non-solid lesions) may be difficult. Detection and characterization on CT is mainly based on two parameters: (1) differences in X-ray attenuation and (2) differences in enhancement. On contrast-enhanced CT images, cysts appear grayish compared to the enhanced liver. On contrast-enhanced MR images, cysts appear almost as signal voids (very dark) compared to the enhanced liver. This suggests that MRI is as sensitive to gadolinium as CT is for iodine contrast media. At US, cysts appear very dark with sharp margins and increased sound transmission through the lesion, although with the application of real-time image optimization possibilities such as beam-steering, increased sound transmission may not be obvious. In addition, in many centers it is common practice to obtain confirmation of US findings at CT or MRI, especially in patients with an underlying malignancy.

Differential Diagnosis

At MR imaging, typical cysts will have no differential diagnosis. At US and CT, smaller lesions may have differential diagnosis with solid liver lesions, such as metastases.

Management

MR imaging often plays a decisive role in the management of patients with small hepatic cysts, particularly if there is an underlying malignancy.

Literature

1. Schwartz LH, Gandras EJ, Colangelo SM, et al. (1999) Prevalence and importance of small hepatic lesions found at CT in patients with cancer. Radiology 210:71–74
2. Haider MA, Amital MM, Rappaport DC, et al. (2002) Multi-detector row helical CT in preoperative assessment of small (1.5 cm) liver metastases: is thinner collimation better? Radiology 225:137–142
3. Hussain SM, Semelka RC (2005) Hepatic imaging: comparison of modalities. Radiol Clin N Am 43:929–947

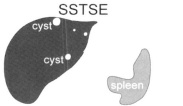
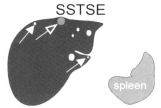
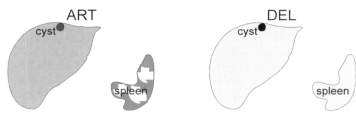

Fig. 5.1. Cysts, drawings. SSTSE: cysts are very bright with sharp demarcations; SSTSE: at a slightly higher anatomic level, a number of smaller subcapsular cysts (*solid arrows*) can be seen due to high intrinsic tissue con- trast; one of the larger cysts shows lower signal due to partial volume (*open arrow*); ART: smaller cysts are not visible; one of the larger cysts shows no enhancement; DEL: the larger cyst remains unenhanced

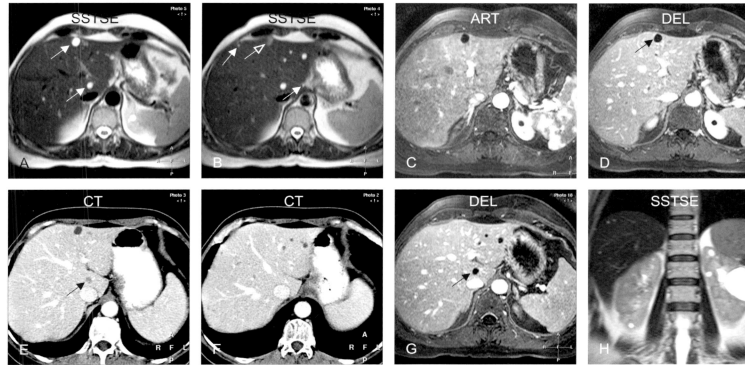

Fig. 5.2. Cysts, multiple liver and renal cysts, MRI and CT findings. A Axial T2-w SSTSE image (SSTSE): Two larger (*arrows*) and several smaller cysts are visible with high signal and sharp demarcation. **B** Axial SSTSE image (SSTSE): At a slightly higher anatomic level, a number of smaller subcapsular cysts (*solid arrows*) can be seen due to high intrinsic tissue contrast. One of the larger cysts shows lower signal due to partial volume (*open arrow*). **C** Axial arterial phase image (ART): One of the larger cysts shows no enhancement. **D** Axial delayed phase image (DEL): The cyst remains unenhanced (*arrow*).

E CT in the portal phase (CT): The larger subcapsular cyst is visible with sharp margins whereas the other cyst (*arrow*) is not well visible due to partial volume. **F** CT in the portal phase at a higher level (CT): Several smaller hypodense lesions are visible („too small to be characterized"). **G** Axial delayed phase image (DEL): The cyst with the partial volume on CT is well visible with sharp demarcation (*arrow*). **H** Coronal SSTSE image (SSTSE): Note multiple hepatic as well as bilateral renal cysts are also present

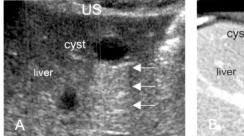
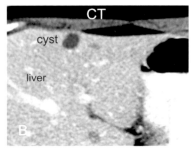
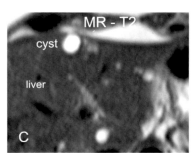
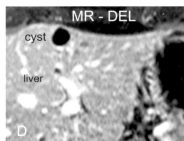

Fig. 5.3. Cyst, US, CT, and MRI findings. A Ultrasound (US) shows a typical hepatic cyst with sharp margins and increased sound transmission through the lesion (*arrows*), indicating its non-solid nature. **B** Computer tomography after contrast in the portal phase (CT) shows an unenhanced cyst with sharp margins. **C** A strongly T2-weighted SSTSE image (MR-T2) shows the cyst as a very bright lesion. **D** T1-weighted image after contrast in the delayed phase GRE (MR-DEL) shows the unenhanced cyst. Note that the cyst appears much darker compared to the liver than on the CT image

6 Cyst IV – Adult Polycystic Liver Disease

One of the most common extrarenal manifestations of adult polycystic kidney disease (APKD) is hepatic cysts, which occur with increasing frequency with advanced age and loss of renal function. Some refer to this condition as adult polycystic liver disease (APLD), which occurs in 34–88% of patients with APKD. Few patients with APLD do not have associated renal cysts. Hepatic cysts usually remain asymptomatic. Some of them develop complications including (1) cyst infection or hemorrhage; (2) biliary obstruction; and (3) portal hypertension. With improved management of the end-stage renal disease, hemodialysis, and renal transplantation, patients with APKD will have increased life expectancy. As a result, complications associated with hepatic cysts may become more common.

MR Imaging Versus Computed Tomography and Ultrasound

At MR imaging, multiple hepatic cysts can be characterized based on a unique combination of findings including low signal intensity on T1-weighted sequences, very bright signal on T2-weighted sequences with sharp margins, and absence of enhancement on all phases of dynamic gadolinium-enhanced including on delayed phase images. Cysts complicated with hemorrhage contain fluid-fluid levels or diffuse high signal intensity on (fat-suppressed) T1-weighted sequences. Hemorrhage is particularly present in renal cysts (Figs. 6.1, 6.2). CT can also visualize liver and renal cysts but hemorrhagic cysts may be difficult to detect on CT examinations (Fig. 6.3). MR imaging is also preferred to CT in this patient group with renal dysfunction. Infected cysts will have imaging features of a pyogenic liver abscess with intraluminal debris and an enhancing wall (see also abscess p. 2).

Differential Diagnosis

Other conditions that present with multiple cystic lesions in the liver include biliary hamartomas (smaller cysts; incidental finding without APKD) and various types of Caroli's disease (cysts located along the biliary tree and should communicate with adjacent bile ducts).

Management

Asymptomatic patients do not require any specific therapy. Optimal management of symptomatic patients with APKD is unclear. Percutaneous drainage is suitable for patients with single dominant cysts and is associated with universal recurrence of symptoms. Other treatment options such as cyst fenestration with or without resection provide unsatisfactory results as well. Orthotopic liver transplantation appears to be a more promising treatment option for patients with diffuse liver involvement with significant comorbid conditions.

Literature

1. Mosetti MA, Leonardou P, Motohara T, Kanematsu M, Armao D, Semelka RC (2003) Autosomal dominant polycystic kidney disease: MR imaging evaluation using current techniques. J Magn Reson Imaging 18:210–215
2. Itai Y, Ebihara R, Eguchi N, et al. (1995) Hepatobiliary cysts in patients with autosomal dominant polycystic kidney disease: prevalence and CT findings. AJR Am J Roentgenol 164:339–342
3. Swenson K, Seu P, Kinkhabwala M, et al. (1998) Liver transplantation for adult polycystic liver disease. Hepatology 28:412–415

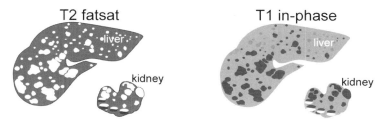

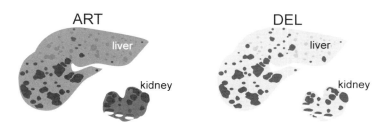

Fig. 6.1. Cysts, drawings. T2 fatsat: cysts are much brighter with sharp demarcation to the liver. Note also renal cysts. **T1 in-phase:** cysts are hypointense to the liver. Some of the renal cysts have in part high signal due to hemorrhage (fluid-fluid levels). Note that these parts of the cysts are darker on T2 fatsat. **ART:** cysts show no enhancement; **DEL:** cysts remain unenhanced

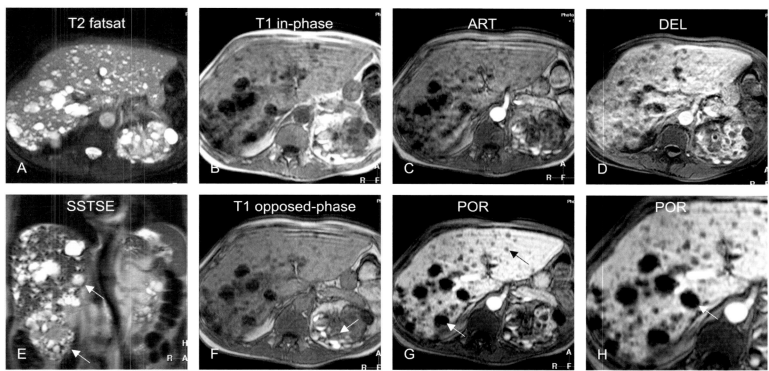

Fig. 6.2. Cysts, multiple, simple liver and complicated renal. A Axial fat-suppressed T2-w TSE image (T2 fatsat): Multiple simple liver and renal cysts are much brighter than the surrounding liver with sharp demarcation. The complicated renal cysts with hemorrhage have darker parts. **B** Axial in-phase T1-w GRE (T1 in-phase): Hepatic cysts are hypointense to the liver. Note that parts of the complicated renal cysts are bright due to hemorrhage (fluid-fluid levels). **C** Axial arterial phase GRE image (ART): The cysts show no enhancement. **D** Axial delayed phase GRE image (DEL): The cysts remain unenhanced. **E** Coronal T2-w SSTSE image (T2 coronal): The hepatic and renal cysts are visible (*arrows*). **F** Axial opposed-phase GRE image (T1 opposed-phase) contains less artifacts than the in-phase image. The renal cysts with hemorrhage are well visible (*arrow*). **G** Axial portal phase GRE image (POR): The cysts show no enhancement (*arrows*). **H** A detailed view from the axial delayed phase post-Gd 2D T1-w GRE image (POR): The cysts remain unenhanced with sharp demarcation to the surrounding liver (*arrow*)

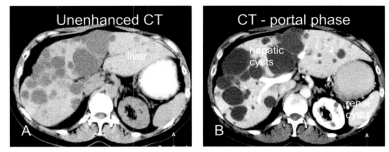
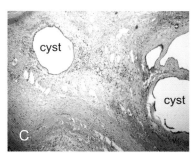
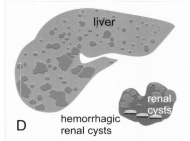

Fig. 6.3. Cysts, CT, histopathology, and a drawing. A Unenhanced CT (another patient) shows multiple hepatic cysts. **B** CT in the portal phase shows no enhancement of the cysts. Note also cysts in the left kidney. **C** Photomicrograph shows multiple cysts with variable size. H&E, ×100. **D** Drawing shows multiple simple liver, and simple and hemorrhagic renal cysts

7 Cystadenoma / Cystadenocarcinoma

Cystic neoplasms, including biliary cystadenomas and cystadeno-carcinomas, are estimated to comprise approximately 5% of liver cysts. Cystadenomas occur predominantly in middle-aged women (41–53 years) and present as incidental findings at imaging. Cystadenomas are often diagnosed incorrectly as simple cysts and treated with aspiration or incomplete excision, which results in recurrence or persistent cyst. The potential for malignant transformation into a cystadenocarcinoma is documented. Biliary cystadenocarcinomas are rare and present almost invariably with symptoms at an older age (around 60 years).

MR Imaging

Cystadenomas appear as multilocular cystic lesions with low signal intensity on T1-weighted sequences, high signal intensity on T2-weighted sequences, and enhancement of the multiple septa in the delayed phase of the dynamic gadolinium-enhanced images. Cystadenoma cannot be distinguished with certainty from cystadenocarcinoma at imaging. Cystadenocarcinomas though tend to have thick and coarse septa with soft tissue nodules. The cystic component may show variable signal intensity on T1- and T2-weighted sequences due to the variable amount of mucinous fluid. The soft tissue nodules may show variable early to late persistent enhancement (Figs. 7.1–7.3). At CT, the presence of thick and coarse septal calcifications may suggest malignancy.

Differential Diagnosis

Differential diagnosis of a large multiloculated cystic liver lesion may include pyogenic abscess, echinococcus cyst, and cystic metastases.

Pathology

Cystadenomas are multilocular with benign cuboidal to columnar epithelium and often contain densely cellular spindle cell („ovarian-like") stromata. Most lesions are lined with mucinous epithelium. Cystadenocarcinomas are also multilocular with malignancy in situ (minority) or invasive tubulopapillary or solid epithelial components; in addition, parts of preexisting cystadenoma may coexist.

Management

Cystadenomas and cystadenocarcinomas require complex excision to prevent recurrence and possible malignant transformation. Most cases will recur after aspiration only or partial resection.

Literature

1. Devaney K, Goodman ZD, Ishak KG (1994) Hepatobiliary cystadenoma and cysadenocarcinoma. A light microscopic and immunohistochemical study of 70 patients. Am J Surg Pathol 18:1078–1091
2. Korobkin M, Stephens DH, Lee JK, et al. (1989) Biliary cystadenoma and cystadenocarcinoma: CT and sonographic findings. AJR Am J Roengenol 153:507–511
3. Vogt DP, Henderson JM, Chmielewski E (2005) Cystadenoma and cystadenocarcinoma of the liver: a single center experience. J Am Coll Surg 200:727–733
4. Ishak KG, Willis GW, Cummins SD, et al. (1977) Biliary cystadenoma and cystadenocarcinoma. Cancer 39:322–338

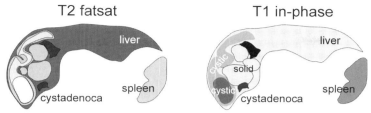
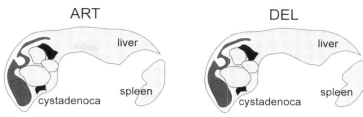

Fig. 7.1. Cystadenocarcinoma, drawings. T2 fatsat: a large lesion with solid and cystic areas is present in the right liver; **T1 in-phase:** the cystic areas have variable signal intensity probably due to variable fluid content (more or less protein content); **ART:** most of the solid component and the thick irregular wall of the cystic component show early enhancement; **DEL:** the enhanced areas retain their contrast

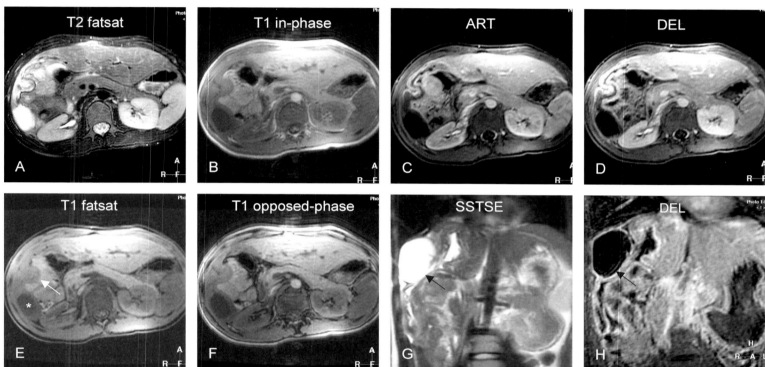

Fig. 7.2. Cystadenocarcinoma, solid and cystic lesion. A Axial T2-w fat suppressed TSE image (T2 fatsat): A large tumor is visible within the right liver with cystic and solid components with respectively high and low signal intensity. **B** Axial in-phase T1-w GRE (T1 in-phase): Tumor shows cystic areas with variable signal intensity. **C** Axial arterial phase post-Gd 2D T1-w GRE image (ART): The solid areas show intense enhancement. **D** Axial delayed phase post-Gd 2D T1-w GRE image (DEL): The solid areas remain enhanced. **E** Axial fat-suppressed T1-w GRE image (T1 fatsat): Tumor shows cystic areas with low (*) and intermediate (*arrow*) signal intensity. **F** Axial opposed-phase GRE image (T1 opposed-phase): Tumor shows no evidence of fat. **G** Coronal SSTSE image (SSTSE): the cystic areas are very bright (*arrow*) and solid parts are isointense with the liver. **H** Coronal delayed phase GRE image (DEL): The cystic components (*arrow*) are surrounded by thick irregular walls

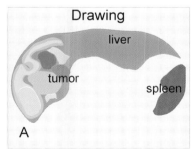
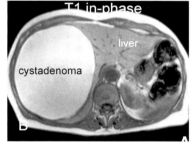
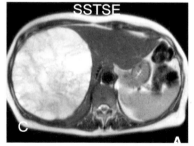
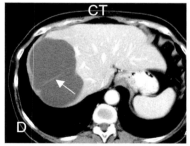

Fig. 7.3. Cystadenocarcinoma (drawing of patient above), and cystadenomas (two different patients). A Drawing illustrates the complexity of the tumor with cystic and solid components. **B** T1-weighted image shows a large lesion with high signal due to mucinous contents. **C** T2-weighted image shows multilocular lesion with slightly variable high signal. No enhancing solid components were present (not shown). **D** CT from another patient shows a thick septum (*arrow*) within a cystic lesion

8 Hemangioma I – Typical Small

Hemangiomas are the most common benign hepatic lesions, with an incidence between 0.4% and 20% in normal subjects, and with a strong female preponderance. The male-to-female ratio is about 1:5. Autopsy studies suggest that many hemangiomas are small (around 5 mm); therefore, the real prevalence of liver hemangiomas probably exceeds the number found by imaging studies. At imaging, hemangiomas are often found as incidental findings or during staging of (colorectal) malignancy. Small lesions may be difficult to characterize at US and CT.

MR Imaging Findings

At MR imaging, small hemangiomas have a characteristic appearance. MRI is more specific than CT and shows hemangiomas as hypointense on T1- and moderately hyperintense on T2-weighted images. Hemangiomas, like cysts, maintain their high signal on sequences with long TE values (> 120 ms). Most of the small hemangiomas show typical peripheral nodular (or discontinuous ring-shaped) enhancement in the arterial and portal phases. The smaller the lesion the smaller the enhanced peripheral nodule will be. In the delayed phase, most hemangiomas retain contrast longer than the surrounding normal liver tissue (Figs. 8.1–8.3). A combination of moderately high signal on T2-weighted images and peripheral nodular enhancement is very specific, and therefore even very small lesions can be detected and characterized with certainty using state-of-the-art MR imaging. Several groups have shown that an accurate diagnosis usually can be reached with MRI in 90–94% of patients. In our experience with the use of current faster sequences, accuracy is probably much higher and reaches almost 100%. Therefore, a biopsy is not necessary in the majority of lesions.

Differential Diagnosis

For typical small hemangiomas with high signal on T2 and peripheral nodular enhancement, there is no differential diagnosis. For atypical cases (either the signal intensity or the enhancement pattern is not quite typical), chemotherapy-treated or mucinous metastases may be considered. Very small hemangiomas may show (rapid) enhancement of the entire lesion in the arterial phase and may raise a differential diagnostic issue with arterioportal shunts and early enhancing neoplasms (see also flash-filling hemangioma on p. 24).

Treatment

Typical small hemangiomas do not need any treatment or follow-up with imaging.

Literature

1. McFarland EG, Mayo-Smith WW, Saini S, et al. (1994) Hepatic hemangiomas and malignant tumors: improved differentiation with heavily T2-weighted conventional spin-echo MR imaging. Radiology 193:43–47
2. Mitchell DG, Saini S, Weinreb J, et al. (1994) Hepatic metastases and cavernous hemangiomas: Distinction with standard- and triple-dose gadoteridol-enhanced MR imaging. Radiology 193:49–57
3. Hussain SM, Semelka RC (2005) Liver masses. Magn Reson Imaging Clin N Am 13:255–275

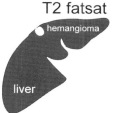
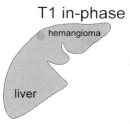
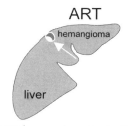
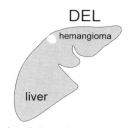

Fig. 8.1. Hemangioma, small, drawings. T2 fatsat: hemangioma is markedly hyperintense to the liver; **T1 in-phase**: hemangioma is hypointense to the liver; **ART**: hemangioma typically shows a peripheral nodular enhancement (*arrow*); **DEL**: hemangioma shows complete homogeneous enhancement

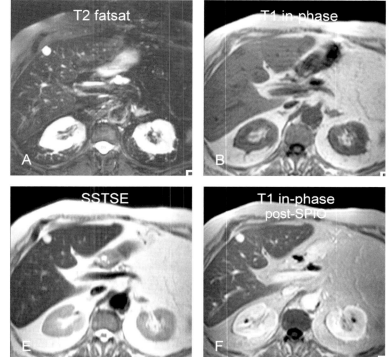
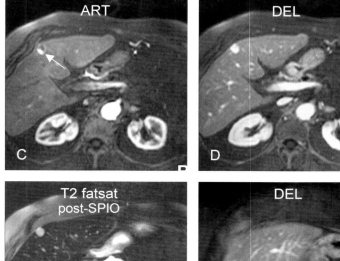

Fig. 8.2. Hemangioma, small, typical MRI findings in a patient with suspected liver metastasis. A Axial fat-suppressed T2-w TSE image (T2 fatsat): Hemangioma is hyperintense to the liver. **B** Axial in-phase image (T1 in-phase): Hemangioma is hypointense to the liver. **C** Axial arterial phase image (ART): Hemangioma shows typical peripheral nodular enhancement (*arrow*). **D** Axial delayed phase image (DEL): Hemangioma shows persistent homogeneous enhancement. **E** Axial SSTSE image (TE = 120 ms) (SSTSE): Hemangioma remains bright, which indicates its non-solid nature. **F** Axial in-phase image after gadolinium and uptake of superparamagnetic iron oxide (SPIO) (T1 in-phase post-SPIO): Gd-enhanced hemangioma appears even brighter in darker liver due to T2* effect caused by the uptake of SPIO into Kupffer cells of the liver. **G** Axial TSE image (T2 fatsat post-SPIO): Unlike the liver, hemangioma does not contain Kupffer cells and remains bright. **H** Coronal delayed phase image (DEL): Hemangioma shows persistent homogeneous enhancement with sharp margins (*arrow*)

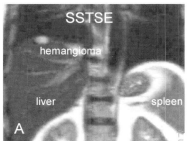
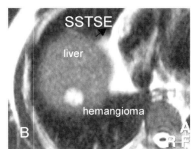
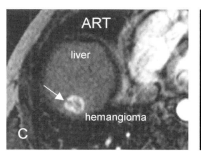
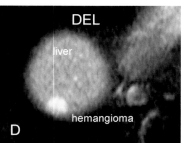

Fig. 8.3. Hemangioma, small, MRI findings. A Axial SSTSE image (TE = 80 ms): a bright hemangioma is visible in subphrenic location. **B** Axial SSTSE image (TE = 120 ms): hemangioma remains bright because of high fluid content. **C** Axial arterial phase image: Hemangioma shows predominantly peripheral enhancement that is separated at several points and appears as broken ring (*arrow*). **D** Axial delayed phase image: Hemangioma shows complete homogeneous and persistent enhancement

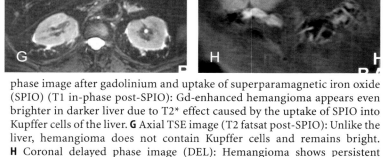

9 Hemangioma II – Typical Medium-Sized with Description of Pathology

Hemangiomas are the most common benign hepatic lesions and occur more often in women. Medium-sized hemangiomas are commonly described on imaging studies because these lesions can be detected and characterized on cross-sectional imaging modalities with confidence.

MR Imaging Findings

At MR imaging, medium-sized hemangiomas have a characteristic morphology and appearance. These lesions are often lobulated with sharp margins. MRI is more specific than CT and shows hemangiomas as hypointense on T1- and moderately hyperintense on T2-weighted images. Medium-sized hemangiomas maintain their high signal on sequences with long TE values (> 120 ms). Most lesions show typical peripheral nodular enhancement in the arterial and portal phases. In the delayed phase, the enhanced parts within the lesion retain contrast longer than the surrounding normal liver tissue. Many lesions may fill-in completely but this is not required for confident diagnosis in typical cases. A combination of moderately high signal on T2-weighted images and peripheral nodular enhancement is very specific and can be considered diagnostic (Figs. 9.1 – 9.3). The findings on delayed images may have added value in atypical cases.

Differential Diagnosis

For typical medium-sized hemangiomas with high signal on T2 and peripheral nodular enhancement, there is no differential diagnosis. For atypical cases (if either the signal intensity or the enhancement pattern is not quite typical), solid or other vascular lesions with high fluid content may be considered. These may include treated or mucinous metastases and rarely angiosarcoma (may show overlapping features on T2-weighted images but with low signal fibrosis and high signal of hemorrhage on T1-weighted images; peripheral nodular enhancement may not progress toward the center; a combination of these unusual signs should be mistrusted and the lesions should be followed or biopsied).

Pathology

At gross pathology, hemangiomas are lobulated with sharp margins to the liver and often show large vascular spaces. At histology, hemangiomas show large cavernous vascular spaces lined with a single layer of endothelial cells and separated by various amounts of fibrosis tissue and inflammatory cells (tumor matrix).

Treatment

Typical medium-sized hemangiomas do not need any treatment or follow-up with imaging.

Literature

1. Mitchell DG, Saini S, Weinreb J, et al. (1994) Hepatic metastases and cavernous hemangiomas: Distinction with standard- and triple-dose gadoteridol-enhanced MR imaging. Radiology 193:49 – 57
2. Semelka RC, Brown ED, Ascher SM, et al. (1994) Hepatic hemangiomas: a multi-institutional study of appearance on T2-weighted and serial gadolinium-enhanced gradient-echo MR images. Radiology 192:401 – 406
3. Worawattanakul S, Semelka RC, Kelekis NL, Woosley JT (1997) Angiosarcoma of the liver: MR imaging pre- and post-chemotherapy. Magn Reson Imaging 15:613 – 617

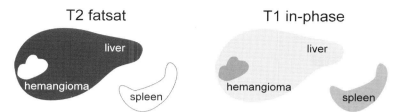
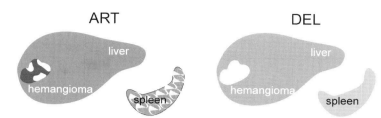

Fig. 9.1. Hemangioma, drawings. T2 fatsat: hemangioma is markedly hyperintense to the liver; **T1 in-phase:** hemangioma is hypointense to the liver; **ART:** hemangioma typically shows a peripheral nodular enhancement in the arterial phase; **DEL:** hemangioma becomes completely enhanced and retains its contrast

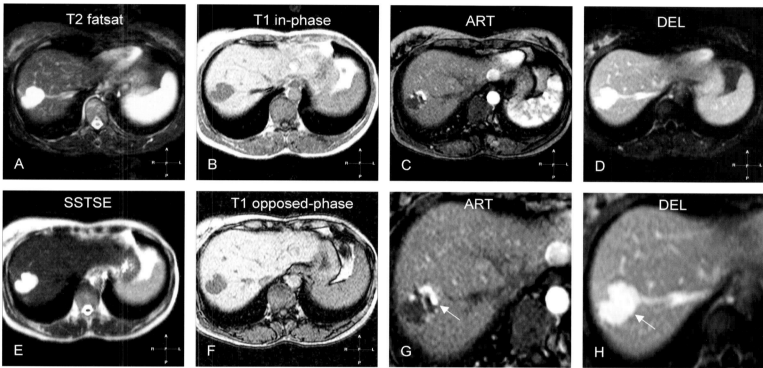

Fig. 9.2. Hemangioma, typical MRI findings. A Axial fat-suppressed T2-w TSE image (T2 fatsat): Hemangioma is lobulated with high signal intensity to the liver. **B** Axial in-phase T1-w GRE (T1 in-phase): Hemangioma is hypointense to the liver. **C** Axial arterial phase post-Gd 2D T1-w GRE image (ART): Hemangioma shows typical peripheral nodular enhancement. **D** Axial delayed phase GRE image (DEL): Hemangioma shows homogeneous enhancement of the entire lesion (i.e., retainment of contrast in enhanced areas). **E** Axial T2-w SSTSE image with TE of 120 ms (SSTSE): Hemangioma remains with high signal on longer TE, which is typical for non-solid lesions such as cysts and hemangiomas. **F** Axial opposed-phase 2D T1-w GRE image (T1 opposed-phase): Hemangioma has a low signal compared to the liver. **G** A detailed view from the arterial phase shows more clearly the peripheral nodular enhancement (*arrow*). **H** A detailed view from the axial image in delayed phase shows the homogeneously enhanced hemangioma with lobulated contours (*arrow*)

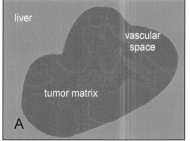
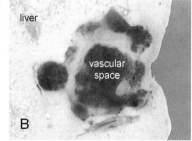
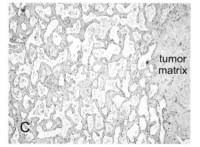
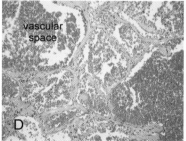

Fig. 9.3. Hemangioma, drawing and pathology. A Drawing: hemangioma is composed of vascular spaces separated by tumor matrix. **B** Gross pathology (different patient): hemangioma is lobulated with sharp margins and large vascular spaces. **C** Photomicrograph shows numerous cavernous vascular spaces lined with a single layer of epithelial cells, separated by fibrosis and inflammatory cells (tumor matrix). H&E, × 100. **D** Photomicrograph shows in more detail the vascular spaces and the tumor matrix. H&E, × 200

10 Hemangioma III – Typical Giant

Giant hemangiomas are less common than their smaller counterparts. The exact definition of a giant hemangioma is not quite clear. Most reports consider lesions larger than 6 cm as giant hemangiomas, whereas others consider a diameter > 10 cm as the criterion. Giant hemangiomas typically present with symptoms and signs that vary from slight abdominal discomfort to life-threatening spontaneous rupture. Giant hemangioma may compress surrounding vessels and bile ducts.

MR Imaging Findings

At MR imaging, giant hemangiomas appear as large lesions with well-defined margins and predominantly high signal on T2-weighted sequences, low signal on T1-weighted sequences, and irregular peripheral (somewhat nodular or flame-like) enhancement during the arterial and portal phase of dynamic gadolinium-enhanced imaging. Usually one or more central scars may be present which are even brighter than the remainder of the lesions. The lesions often show persistent enhancement with unenhanced central scar (even after 5–10 min after injection of gadolinium). Central scar consists of myxoid tissue with poor cellularity and vascularity. Some lesions may contain areas with thrombus or fibrosis with lower signal on T2-weighted sequences and somewhat heterogeneous enhancement (Figs. 10.1–10.3).

Differential Diagnosis

For typical giant hemangiomas with (1) large size (> 6 cm); (2) high signal on T2 and a brighter central scar; (3) discontinuous peripheral enhancement with progressive enlargement and coalescence of the enhancing parts, and (4) persistent enhancement in the delayed phase with well-defined margin, there is no differential diagnosis. Giant hemangiomas, though, may have some overlapping features with other primary liver lesions with a central scar and secondary liver lesions that may replace the entire liver parenchyma such as diffuse ovarian carcinoma metastases. On CT, giant hemangioma may have similarities with hepatocellular carcinoma in a non-cirrhotic liver.

Management

Typical giant hemangiomas without any symptoms do not need any treatment, and follow-up depends on clinical history and imaging findings. For management of symptomatic lesions, see the next case.

Literature

1. Danet IM, Semelka RC, Braga L, et al. (2003) Giant hemangioma of the liver: MR imaging characteristics in 24 patients. Magn Reson Imaging 21:95–101
2. Terkivatan T, Vrijland WW, Den Hoed PT, De Man RA, Hussain SM, et al. (2002) Size of lesion is not a criterion for resection during management of giant liver haemangioma. Br J Surg 89:1240–1244
3. Adam YG, Huvos AG, Fortner JG (1970) Giant hemangiomas of the liver. Ann Surg 172:239–245

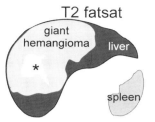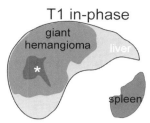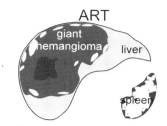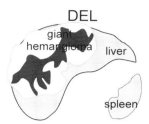

Fig. 10.1. Hemangioma, giant with a mid-size central scar, drawings. T2 fatsat: giant hemangioma is hyperintense to the liver with a brighter central scar (*); **T1 in-phase:** hemangioma is hypointense to the liver with a more darker

central scar (*); **ART:** hemangioma shows a peripheral nodular enhancement; **DEL:** most of the giant hemangioma becomes enhanced except the central area including the central scar

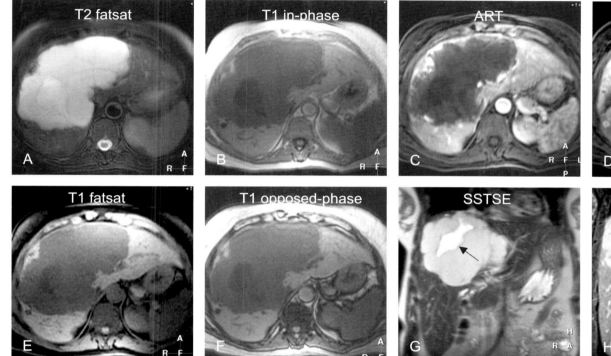

Fig. 10.2. Hemangioma, giant with a mid-size central scar, typical MRI findings. **A** Axial TSE image (T2 fatsat): Giant hemangioma is lobulated and hyperintense to the liver with a brighter central scar. **B** Axial in-phase image (T1 in-phase): Hemangioma is hypointense to the liver with a darker central scar. **C** Axial arterial phase image (ART): Hemangioma shows a peripheral nodular enhancement. **D** Axial delayed phase image (DEL): Giant hemangioma shows homogeneous persistent enhancement of the entire lesion except the

central part including the central scar. **E** Axial fat-suppressed T1-w GRE image (T1 fatsat): Hemangioma has sharp margins to the liver. **F** Axial opposed-phase image (T1 opposed-phase): No fatty infiltration is present. **G** Coronal SSTSE image (SSTSE) of the hemangioma with a higher signal central scar (*arrow*). **H** Coronal delayed phase image (DEL) shows unenhanced bow-tie-shaped central scar (*arrow*)

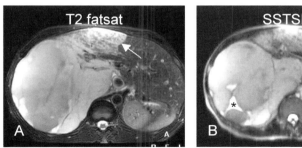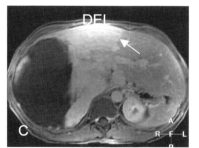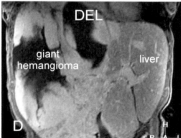

Fig. 10.3. Hemangioma, giant with an atypical feature (another patient). A Axial TSE image (T2 fatsat): Giant hemangioma contains an area that appears heterogeneous (*arrow*). **B** Axial SSTSE image (SSTSE): Hemangioma shows a bright eccentric („central") scar (*). **C** Axial delayed phase image (DEL):

Most of the lesion shows persistent homogeneous enhancement, including the part heterogeneous at T2 (*arrow*). **D** Coronal delayed phase image (DEL): Most of the lesion shows homogeneous persistent enhancement

11 Hemangioma IV – Giant Type with a Large Central Scar

Giant hemangiomas may show variability in the size of the lesion as well as the size and appearance of the central scar. Long-standing lesions may cause compensatory hypertrophy of the unaffected liver. In addition, giant hemangiomas may displace the liver veins and compress the inferior vena cava. In addition, left-sided lesions may displace and compress the stomach and cause symptoms.

MR Imaging Findings

At MR imaging, giant hemangiomas appear as large lesions with well-defined margins and predominantly high signal on T2-weighted sequences, low signal on T1-weighted sequences, and irregular peripheral enhancement during the arterial and portal phase of dynamic gadolinium-enhanced imaging. The size and particularly the T2 appearance of the central scar relative to the remainder of the lesion may vary. The central scar may contain areas with lower signal intensity on T2-weighted sequences (Figs. 11.1, 11.2). The brighter areas with the central scar most likely correspond to the myxoid tissue and the darker areas suggest the presence of fibrosis. In some cases, the central scar may even be larger than the periphery of the lesion. This suggests that the central scar may have been formed within the central vascular channels of the lesion after myxoid changes that eventually change into fibrosis. Despite this variability on T2-weighted images, the enhancement pattern should be quite characteristic on the dynamic gadolinium-enhanced images (Fig. 11.3). Lack of this enhancement pattern in combination with the absence of well-defined margins of the lesion and central scar should raise doubts about the benign nature of the lesion. Patients with such lesions should have a follow-up examination at 3–6 months or a biopsy.

Pathology

At pathology, giant hemangiomas essentially do not differ from smaller hemangiomas. However, giant hemangiomas may have (areas with) more thrombus and fibrosis. Central scar consists of myxoid tissue with poor cellularity and vascularity.

Management

Symptomatic giant hemangiomas may be treated surgically, especially causing inflammatory syndrome or Kassabach-Merritt syndrome (disseminated intravascular coagulopathy). In this respect, size of the lesion is often not a criterion for resection.

Literature

1. Valls C, Renee M, Gill M, et al. (1996) Giant hemangioma of the liver: atypical CT and MR findings. Eur Radiol 6:448–470
2. Mendez Romero A, Wunderink W, Hussain SM, et al. (2006) Stereotactic body radiation therapy for primary and metastatic liver tumors: A single institution phase I–II study. Acta Oncol 45:831–837
3. van Gorcum M, van Buuren HR, Hussain SM, et al. (2005) Fever as a sign of inflammatory syndrome in a female patient with hepatic hemangioma. Ned Tijdschr Geneeskd 149:1227–1230

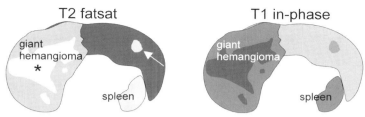 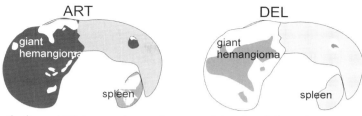

Fig. 11.1. Hemangioma, giant, drawings. **T2 fatsat**: giant hemangioma is hyperintense to the liver with a brighter central scar (*); note also a smaller additional hemangioma (*arrow*); **T1 in-phase**: hemangiomas are hypointense to the liver; **ART**: hemangiomas show a peripheral nodular enhancement; **DEL**: most of the giant hemangioma becomes enhanced except for the central scar. Smaller hemangioma is almost completely enhanced

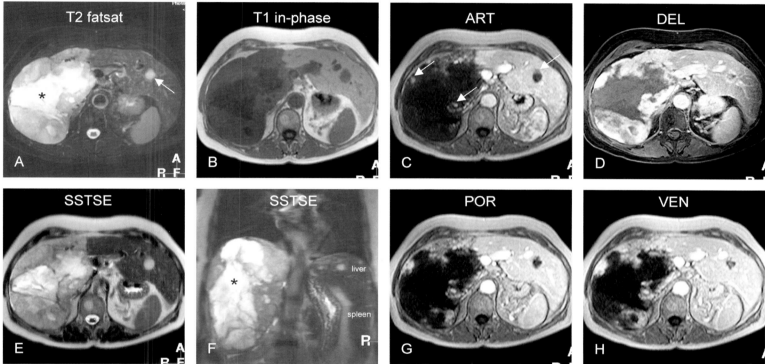

Fig. 11.2. Hemangioma, giant type, typical MRI findings. **A** Axial fat-suppressed T2-w TSE image (T2 fatsat): Giant hemangioma is lobulated and hyperintense to the liver with a brighter central scar (*). Note also a smaller hemangioma (*arrow*) with compensatory liver hypertrophy. **B** Axial T1-w image (T1 in-phase): Hemangioma is hypointense to the liver with a darker central scar. **C** Axial arterial phase image (ART): Hemangiomas show peripheral nodular enhancement (*arrows*). **D** Axial delayed phase image (DEL): Giant hemangioma shows persistent homogeneous enhancement except for the central scar. **E** Axial SSTSE image with a TE of 120 ms (SSTSE): Hemangioma retains its high signal. **F** Coronal SSTSE image (SSTSE): Giant hemangioma occupies the entire right liver with a large central scar (*). **G** Axial portal phase image (POR): Peripheral nodular enhancement has increased. **H** Axial venous phase image (VEN) shows further progression of the enhancement

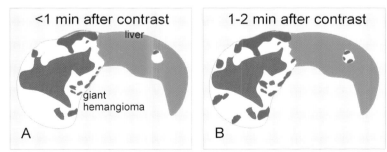 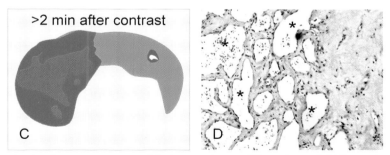

Fig. 11.3. Giant hemangioma, enhancement pattern and histology. **A** Within the first minute after injection of gadolinium, peripheral nodules appear. **B** Between 1 and 2 min, the nodules become larger and coalesce. **C** More than 2 min after contrast most of the hemangioma will be enhanced. **D** Photomicrograph shows the vascular spaces (*) that are gradually filled with contrast medium during dynamic examination. H&E, × 100

12 Hemangioma V – Atypical, Flash-Filling with Perilesional Enhancement

Hemangiomas can show a spectrum of atypical findings at imaging including: (1) unusual appearance (echogenic or hypoechoic border) at US mimicking metastases; (2) heterogeneous appearance, for instance due to hemorrhage or calcification; (3) hyalinization of particularly small lesions may cause low signal on T2-weighted images and atypical enhancement pattern at CT and MR imaging; and (4) rapidly enhancing lesions with or without perilesional enhancement or shunting. Rapid enhancement can be seen in a subset of (usually small) hemangiomas. Such lesions may be more of a diagnostic issue at CT than MR imaging.

MR Imaging Findings

At MR imaging, rapidly enhancing (or flash-filling) hemangiomas show a rapid and diffuse enhancement of the entire lesion with perilesional enhancement or shunting in a majority of the cases in the arterial phase, although the appearance in the delayed phase (with persistent enhancement of the entire lesion) as well as the signal intensity characteristics remain similar to those of the classical type with peripheral nodular enhancement. Flash-filling hemangiomas show low signal intensity on T1-weighted sequences and high signal intensity on T2-weighted sequences with well-defined margins; the lesions retain their high signal on T2-weighted sequences with longer TE (Figs. 12.1, 12.2). Ultrasound and especially (multiphasic) CT are often inconclusive (Fig. 12.3).

Differential Diagnosis

Hypervascular metastases form the most important differential diagnostic problem in the clinical setting. The T2 characteristics in combination with the delayed phase images facilitate the differentiation from hypervascular metastases, which lose their signal on T2-weighted sequences with longer TE and almost invariably show washout of contrast on delayed phase images. In addition, compared to rapidly enhancing hemangiomas, hypervascular metastases show less intense arterial enhancement.

Management

Atypical flash-filling hemangiomas should have a follow-up examination in 3 – 6 months to confirm the diagnosis, particularly in patients with underlying malignancies. Other, less desirable possibilities may include ultrasound-guided biopsy.

Literature

1. Vilgrain V, Boulos L, Vullierme MP, et al. (2000) Imaging of atypical hemangiomas of the liver with pathologic correlation. Radiographics 20:379 – 397
2. Outwater EK, Ito K, Siegelman E, et al. (1997) Rapidly enhancing hepatic hemangiomas at MRI: distinction from malignancies with T2-weighted images. JMRI 7:1033 – 1039
3. Jeong MG, Yu JS, Kim KW (2000) Hepatic cavernous hemangioma: temporal peritumoral enhancement during multiphasic dynamic MR imaging. Radiology 216:692 – 697

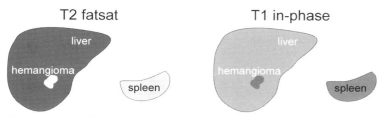
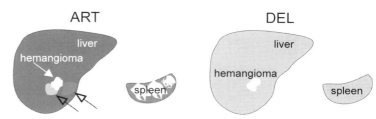

Fig. 12.1. Hemangioma, flash-filling with perilesional enhancement, drawings.
T2 fatsat: hemangioma is markedly hyperintense to the liver; T1 in-phase: hemangioma is hypointense to the liver; ART: hemangioma shows intense homogeneous enhancement in large part (*solid arrow*) with faint perilesional enhancement (*open arrows*); DEL: hemangioma becomes homogeneously enhanced and retains its contrast

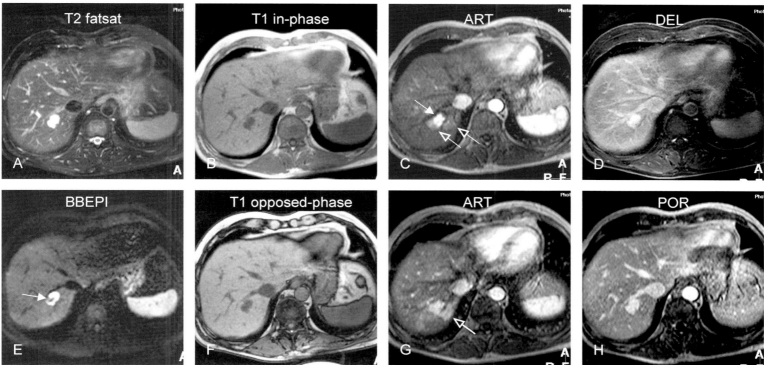

Fig. 12.2. Hemangioma, flash-filling with perilesional enhancement, MRI findings. A Axial fat-suppressed T2-w TSE image (T2 fatsat): Hemangioma is lobulated with high signal intensity to the liver. **B** Axial in-phase T1-w GRE (T1 in-phase): Hemangioma is hypointense to the liver. **C** Axial early arterial phase GRE image (ART): Hemangioma shows intense homogeneous enhancement in large part (*solid arrow*) and faint perilesional enhancement (*open arrows*). **D** Axial delayed phase GRE image (DEL): hemangioma shows homogeneous enhancement of the entire lesion. **E** Axial black-blood echo-planar imaging (BBEPI) with flow sensitive diffusion gradients shows signal void within hemangioma indicating presence of high flow (*arrow*). **F** Axial opposed-phase image (T1 opposed-phase): Hemangioma has a low signal compared to the liver. **G** Axial late arterial phase GRE image (ART) shows increase in perilesional enhancement (*open arrow*). **H** Axial portal phase GRE image (DEL): The increased perilesional enhancement is no longer present and the liver has become homogeneous

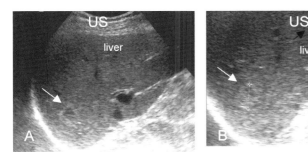
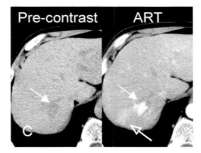
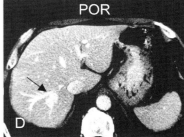

Fig. 12.3. Hemangioma, US and triphasic CT in a patient known to have lung carcinoma. A, B US was performed because of abnormal liver function tests and showed a lesion (*arrow*). **C** Subsequent triphasic CT: CT before contrast shows a hypodense lesion (*arrow*) with early arterial enhancement as well as perilesional enhancement in the arterial phase (*open arrow*). **D** CT in the portal phase shows homogeneous persistent enhancement of the lesion. CT findings were inconclusive; therefore MRI was advised (shown above)

13 Hemangioma VI – Multiple with Perilesional Enhancement

Hemangiomas may be multiple in up to 10% of cases. Multiple hemangiomas generally consist of a few scattered lesions. They often have atypical imaging features, including unusual appearance at US and CT, with or without perilesional enhancement or wedge-shaped transient arterial enhancement. Some lesions may be exophytic and may contain fibrotic septa. These findings in combination with multiplicity may mimic metastases, particularly at US and (single-phase) CT. Distinction from hepatic metastases is critical to avoid improper patient management.

MR Imaging Findings

At MR imaging, multiple hemangiomas show low signal intensity on T1-weighted sequences and high signal intensity on T2-weighted sequences with well-defined margins; the surrounding liver may show signs of diffuse fatty infiltration. In the arterial phase, the lesions show variable enhancement including the typical peripheral nodular enhancement in some lesions, homogeneous enhancement in other lesions, with or without perilesional or wedge-shaped enhancement. In the delayed phase, all lesions show invariably persistent enhancement of the entire lesion with sharp margins with complete homogeneous enhancement of the surrounding liver (Figs. 13.1, 13.2). In some lesions, the presence of flow within some lesions may further improve the specificity of MR imaging (see Fig. 13.2E).

Differential Diagnosis

Multiplicity of hepatic lesions is often associated with liver metastases. Due to the lack of consistent soft tissue characteristics and routine multiphasic contrast-enhanced examinations, ultrasound and CT are often inconclusive in patients with multiple hepatic hemangiomas (Fig. 13.3). At MR imaging, a combination of high signal on T2-weighted images and persistent enhancement in the delayed phase facilitate the differentiation from (hypervascular) metastases.

Management

Based on MR imaging, unnecessary biopsies and diagnostic delay can be avoided.

Literature

1. Vilgrain V, Boulus L, Vullierme MP, et al. (2000) Imaging of atypical hemangiomas of the liver with pathologic correlation. Radiographics 20:379–397
2. Mitchell DG, Saini S, Weinreb J, et al. (1994) Hepatic metastases and cavernous hemangiomas: distinction with standard and triple-dose gadoteridol-enhanced MR imaging. Radiology 193:49–57
3. Jang HJ, Kim TK, Park SJ, et al. (2003) Hepatic hemangioma: atypical appearances on CT, MR imaging, and sonography. AJR Am J Roentgenol 180:135–141

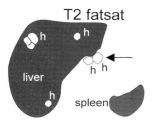
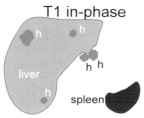
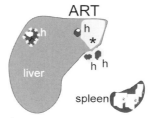
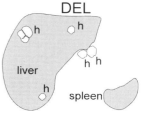

Fig. 13.1. Hemangioma, multiple, drawings. T2 fatsat: hemangiomas (*h*) appear very bright due to iron deposition in the liver and the spleen; two lesions are exophytic (*arrow*); **T1 in-phase:** hemangiomas are hypointense; the spleen appears very dark due to iron deposition; **ART:** hemangiomas typically show a peripheral nodular enhancement; wedge-shaped enhancement (*), **DEL:** hemangiomas retain contrast

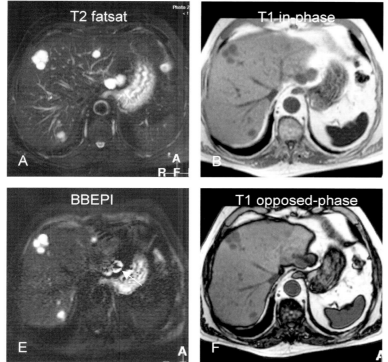
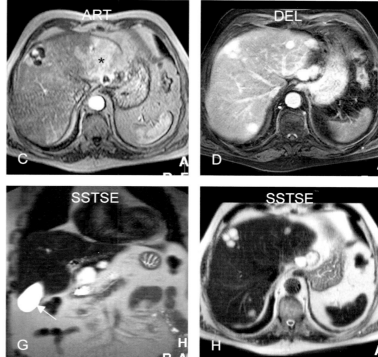

Fig. 13.2. Hemangioma, multiple, MRI findings. A Axial TSE image (T2 fatsat): Hemangiomas appear very bright with the abnormally darker liver and spleen due to iron deposition. Note that two lesions are exophytic (*arrow*). **B** Axial in-phase image (T1 in-phase): Hemangiomas are hypointense; the spleen appears very dark due to iron deposition. **C** Axial arterial phase image (ART): Hemangiomas show typical peripheral nodular enhancement. Note a wedge-shaped enhancement (*). **D** Axial delayed phase image (DEL): Hemangiomas retain contrast. **E** Axial flow-sensitive black-blood EPI image (BBEPI): The exophytic hemangiomas show central darkening due to flow (bulk motion), which is confirmatory for exophytic hemangiomas (*arrow*). **F** Axial opposed-phase image (T1 opposed-phase): The liver shows mild diffuse steatosis. **G** Coronal and **H** axial SSTSE images (SSTSE): Due to the dark liver, hemangiomas appear more like high fluid-containing structures such as cysts (compare to the fluid in the gallbladder, *arrow*)

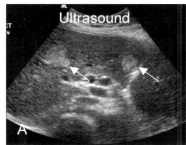
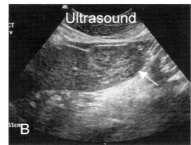
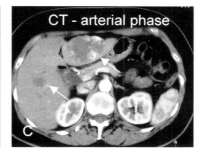
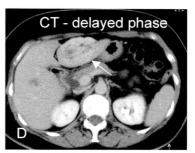

Fig. 13.3. Hemangioma, multiple (another patient known with colon carcinoma and misdiagnosed at CT with multiple metastases), ultrasound and CT findings. A US shows two echogenic lesions (*arrows*). **B** US shows a third lesion with mixed appearance (*arrow*). **C** Subsequent CT in the arterial phase: Two hemangiomas show peripheral nodular enhancement (*arrows*), which were mistaken for metastases. **D** CT in delayed phase: At least the larger lesion shows persistent enhancement, which is typical for an hemangioma

14 Hemorrhage

Liver-related hemorrhage or bleeding may be located within the liver (intrahepatic) or outside the liver (subcapsular or extracapsular). The location of the hemorrhage may be related to the mechanism of injury or volume of blood. Most collections occur after penetrating trauma or as a complication of interventional or surgical procedure. Spontaneous liver-related hemorrhage is a well known complication of solid liver lesions (see next case, p. 30). In addition, it can occur in coagulation disorders, during anticoagulation therapy, or as a complication of HELLP (hemolysis, elevated liver enzymes, low platelets) syndrome.

MR Imaging Findings

The MR imaging appearance of hemorrhage is related to the presence of different stages of blood breakdown products within the collections. Acute hemorrhage (within 2 – 3 days) shows fluid signal intensity behavior that is consistent with intracellular deoxyhemoglobin: fluid collection is homogeneous, and low on T1- as well as markedly low on T2-weighted images. Subacute hemorrhage (within 3 – 5 days) shows fluid signal intensity behavior that indicates the presence of intracellular methemoglobin: fluid collection is intermediate to bright on T1- and dark on T2-weighted images. In later stages, hemorrhage may have a T1 bright central part (intracellular methemoglobin) with a T1 as well as a T2 dark rim of hemosiderin (Figs. 14.1 – 14.3). Gradually, hemorrhage may resolve completely or remain visible as a focal abnormality predominantly composed of hemosiderin. Dark fluid collection on T2 is a distinctive feature of (sub)acute hemorrhage, which is particularly important in patients with suspected HELLP syndrome. CT and US findings of hemorrhage are often non-specific and may not provide adequate information.

Differential Diagnosis

In ambiguous cases, the differential diagnosis may include: (1) pyogenic liver abscess (recent hemoglobin levels as well as clinical history important); (2) cystic neoplasm (look for the enhancing wall and solid structures); and (3) solid tumor with hemorrhage (see p. 30).

Management

If hemorrhage occurs as a complication of a procedure, follow-up with imaging is recommended. If hemorrhage is a result of an underlying disease or condition, it is obvious that the focus of treatment will be the underlying cause.

Literature

1. Balci NC, Semelka RC, Noone TC, Ascher SM (1999) Acute and subacute liver-related hemorrhage: MR findings. Magn Reson Imaging 17: 207 – 211
2. McGill DB, Rakela J, Zinsmeister AR, et al. (1990) A 21 year experience with major hemorrhage after percutaneous liver biopsy. Gastroenterology 99:1396 – 1400
3. Schroeder MD, Brandsetter MD, Vogelsang H, et al. (1997) Massive intrahepatic hemorrhage as first manifestation of PAN. Hepatogastroenterology 44:148 – 152

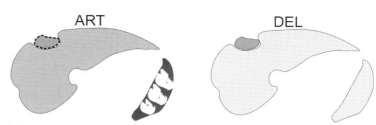

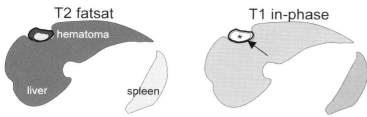

Fig. 14.1. Hematoma, drawings. T2 fatsat: hematoma shows a bright (fluid-like) area centrally with a dark rim mainly composed of hemosiderin; **T1 in-phase**: hematoma shows high signal centrally mainly caused by methemo- globin (*), which is surrounded by a dark rim of hemosiderin (*arrow*); **ART**: hematoma shows no enhancement; **DEL**: hematoma remains unenhanced

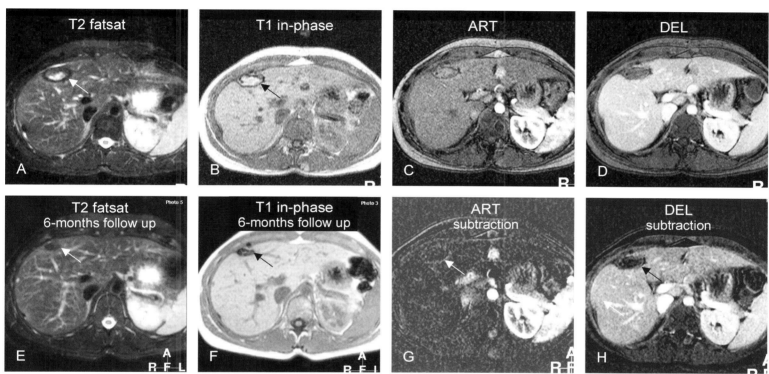

Fig. 14.2. Hemorrhage, typical MRI findings. A Axial fat-suppressed T2-w TSE image (T2 fatsat) shows a hematoma (*arrow*) with high signal centrally and a thick dark rim (representing mainly hemosiderin). **B** Axial in-phase image (T1 in-phase): The hematoma is typically bright centrally (*) due to the T1-shortening effect of methemoglobin and the dark rim is caused by he- mosiderin (*arrow*). **C** Axial GRE image in the arterial phase (ART): The en- hancement is difficult to assess due to the high signal prior to the contrast injection. **D** Axial delayed phase (DEL): The hematoma appears to remain unenhanced. **E** Axial TSE image (T2 fatsat at 6 months) shows the hematoma with decreased size and signal (*arrow*). **F** Axial in-phase image (T1 in-phase at 6 months) shows the hematoma predominantly composed of hemosider- in (*arrow*). **G** A subtraction image (arterial phase) shows convincingly the lack of enhancement (*arrow*). **H** A subtraction image (delayed phase) con- firms that the hematoma remains unenhanced (*arrow*), facilitating its dis- tinctions from a hemorrhagic tumor

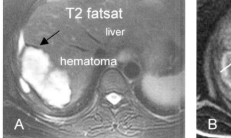

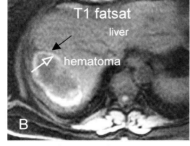

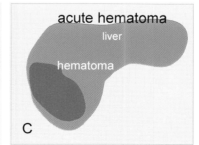

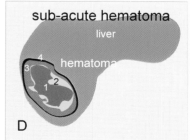

Fig. 14.3. Hemorrhage, MRI appearance and schematic explanation. A, B Hemo- siderin rim appears dark on T2 as well as on T1 (susceptibility effect), which is followed by another rim with very bright signal on T1 (*open arrow*) due to T1 shortening of methemoglobin. **C** Acute hematoma behaves very similarly to simple fluid at MR imaging. **D** Subacute hematoma is often composed of (1) oxyhemoglobin; (2) deoxyhemoglobin; (3) methemoglobin; and (4) he- mosiderin, with a characteristic combination of signal intensities

15 Hemorrhage – Within a Solid Tumor

Several solid liver lesions, including hepatocellular adenomas, hepatocellular carcinomas, and some (neuroendocrine) liver metastases, may show hemorrhage. The distinction between hemorrhage and solid parts may be important for diagnosis, follow-up, and treatment. At US and CT, it may be challenging to make a distinction between the solid and hemorrhagic components of the liver lesion. As hematomas have a distinct appearance, MR imaging is particularly helpful in the identification and distinction of the hemorrhage within liver tumors.

MR Imaging Findings

The MR imaging appearance of hemorrhage is related to the presence of different stages of blood breakdown products within the collections (please see Chap. 14). Particularly subacute hemorrhage shows fluid signal intensity behavior that indicates the presence of intracellular methemoglobin: fluid collection is intermediate to bright on T1- and dark on T2-weighted images. Particularly solid liver lesions will have predominantly low signal intensity on T1-weighted images, whereas hemorrhage will stand out with high signal intensity. This is especially the case on the T1-weighted sequences with fat suppression. Solid liver lesions often have increased heterogeneous signal intensity on T2-weighted images and show variable enhancement after injection of gadolinium. The combination of findings on T1- and T2-weighted, and contrast-enhanced, images facilitates distinction with a high level of confidence (Figs. 15.1, 15.3). At US and CT, distinguishing between hemorrhage and various solid components may be difficult (Fig. 15.3).

Differential Diagnosis

Other common liver lesions that may show high signal on T1-weighted sequences include fat containing lesions such as hepatocellular adenomas and carcinomas (apply chemical shift imaging and/or fat suppression for distinction from hemorrhage), melanoma metastases (apply fat suppression for distinction), and protein-containing liver lesion (usually less bright than hemorrhage).

Literature

1. Casillas VJ, Amendola MA, Gascue A, et al. (2000) Imaging of nontraumatic hemorrhagic hepatic lesions. Radiographics 20:367–378
2. Prasad SR, Wang H, Rosas H, et al. (2005) Fat-containing lesions of the liver: radiologic-pathologic correlation. Radiographics 25:321–331
3. Kelekis NL, Semelka RC, Woosley JT (1996) Malignant lesions of the liver with high signal on T1-weighted MR images. J Magn Reson Imaging 6: 291–294

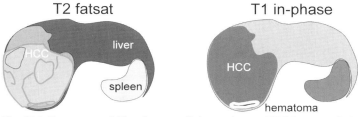

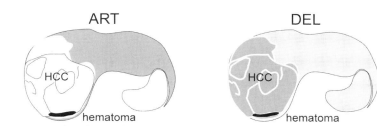

Fig. 15.1. Hematoma within a hepatocellular carcinoma (HCC) in a non-cirrhotic liver, drawings. T2 fatsat: large HCC is visible without detectable hematoma; **T1 in-phase:** hematoma is very bright compared to other tissues, due to the presence of methemoglobin; **ART:** hematoma shows no enhancement; HCC shows heterogeneous enhancement; **DEL:** hematoma remains unenhanced; HCC shows washout with enhanced septae

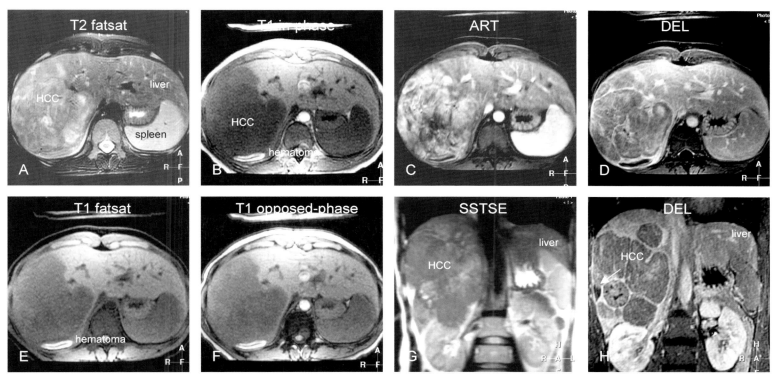

Fig. 15.2. Hematoma within an HCC in a non-cirrhotic liver, MRI findings. A Axial TSE image (T2 fatsat): A large, heterogeneous HCC is visible in a non-cirrhotic liver, without detectable hematoma. **B** Axial in-phase image (T1 in-phase): Hematoma is very bright compared to other tissues, due to the presence of methemoglobin. **C** Axial arterial phase image (ART): Hematoma shows no enhancement; HCC shows intense heterogeneous enhancement. **D** Axial delayed phase image (DEL): Hematoma remains unenhanced; HCC shows washout with multiple enhanced intratumoral septae. **E** Axial fat-sup-pressed T1 GRE image (T1 fatsat): Hematoma appears as the brightest structure in the image, mainly due to fat suppression. **F** Axial opposed-phase image (T1 opposed-phase) shows no sign of fatty infiltration. **G** Coronal single-shot TSE image (SSTSE): Hematoma is not visible within the large HCC. **H** Coronal delayed phase image (DEL): Hematoma remains unenhanced (*arrow*); HCC shows washout with multiple enhanced intratumoral septae

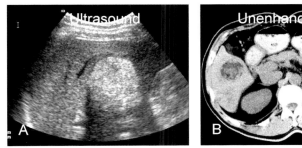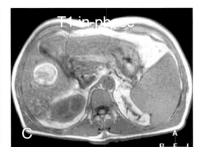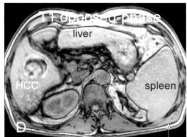

Fig. 15.3. Hemorrhagic and fatty HCC in a cirrhotic liver (another patient), US, CT and MRI findings. A US showed an echogenic indeterminate lesion. **B** Unenhanced CT revealed a fatty lesion and suggested hepatocellular adenoma. **C** T1 in-phase MR image shows a bright lesion in a cirrhotic liver. **D** T1 op-posed-phase image shows signal loss (fatty lesion) with persistent high signal (hematoma); gadolinium-enhanced images (not shown) showed an enhancing solid lesion. Based on MRI, a fatty as well as hemorrhagic HCC was diagnosed

16 Mucinous Metastasis – Mimicking an Hemangioma

Colorectal mucinous carcinoma is a histopathologic subtype of rectal adenocarcinoma, which is characterized by the production of an abundant amount of extracellular mucin. The incidence of the mucinous carcinomas varies between 10% and 20% of the total number of colorectal carcinomas. Mucinous carcinomas are known to be highly infiltrative lesions, which lead to a lower resection rate and a higher postoperative dissemination rate. These factors lead to a poorer prognosis in patients with the mucinous as compared with non-mucinous colorectal carcinomas. Because of higher fluid than solid content with concomitant less vascularity, the liver metastases of colorectal adenocarcinomas may mimic non-solid liver lesions such as cysts and hemangiomas at imaging. Particularly, MR imaging may facilitate the distinction of mucinous liver metastases from benign non-solid liver lesions.

MR Imaging Findings

Because of the abundant extracellular mucin, liver metastases of mucinous colorectal adenocarcinomas typically show predominantly high to very high signal on T2-weighted MR images. On T1-weighted images, the lesions often have unremarkable low signal intensity. After injection of gadolinium, mucinous liver metastases show enhancement of the intratumoral structures, including septa and vessels, in the arterial as well as delayed phases (Figs. 16.1, 16.2). Particularly at CT the enhancement of intratumoral structures may mimic the peripheral nodular enhancement and, in combination with signs such as a traversing vessel, may suggest a benign lesion such as hemangioma (Fig. 16.3A). In our experience, positron emission tomography (PET) may show no abnormal activity and may wrongfully suggest that CT findings are correct (Fig. 16.3B). In such cases, after MR imaging an US-guided biopsy or a resection of the liver lesion may show conclusive evidence of metastasis.

Pathology

At gross pathology, the lesions appear as solid pink lesions with sharp demarcation to the surrounding liver. At histology, the lesions show large spaces filled with abundant mucin. These spaces are interspersed with large septa containing vessels (Fig. 16.3C, D).

Literature

1. Wu CS, Tung SY, Chen PC, Kuo YC (1996) Clinicopathologic study of colorectal mucinous carcinoma in Taiwan: a multivariate analysis. J Gastroenterol Hepatol 11:77–81
2. Ueda K, Matsui O, Nobata K, Takashima T (1996) Mucinous carcinoma of the liver mimicking cavernous hemangioma on pre- and postcontrast MR imaging [letter]. Am J Roentgenol 166:468–469
3. Outwater EK, Tomaszewski JE, Daly JM, Kressel HY (1991) Hepatic colorectal metastases; correlation of MR imaging and pathology. Radiology 180:327–332

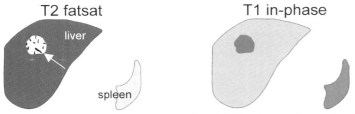
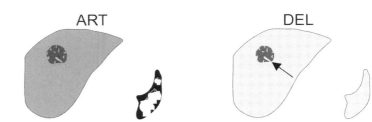

Fig. 16.1. Mucinous colorectal metastasis mimicking hemangioma, drawings. **T2 fatsat:** metastasis is very bright containing low intensity structures, including a traversing vessel (*arrow*); **T1 in-phase:** metastasis is hypointense to the liver; **ART:** metastasis shows enhancement of low intensity structures and vessel; **DEL:** metastasis shows increased enhancement of the intratumoral structures and the vessel (*arrow*)

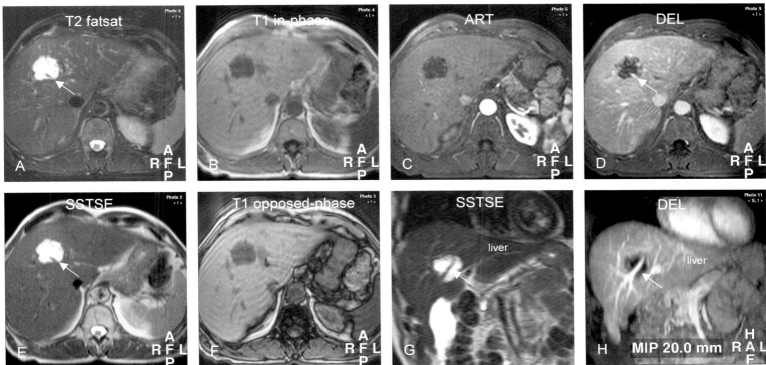

Fig. 16.2. Mucinous colorectal metastasis mimicking hemangioma at CT: MRI findings. A Axial TSE image (T2 fatsat): Lesion is very bright and contains low intensity structures and a traversing vessel (*arrow*). **B** Axial in-phase image (T1 in-phase): Metastasis is hypointense to the liver. **C** Axial arterial phase image (ART): Intratumoral structures, including the vessel, show some enhancement; transversing vessel is often considered a sign of benign lesions. **D** Axial delayed phase image (DEL): Intratumoral structures and the traversing vessel (*arrow*) are more enhanced. **E** Axial SSTSE image with a TE of 120 ms: metastasis retains its signal, which is a common finding of hemangioma and cysts. **F** Axial opposed-phase image (T1 opposed-phase) shows no change in the aspect of the liver, nor of the lesion. **G** Coronal SSTSE (SSTSE) shows metastasis with the traversing vessel (*arrow*). **H** Maximum intensity projection (MIP) of the delayed phase (DEL) provides an overview of the traversing liver vein (*arrow*)

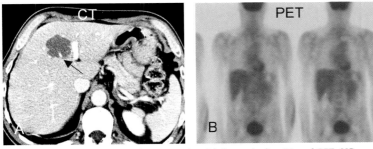
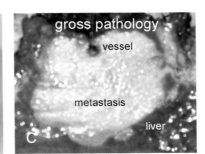
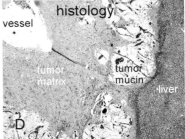

Fig. 16.3. Mucinous colorectal metastasis with inconclusive CT and PET; MR-pathology correlation. A CT shows little enhancement, and in combination with the traversing vessel (*arrow*), the lesion was considered benign. **B** Positron emission tomography (PET) showed normal uptake in the liver. **C** Based on MR imaging, the lesion was biopsied and then resected. Pathology confirmed a metastasis with a traversing vessel. **D** Photomicrograph shows the metastasis composed of tumor matrix, pools of mucin, and a traversing vessel. H&E stain, × 100

Solid Liver Lesions

II

Metastases: Colorectal

IIA

17 Colorectal Metastases I – Typical Lesion

Metastases are the most common malignant tumors of the liver in Western countries. Liver metastases usually appear as solitary or multiple lesions. Unlike many other cancers, the presence of distant metastases from colorectal cancer does not preclude curative treatment. About 25% of patients with colorectal liver metastases have no other distant metastases. Of these 10–25% are candidates for surgical resection. For the 75–90% of patients with liver metastases who are not amenable to surgery, several new minimally invasive treatments are available such as radiofrequency ablation, stereotactic radiation therapy, and systemic chemotherapy.

MR Imaging Findings

At MR imaging, most colorectal carcinoma liver metastases have a target-like appearance. The lesions have predominantly low signal intensity on T1-weighted images and moderately high signal intensity on T2-weighted images with fat suppression. On T2-weighted images, the internal tumor anatomy has a target-like configuration: (a) the highest (fluid-like) signal intensity is in the center of the lesion due to coagulative necrosis; (b) there is a lower signal intensity in a relatively broad zone outside the center due to the presence of desmoplastic reaction, which mainly forms the tumor matrix; and (c) again there is a slightly higher signal intensity in the outermost zone (growing edge) due to more compact tumor cells with more vessels and less desmoplasia. The growing edge of the colorectal metastases is usually very thin. Some lesions may also be surrounded by edema within the surrounding compressed liver parenchyma. After administration of gadolinium, most colorectal metastases show an irregular continuous ring-shaped (as opposed to the broken ring or peripheral nodular enhancement of hemangioma) enhancement in the arterial phase. This ring-shaped enhancement represents the vascularized growing edge of the lesion. In the portal and delayed phase the metastases often show washout in the outer parts with progressive enhancement toward the center of the lesions (Figs. 17.1–17.3). Larger lesions may show heterogeneous, cauliflower like enhancement.

Differential Diagnosis

Benign (small) liver lesions such as cysts (see p. 6), biliary hamartomas (see p. 4), hemangiomas (see p. 18), and focal nodular hyperplasia (see p. 116) are common liver entities, which may coexist with the metastatic lesions and form a common differential diagnostic problem. State-of-the-art MR imaging is highly accurate in distinguishing malignant from benign liver lesions.

Literature

1. Outwater E, Tomaszewski JE, Daly JM, et al. (1991) Hepatic colorectal metastases: Correlation of MR imaging and pathologic appearance. Radiology 180:327–332
2. Semelka RC, Cance WG, Marcos HB, et al. (1999) Liver metastases: comparison of current MR techniques and spiral CT during arterial portography for detection in 20 surgically staged cases. Radiology 213:86–91
3. Hussain SM, Semelka RC (2005) Liver masses. Magn Reson Imaging Clin N Am 13:255–275

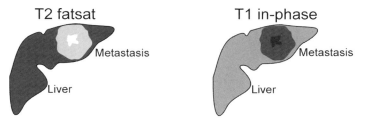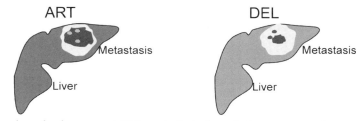

Fig. 17.1. Metastasis, colorectal, drawings. T2 fatsat: metastasis is predominantly hyperintense to the liver with a brighter center; **T1 in-phase**: metastasis is hypointense to the liver; **ART**: metastasis shows a typical irregular ring-shaped enhancement; **DEL**: metastasis shows heterogeneous enhancement

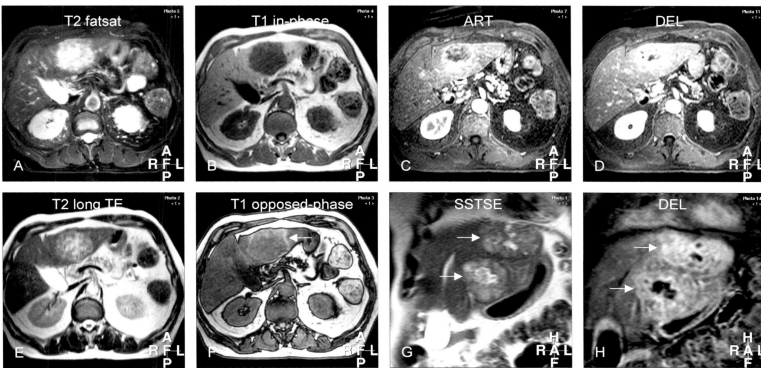

Fig. 17.2. Metastasis, colorectal, MRI findings. A Axial fatsat T2-w turbo spin echo (TSE) image (T2 fatsat): Metastasis is predominantly hyperintense to the liver with a brighter center. **B** Axial in-phase T1-w gradient recalled echo (GRE) (T1 in-phase): Metastasis is hypointense to the liver. **C** Axial arterial phase post-Gd 3D T1-w GRE image (ART): Metastasis shows typical irregular ring-shaped enhancement. **D** Axial delayed phase image (DEL): metastasis becomes more heterogeneous. **E** Axial T2-w single-shot TSE (SSTSE) image with an echo time (TE) of 120 ms (T2 longer TE): Metastasis shows a lower signal in the outer parts indicating the solid nature. **F** Axial opposed-phase T1-w GRE image (T1 opposed-phase) shows a signal drop in the liver indicating steatosis. Metastasis becomes isointense with persistent high perifocal signal due to compressed liver (*arrow*). **G** Coronal T2-w SSTSE (SSTSE) shows two identical metastases with typical tumor anatomy (*arrows*). **H** Coronal delayed phase image (DEL) clearly shows the less enhanced central parts of the metastases (*arrows*)

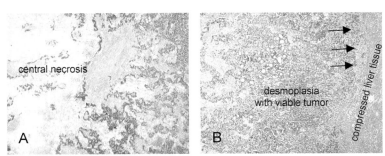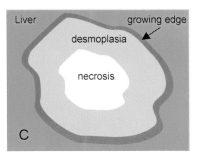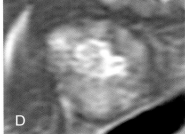

Fig. 17.3. Metastasis, colorectal, tumor anatomy. A Photomicrograph from the central part of a metastasis shows the less vascularized coagulative necrosis. H&E, ×100. **B** Photomicrograph from the outer part shows the desmoplasia with viable tumor tissue and the growing edge (*arrows*). H&E, ×100. **C** Drawing illustrates the tumor anatomy. **D** A detailed view of the axial SSTSE image shows the metastasis anatomy in-vivo

18 Colorectal Metastases II – Typical Multiple Lesions

Colorectal metastases can occur as multiple lesions. Unlike many other cancers, the presence of multiple colorectal metastases does not preclude curative treatment. Therefore, it is important to detect and characterize the liver lesions with the best possible imaging modality available today. MR imaging should be the modality of choice because it can make a distinction between very small metastases and benign liver lesions such as small cysts and hemangiomas. In addition, the ability of MR imaging to detect and characterize diffuse parenchymal liver disease is unparalleled.

MR Imaging Findings

At MR imaging, the individual lesions in the setting of multiple liver metastases will often demonstrate a typical MR imaging appearance as described in the previous chapter: the lesions have a target-like appearance on T2-weighted images and show irregular continuous ring-shaped enhancement in the arterial phase (see Chap. 17 for detailed description). In the context of multiple liver metastases, the liver parenchyma may show changes due to the presence of variable fatty infiltration, edema, and mild biliary dilatation. Due to these and other changes like vascular compression and obstruction, transient perilesional or (sub)segmental parenchymal enhancement may be present (Figs. 18.1–18.3).

Differential Diagnosis

Especially at ultrasound (US) and computed tomography (CT), very small multiple colorectal liver metastases may coalesce and mimic diffuse parenchymal liver disease. The impression of diffuse liver disease may even become more confusing by concurrent diffuse fatty infiltration. In general, within fatty livers the individual lesions are difficult to recognize at CT. MR imaging – based on the high intrinsic soft tissue contrast of T2-weighted images, the application of chemical shift imaging, and the strong T1 shortening effect of gadolinium on contrast-enhanced images – facilitates the detection and characterization of multiple colorectal metastases even in the presence of diffuse parenchymal changes caused by fatty infiltration and edema.

Literature

1. Semelka RC, Cance WG, Marcos HB, et al. (1999) Liver metastases: comparison of current MR techniques and spiral CT during arterial portography for detection in 20 surgically staged cases. Radiology 213:86–91
2. Seneterre E, Taorel P, Bouvier Y, et al. (1996) Detection of hepatic metastases: ferumoxides-enhanced MR imaging versus unenhanced MR imaging and CT during arterio-portography. Radiology 200:785–792
3. Outwater E, Tomaszewski JE, Daly JM, et al. (1991) Hepatic colorectal metastases: Correlation of MR imaging and pathologic appearance. Radiology 180:327–332

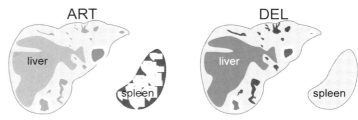
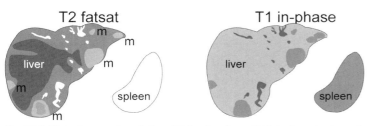

Fig. 18.1. Metastases, colorectal, multiple, drawings. T2 fatsat: metastases (*m*) are surrounded by the high signal intensity edema. Dilated bile ducts are very bright and the normal liver is darker; **T1 in-phase:** metastases and the bile ducts are hypointense to the liver; **ART:** metastases show typical irregular ring-shaped enhancement, with diffuse increased enhancement around bile ducts; **DEL:** persistent enhancement indicates diffuse disease

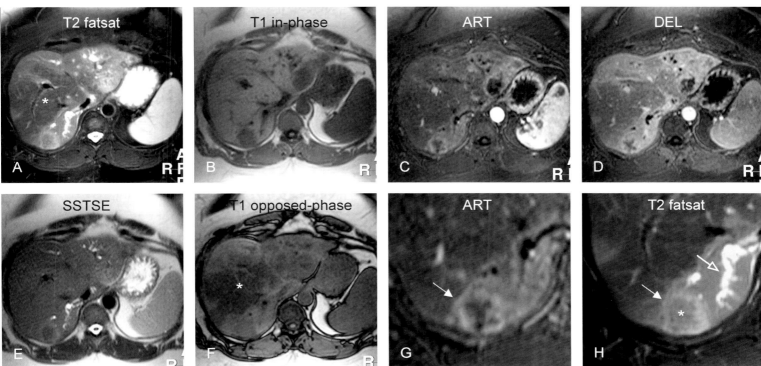

Fig. 18.2. Metastases, colorectal, multiple, steatosis, dilated bile ducts, MRI findings. A Axial TSE image (T2 fatsat): Metastases (*m*) are surrounded by the high signal intensity liver edema and dilated bile ducts. The normal liver is much darker (*). **B** Axial in-phase image (T1 in-phase): Metastases and the bile ducts are hypointense to the liver. **C** Axial arterial phase image (ART): Metastases show typical irregular ring-shaped enhancement with increased diffuse enhancement around the dilated bile ducts. **D** Axial delayed phase image (DEL): Persistent enhancement indicates diffuse metastatic or inflammatory (cholangitis) disease. **E** Axial SSTSE image: The findings are less apparent than on the T2 fatsat image. **F** Axial opposed-phase image (T1 opposed-phase) shows diffuse steatosis centrally (*). **G** A detailed view of the arterial phase image shows the typical irregular ring-shaped enhancement of mainly the growing edge of the lesion (*arrow*). **H** A detailed view of the T2 fatsat image shows the growing edge of the lesion brighter (*arrow*) than the central part (*). Dilated bile duct (*open arrow*)

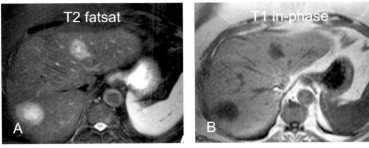
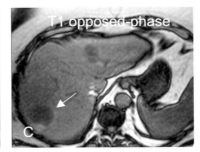
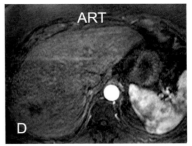

Fig. 18.3. Metastases, colorectal, multiple, steatosis, MRI findings (another patient). A Axial TSE image (T2 fatsat): Metastases are hyperintense to the liver with a typical target-configuration. **B** Axial in-phase image (T1 in-phase): Metastases are hypointense to the liver. **C** Axial opposed-phase image (T1 opposed-phase): Mild diffuse steatosis causes faint high perilesional signal due to compressed non-fatty liver tissue (*arrow*). **D** Axial arterial phase image (ART): Metastases show typical irregular ring-shaped enhancement

19 Colorectal Metastases III – Metastasis Versus Cyst

Benign liver lesions are common; the exact prevalence is unknown, but some studies suggest that benign liver masses may be found in more than 20 % of the general population. Recent studies suggest that small (< 15 mm) liver lesions seen at CT are benign in more than 80 % of patients with known malignancy. With the application of multi-row detector CT and thinner collimation, it is likely that more liver lesions will be detected that will need additional imaging for characterization, most likely with MR imaging. As colorectal liver metastases are the most common malignant liver lesions, they may concur with other common benign liver lesions such as cysts and hemangiomas. It is particularly important to distinguish benign from metastatic and primary malignant lesions.

MR Imaging Findings

At MR imaging, cysts are low in signal intensity on T1-weighted images, high in signal intensity on T2-weighted images, and retain signal intensity on longer echo time (e.g., > 120 ms) T2-weighted images. After injection of contrast, cysts do not show any enhancement. Delayed contrast-enhanced imaging may be useful to ensure that lesions are cysts and not poorly vascularized metastases that show gradual enhancement. T2-weighted sequences with long TE in combination with delayed phase images are especially effective at showing small (≤ 5 mm) cysts. Colorectal metastases often have a typical target-like appearance on T2-weighted images and show irregular ring-shaped enhancement after injection of gadolinium (Figs. 19.1 – 19.3).

Management

In the United States, more than 50 % of patients (in 1998, 56,000 of 131,600 patients) who die from colorectal cancer have liver metastases at autopsy. Of those who have colorectal liver metastases, 10 – 25 % are candidates for surgical resection, and the 5-year survival rate following resection of isolated colorectal liver metastases can be as high as 38 %. Without any treatment, the survival rate is less than 1 %. For the remaining 75 – 90 % of patients with liver metastases who are not amenable to surgery, several new therapies have been developed.

Literature

1. Karhunen PJ (1986) Benign hepatic tumours and tumour-like conditions in men. J Clin Pathol 39:183 – 188
2. Schwartz LH, Gandras EJ, Colangelo SM, et al. (1999) Prevalence and importance of small hepatic lesions found at CT in patients with cancer. Radiology 210:71 – 74
3. Haider MA, Amital MM, Rappaport DC, et al. (2002) Multi-detector row helical CT in preoperative assessment of small (1.5 cm) liver metastases: is thinner collimation better? Radiology 225:137 – 142
4. Yoon SS, Tanabe TK (1999) Surgical treatment and other regional treatments for colorectal cancer liver metastases. Oncologist 4:197 – 208

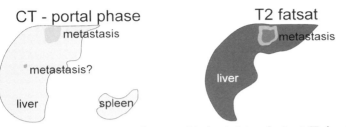
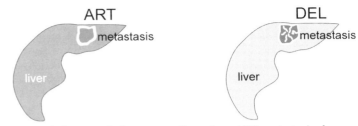

Fig. 19.1. Metastasis, colorectal, a second lesion indeterminate at CT, drawings. CT in portal phase: metastasis is hypodense with faint enhancement; the second lesion was said to be too small to characterize with certainty; T2 fat-sat: metastasis has a typical target configuration; ART: metastasis shows a typical irregular ring-shaped enhancement; DEL: metastasis shows heterogeneous enhancement

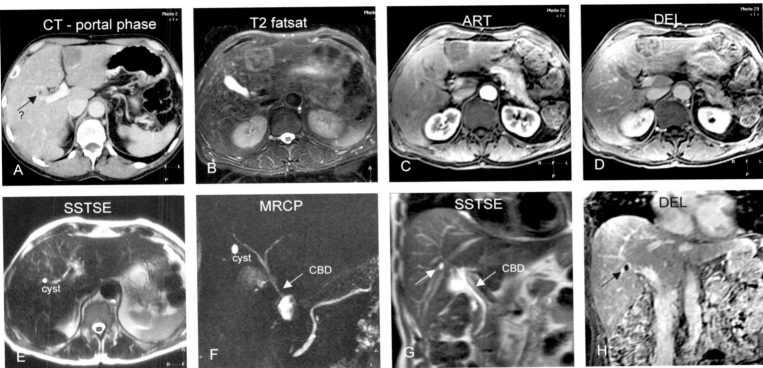

Fig. 19.2. Metastasis, colorectal, a second lesion indeterminate at CT, MRI findings. A Axial CT in portal phase shows the metastasis in the left liver as a hypodense lesion with faint enhancement. A second lesion in the right liver was considered to be too small to characterize. B Axial TSE image (T2 fatsat): Metastasis is predominantly hyperintense with a typical target configuration. C Axial arterial phase image (ART): Metastasis shows typical irregular ring-shaped enhancement. D Axial delayed phase image (DEL): Metastasis becomes heterogeneous. E Axial SSTSE image with a TE of 120 ms at a different anatomic level shows the second lesion as a typical cyst with very high signal intensity. F Magnetic resonance cholangiopancreatography (MRCP) with a TE of about 1000 ms confirms the presence of a very bright, fluid containing cyst (CBD common bile duct). G Coronal SSTSE (SSTSE) shows the cyst within the right liver (arrow) and its relationship to the biliary tree. H Coronal delayed phase image (DEL) clearly shows the unenhanced small cyst (arrow)

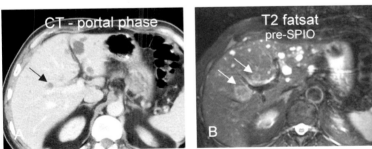
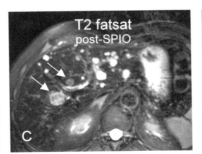
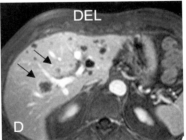

Fig. 19.3. Metastases, colorectal, multiple lesions in another patient with indeterminate CT, MRI findings. A Axial CT in portal phase shows possible growth in one of the lesions that was considered to be a cyst (arrow) like several other liver lesions. B Axial TSE image (T2 fatsat) prior to the uptake of superparamagnetic iron oxide (SPIO): shows two metastases with typical target configuration (arrows) and a lower signal than multiple liver cysts. C Axial TSE image (T2 fatsat) after the uptake of SPIO confirms the metastases (arrows) in a much darker liver. D Axial delayed phase image (DEL): Metastases have a typical ring-shaped enhancement (arrows)

20 Colorectal Metastases IV – Metastasis Versus Hemangiomas

Colorectal metastases may concur with hemangiomas in the liver. Especially small hemangiomas and hemangiomas with atypical features like unusual (perilesional) enhancement, shunting, inflammation, intratumoral hemorrhage, and compression by adjacent structures may cause difficulty in diagnosis at US and CT. Based on T1- and T2-weighted and routine dynamic gadolinium-enhanced sequences, MR imaging has the ability to make an accurate diagnosis in the majority of cases and hence to expedite the patient management.

MR Imaging Findings

At MR imaging, colorectal metastases often have a typical target-like appearance on T2-weighted images with moderately high signal intensity, and show irregular, continuous, ring-shaped enhancement in the arterial phase after injection of gadolinium, and washout in the delayed phase (see also Chap. 17 for a detailed description). Typical hemangiomas are hypointense on T1- and moderately hyperintense on T2-weighted images, and show peripheral nodular enhancement. The smaller the lesion the smaller the enhanced peripheral nodules will be. In the delayed phase, most hemangiomas show persistent enhancement as opposed to metastases, which show washout in delayed phase. Therefore, a combination of T2-weighted images and enhancement pattern is very specific, and allows characterization of even very small liver lesions (Figs. 20.1 – 20.3). In a majority of such cases, biopsy may technically be challenging and is often unnecessary.

Management

State-of-the-art MR imaging allows a distinction between metastases and concurrent hemangiomas with high accuracy and can avoid unnecessary costs and delays in patient management. Currently, most centers apply a very aggressive approach toward colorectal liver metastases. Confident imaging diagnoses play an essential role in guiding such approaches. In this context, MR imaging plays a pivotal role in the management of patients with liver lesions.

Literature

1. Hussain SM, Semelka RC (2005) Liver masses. Magn Reson Imaging Clin N Am 13:255–275
2. Vilgrain V, Boulos L, Vullierme MP, et al. (2000) Imaging of atypical hemangiomas of the liver with pathologic correlation. Radiographics 20:379–397
3. Semelka RC, Brown ED, Ascher SM, et al. (1994) Hepatic hemangiomas: A multi-institutional study of appearance on T2-weighted and serial gadolinium-enhanced gradient-echo MR images. Radiology 192:401–406

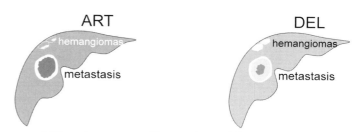
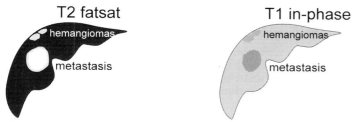

Fig. 20.1. Metastasis, with concurrent hemangiomas, drawings. **T2 fatsat:** metastasis and hemangiomas are hyperintense to the liver; **T1 in-phase:** lesions are hypointense to the liver; **ART:** metastasis shows an irregular ring-shaped enhancement. The enhancement of hemangiomas is less obvious. **DEL:** metastasis shows heterogeneous and persistent rim enhancement. Hemangiomas show homogeneous enhancement

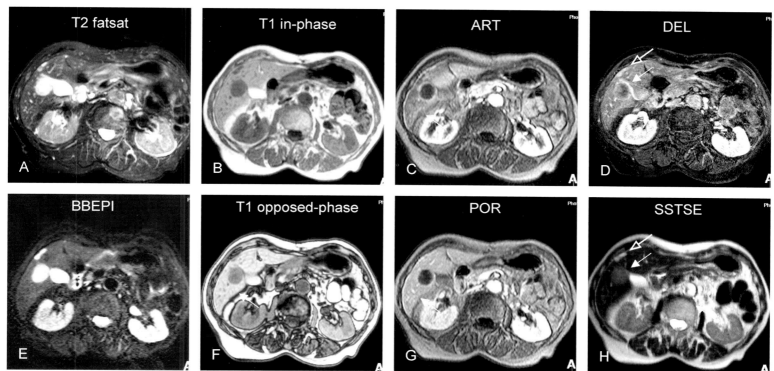

Fig. 20.2. Metastasis, with concurrent hemangiomas, MRI findings. A Axial fatsat T2-w TSE image (T2 fatsat): Metastasis and hemangiomas are hyperintense to the liver. **B** Axial in-phase T1-w image (T1 in-phase): Metastasis and hemangiomas are hypointense to the liver. **C** Axial arterial phase image (ART): Metastasis shows irregular ring-shaped enhancement. The enhancement of the hemangiomas is less obvious. **D** Axial delayed phase image (DEL): Metastasis shows heterogeneous and persistent ring-shaped enhancement (*solid arrow*). Hemangiomas show homogeneous enhancement (*open arrow*).

E Axial black-blood echoplanar imaging (BBEPI): Better conspicuity of the lesions is mainly due to the darker vessels. **F** Axial opposed-phase T1-w GRE image (T1 opposed-phase) shows no sign of fatty infiltration. **G** Axial portal phase image (POR): Hemangiomas have almost become isointense due to the progressing enhancement. **H** Axial SSTSE with a long TE of 120 ms shows the solid metastasis much darker (*solid arrow*) than the non-solid hemangiomas (*open arrow*)

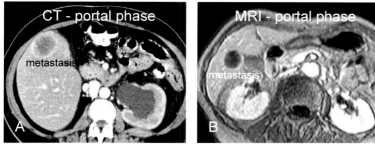
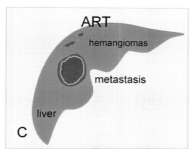
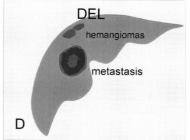

Fig. 20.3. Metastasis, enhancement pattern on CT and MRI, and drawings. A CT in the portal phase shows a thick irregular ring-shaped enhancement. Note also the left-sided hydronephrosis caused by a recurrent colorectal tumor in the pelvic cavity. **B** MRI in the portal phase shows a similar enhancement pattern. **C** Drawing illustrates the ring-shaped versus peripheral nodular enhancement. **D** Drawing illustrates the persistent ring-shaped (metastasis) and homogeneous enhancement (hemangioma)

21 Liver Metastases V – Large, Mucinous, Mimicking a Primary Liver Lesion

Colorectal metastases are typically small or medium-sized (multiple) liver lesions with target-like configuration and irregular ring-shaped enhancement. Some (colo)rectal liver metastases may have unusual size and aspect, and may cause difficulty in proper diagnosis. For instance, some patients may present with a large, single lesion with compressed surrounding liver parenchyma and mimicking primary liver lesions such as cholangiocarcinomas or hepatocellular carcinomas.

MR Imaging Findings

At MR imaging, large mucinous colorectal liver metastases may not have a target-like appearance, which is a characteristic feature of most non-mucinous colorectal liver metastases. Such lesions usually will have predominantly heterogeneous increased signal intensity on T2-weighted images with sharp margins to the surrounding liver; on the T1-weighted images the lesions will mainly have low signal intensity to the liver. Parts of the lesion may have high signal intensity on T1-weighted images due to the presence of mucin. After injection of gadolinium, the lesion shows heterogeneous enhancement in the arterial phase and some washout with enhancement of a pseudocapsule (Figs. 21.1 – 21.3).

Differential Diagnosis

Some of the features, including (1) a single lesion, (2) large size, (3) heterogeneous enhancement, and (4) some washout, may suggest a primary malignant liver lesion such as cholangiocarcinoma or hepatocellular carcinoma in a non-cirrhotic liver. Clinical information of the underlying (colo)rectal malignancy and possibly mucinous histology may direct the reader in the right direction. If the patient has no underlying colorectal tumor, tumor markers including carcinoembryonic antigen (CEA) and alpha-fetoprotein (AFP) should be determined. If these tumor markers are also negative, a somatostatin-receptor scan should be performed to exclude a neuroendocrine tumor metastasis.

Management

Management will depend on the exact nature of the lesion. In the case of a solitary colorectal metastasis, curative resection should be attempted.

Literature

1. Semelka RC, Cance WG, Marcos HB, et al. (1999) Liver metastases: comparison of current MR techniques and spiral CT during arterial portography for detection in 20 surgically staged cases. Radiology 213:86–91
2. Outwater E, Tomaszewski JE, Daly JM, et al. (1991) Hepatic colorectal metastases: Correlation of MR imaging and pathologic appearance. Radiology 180:327–332
3. Yoon SS, Tanabe TK (1999) Surgical treatment and other regional treatments for colorectal cancer liver metastases. Oncologist 4:197–208

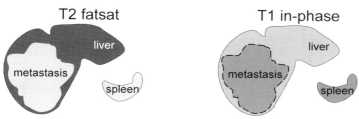
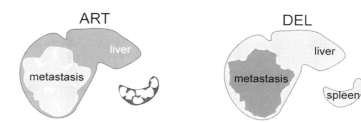

Fig. 21.1. Metastasis, colorectal, mucinous, drawings. T2 fatsat: metastasis is predominantly hyperintense to the liver with a large size and ragged edges; T1 in-phase: metastasis is predominantly hypointense to the liver; ART: me-tastasis shows predominantly heterogeneous intense enhancement; DEL: metastasis shows washout with enhanced discontinuous pseudocapsule

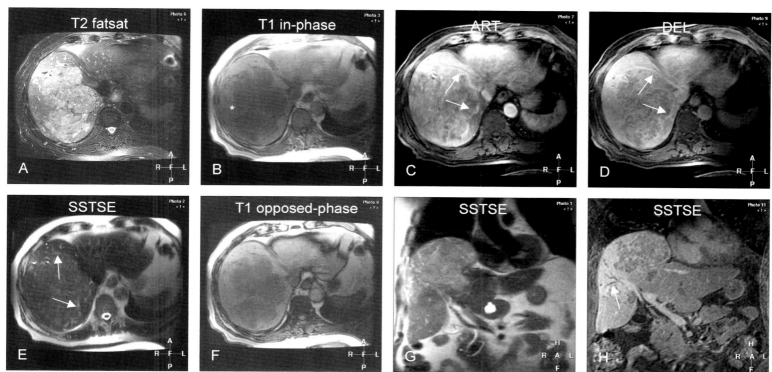

Fig. 21.2. Metastasis, colorectal, mucinous, large, MRI findings. A Axial TSE image (T2 fatsat): Metastasis is predominantly hyperintense to the liver with a large size and ragged edges. **B** Axial in-phase image (T1 in-phase): Metastasis is predominantly hypointense with some brighter areas (*). **C** Axial arterial phase image (ART): Metastasis shows intense heterogeneous enhancement, with some edge enhancement (*arrows*). **D** Axial delayed phase image (DEL): Metastasis shows washout with enhancement of a discontinuous pseudocapsule (*arrows*). **E** Axial SSTSE image (SSTSE): Metastasis shows a partial pseudocapsule with high signal (*arrows*), which is most likely caused by vessels and compressed liver parenchyma. **F** Axial opposed-phase image (T1 opposed-phase) shows no fatty infiltration. **G** Coronal SSTSE image (SSTSE) shows the metastasis bulging into the right hemidiaphragm. **H** Coronal delayed phase image (DEL) shows heterogeneously enhanced metastasis with encased intrahepatic bile ducts (*arrow*)

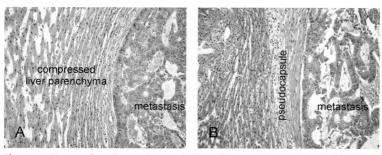
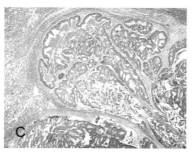
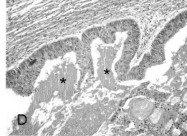

Fig. 21.3. Metastasis, colorectal, large lesion with pseudocapsule and direct MR pathology correlation. A, B Photomicrographs show the metastasis surrounded by compressed liver parenchyma with atrophic hepatocytes, mimicking a thin fibrous capsule. H&E, × 100. **C** Photomicrograph of a large gland surrounded by compressed liver parenchyma. H&E, × 100. **D** Photomicrograph shows the gland that is in part filled with mucin (*). H&E, × 200

22 Colorectal Metastases VI – with Portal Vein and Bile Duct Encasement

Unresectable colorectal liver metastases carry a dismal prognosis. In fact, only 10–25% of colorectal liver metastases are candidates for surgical resection, and the 5-year survival rate following resection of isolated colorectal liver metastases can be as high as 38%. Without any treatment, the survival rate is less than 1%. For the remaining 75–90% of patients with liver metastases who are not amenable to surgery, several new minimally invasive therapies (MIT) have been developed. These include radiofrequency ablation (RFA), percutaneous ethanol injection, percutaneous acetic acid injection, transcatheter arterial chemoembolization, and stereotactic radiotherapy (SRT). There is a large body of data indicating that RFA can reliably treat tumors less than 3 cm in diameter. However, the modality by itself is less effective when applied to larger tumors and tumors in close proximity of vessels. SRT is a novel technique that may be used in patients who cannot be treated with interventional techniques or in conjunction with the other MIT.

MR Imaging Findings

At MR imaging, unresectable liver metastases may present with a number of findings, which include (1) coincidental extrahepatic metastases; (2) all or most segments of the liver affected; (3) vascular invasion or vascular encasement (with or without biliary encasement); and (4) certain anatomic locations rendering the resection technically impossible. Particularly, T2-weighted diffusion-weighted, black-blood echoplanar MR imaging is useful for detection of vascular as well as biliary encasement in combination with a high liver-to-lesion contrast (Figs. 22.1, 22.2). MR imaging is also an excellent modality for follow-up after minimally invasive therapies. The T2-weighted sequences in combination with the dynamic gadolinium-enhanced images allow accurate distinction from nonmalignant parenchymal changes within the liver (Figs. 22.2, 22.3).

Management of Unresectable Liver Lesions

Patients with unresectable liver lesions, usually metastases, may be amenable to systemic chemotherapy (goals: palliation or downstaging); isolated liver perfusion with chemotherapeutic agents (goals: local control or curative-in-attempt); RFA (goals: palliation; downstaging for possible resection; local control while on waiting list for liver transplantation); and stereotactic radiation therapy (palliation or downstaging usually if other MIT options are not applicable).

Literature

1. Weeks SM, Burke C (2005) Local therapeutic treatments for focal liver disease. Radiol Clin N A 43:899–914
2. Mendez Romero A, Wunderink W, Hussain SM, et al. Stereotactic body radiation therapy for primary and metastatic liver tumors: A single institution phase I-II study. Acta Oncol. 2006;45:831–837
3. Yoon SS, Tanabe TK (1999) Surgical treatment and other regional treatments for colorectal cancer liver metastases. Oncologist 4:197–208

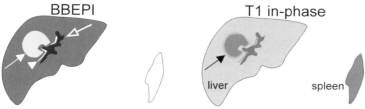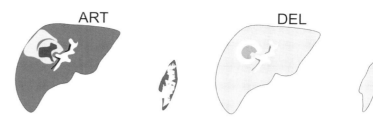

Fig. 22.1. Metastasis, inoperable, drawings. BBEPI: metastasis (*solid arrow*) shows encasement of the bile duct (*arrowhead*) and the portal vein (*open arrow*); **T1 in-phase:** metastasis is surrounded by a bright rim of compressed liver parenchyma (*arrow*); **ART:** metastasis shows ring-shaped and perilesional enhancement; **DEL:** metastasis shows persistent ring-shaped enhancement

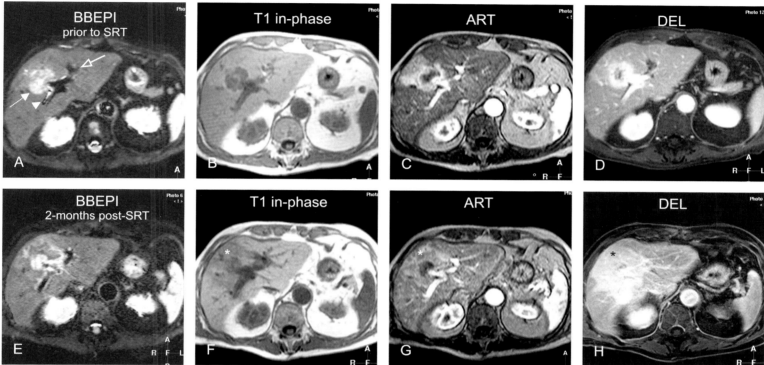

Fig. 22.2. Metastasis, inoperable and treated with stereotactic radiation therapy (SRT), MRI findings. A Axial black-blood EPI (BBEPI): Metastasis (*solid arrow*) shows encasement of the (bright) bile ducts (*arrowhead*) and portal vein with signal void (*open arrow*). **B** Axial in-phase image (T1 in-phase): Metastasis is surrounded by a rim of compressed liver parenchyma. **C** Axial arterial phase GRE image (ART): Metastasis shows ring-shaped and perilesional enhancement. **D** Axial delayed phase image (DEL): Metastasis shows persistent ring enhancement. **E** Axial BBEPI (BBEPI) 2 months after SRT: Metastasis has decreased in size. **F** Axial in-phase image (T1 in-phase): Metastasis is surrounded by a wedge-shaped area of edema (*). **G** Axial arterial phase image (ART): Metastasis shows faint ring-shaped and a large wedge-shaped (*) enhancement. **H** Axial delayed phase image (DEL): Metastasis shows persistent wedge-shaped enhancement (*)

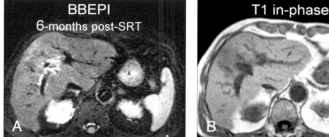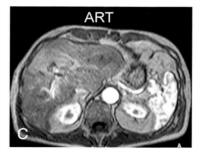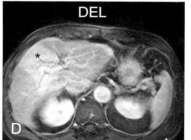

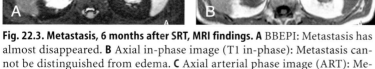

Fig. 22.3. Metastasis, 6 months after SRT, MRI findings. A BBEPI: Metastasis has almost disappeared. **B** Axial in-phase image (T1 in-phase): Metastasis cannot be distinguished from edema. **C** Axial arterial phase image (ART): Metastasis shows negligible enhancement. **D** Axial delayed phase image (DEL): No metastasis is visible within the enhanced wedge-shaped area (*)

23 Colorectal Metastases VII – Recurrent Disease Versus RFA Defect

Increasing numbers of patients with (colorectal) liver metastases undergo surgical resection or minimally invasive therapy and need follow-up with imaging after treatment. There are no strict guidelines for follow-up of such patients. Currently, many centers use laboratory tests (liver function and serum carcinoembryonic antigen, CEA), with or without abdominal ultrasound, for follow-up of patients. Other centers use computed tomography as their main tool for follow-up. In our experience, MR imaging is highly reliable and a versatile imaging technique for detecting and characterizing residual or recurrent liver lesions. In addition, MR imaging allows the differentiation of relevant focal abnormalities from benign tissue changes within the liver.

MR Imaging Findings

At MR imaging, recurrent or residual (colorectal) liver metastases have a distinct appearance. On (fat-suppressed) T2-weighted sequences, these lesions are predominantly higher in signal intensity than the surrounding liver, and often have a target-like appearance which is typical for most colorectal metastases. The lesions show continuous ring-shaped enhancement in the arterial phase, with or without concomitant perilesional or wedge-shaped subsegmental parenchymal enhancement. The latter finding may indicate bile duct and/or portal compression or invasion. In addition, perilesional enhancement with colon cancer may be caused by variable degrees of hepatic parenchymal compression, desmoplastic reaction, and inflammatory infiltrates. Based on the T2 aspect and the enhancement pattern, MR imaging allows reliable differentiation of recurrent or residual disease from benign conditions, for instance after radiofrequency ablation (RFA). In this respect, it should be kept in mind that tissue-specific contrast media may provide confusing results because metastases and non-cancerous tissues behave similarly on post-SPIO images (Figs. 23.1 – 23.3).

Differential Diagnosis

Differential diagnosis may include scar tissue, coagulative necrosis, benign liver lesions such as focal fatty infiltration or focal non-steatosis. State-of-the-art MR imaging combines the findings on the T2-weighted images, chemical shift imaging, and routine arterial and delayed phases after contrast injection. Therefore, MR imaging is more reliable than other imaging modalities.

Literature

1. Braga L, Semelka RC (2005) Magnetic resonance imaging features of focal liver lesions after intervention. Top Magn Reson Imaging 16:99–106
2. Outwater E, Tomaszewski JE, Daly JM, et al. (1991) Hepatic colorectal metastases: Correlation of MR imaging and pathologic appearance. Radiology 180:327–332
3. Abdalla EK, Vauthey JN, Ellis V, et al. (2004) Recurrence and outcomes following hepatic resection, radiofrequency ablation, and combined resection/ablation for colorectal liver metastases. Ann Surg 239:818–825

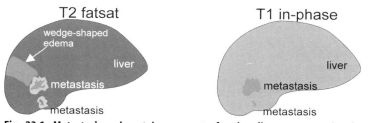
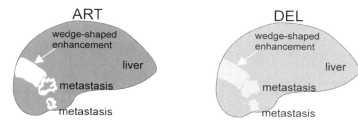

Fig. 23.1. Metastasis, colorectal, recurrent after hemihepatectomy, drawings. **T2 fatsat:** two metastases and wedge-shaped edema are visible; **T1 in-phase:** larger metastasis is better visible than the smaller one; **ART:** metastases show irregular ring-shaped enhancement with wedge-shaped enhancement; **DEL:** metastases become less enhanced

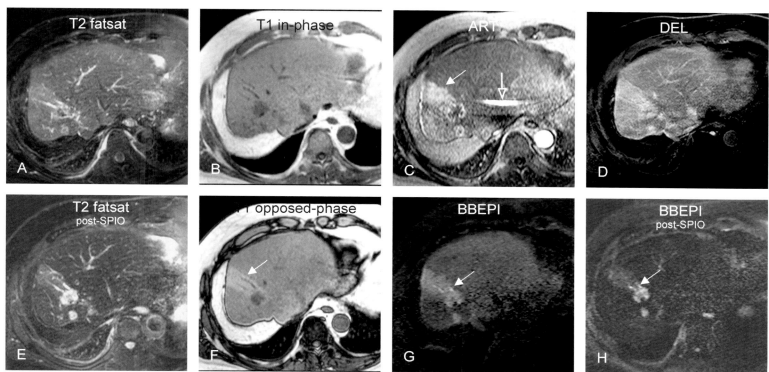

Fig. 23.2. Metastasis, colorectal, recurrent after hemihepatectomy, MRI findings. **A** Axial TSE image (T2 fatsat): Two metastases and wedge-shaped edema are visible. **B** Axial in-phase image (T1 in-phase): Metastasis is hypointense to the liver. **C** Axial arterial phase image (ART): Metastases show irregular ring-shaped enhancement with wedge-shaped enhancement (*solid arrow*). Note the fold-over (SENSE) artifact (*open arrow*). **D** Axial delayed phase image (DEL): Metastases become less enhanced with decreased conspicuity. **E** Axial TSE image after SPIO uptake (T2 fatsat post-SPIO): Metastases show improved conspicuity due to the decreased liver signal; note that the wedge-shaped area also shows SPIO uptake and confirms that it is liver tissue. **F** Axial opposed-phase image (T1 opposed-phase) shows mild diffuse fatty infiltration with fatty sparing (*arrow*). **G** Axial BBEPI before and **H** after uptake of SPIO shows small dilated bile ducts within the wedge-shaped area suggesting segmental bile duct obstruction with decreased portal circulation, fatty sparing, and edema

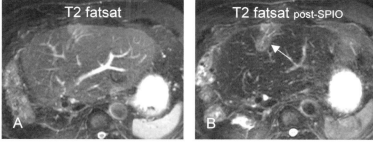
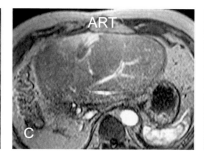
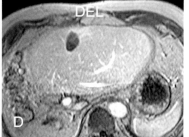

Fig. 23.3. Metastasis, colorectal, radiofrequency ablation (RFA) defect (same patient as above), MRI findings. A Axial TSE image before and **B** after uptake of SPIO shows the oval-shaped RFA defect (*arrow*). **C** Axial arterial phase image: Wedge-shaped enhancement is present around the RFA defect. **D** Axial delayed phase image: RFA defect is well demarcated with a smooth regular rim enhancement due to hyperemia, indicating successful local treatment

Metastases: Non-Colorectal

24 Breast Carcinoma Liver Metastases

Metastatic breast cancer is the most advanced stage (stage IV) of breast cancer. Most commonly it spreads to bone, followed by lung and liver. Approximately 25 % of breast cancers spread first to the bone. In 21 % of cases, the lung is the only site of metastases. The liver is the third most common site for breast cancer. Two-thirds of women with metastatic breast cancer eventually will have liver metastases. Benign lesions are however common in the general population. It is likely that liver lesions will be present on imaging studies in patients with newly diagnosed breast cancer. An unnecessary liver biopsy can be avoided with the application of the state-of-the-art MR imaging of the liver, which can characterize most of the benign lesions as well as the breast carcinoma metastases.

MR Imaging Findings

At MR imaging, breast carcinoma metastases appear low signal intensity on T1-weighted images and moderately high signal intensity on T2-weighted images with fat suppression. On T2-weighted images, the breast carcinoma metastases in the liver may have a target-like configuration, very similar to the colorectal carcinoma metastases. After administration of gadolinium, breast carcinoma metastases may show variable enhancement patterns including an irregular continuous ring-shaped enhancement in the arterial phase. This ring-shaped enhancement reveals the growing edge of the lesion. In the portal and delayed phase the metastases often show washout in the outer parts and a progressive enhancement toward the center of the lesions. Larger lesions may show heterogeneous enhancement. At computed tomography (CT), the breast carcinoma metastases in the liver have a non-specific appearance (Figs. 24.1 – 24.3).

Differential Diagnosis

MR imaging allows the differentiation of metastatic liver lesions from common benign liver lesions such as cysts, hemangiomas, focal nodular hyperplasia, and focal fatty infiltration. Breast carcinoma metastases may have similarities with other metastases including colorectal.

Management

The majority of treatments for metastatic breast cancer focus on alleviating symptoms and may include radiation therapy, chemotherapy, and hormone therapies.

Literature

1. Noon TC, Semelka RC, Balci NC, et al. (1999) Common occurrence of benign liver lesions in patients with newly diagnosed breast cancer investigated by MRI for suspected liver metastases. JMRI 10:165–169
2. Braga L, Semelka RC, Pietrobon L, et al. (2004) Does hypervascularity of liver metastases as detected on MRI predict disease progression in breast cancer patients? AJR Am J Roentgenol 182:1207–1213
3. Zimmerman P, Lu DSK, Yang LY, et al. (2000) Hepatic metastases from breast carcinoma: comparison of noncontrast, arterial-dominant, and portal-dominant phase spiral CT. JCAT 24:197–203

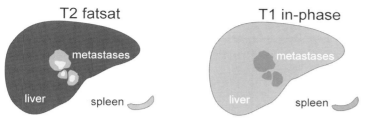
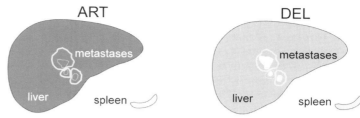

Fig. 24.1. Breast carcinoma metastases, drawings. T2 fatsat: three breast carcinoma metastases are moderately hyperintense with brighter central parts; **T1 in-phase:** metastases are slightly darker than the liver; **ART:** metastases show faint ring-shaped enhancement; **DEL:** metastases show peripheral washout with enhanced central parts

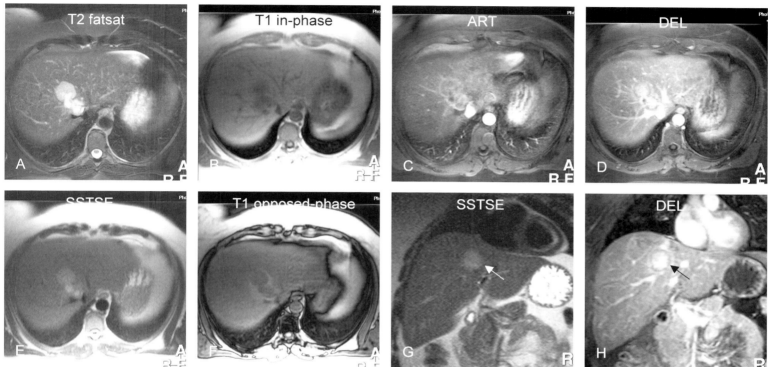

Fig. 24.2. Breast carcinoma metastases, MRI findings. A Axial fatsat T2-w turbo spin echo (TSE) image (T2 fatsat): Three breast carcinoma metastases are moderately hyperintense with brighter central parts, consistent with coagulative necrosis. **B** Axial in-phase gradient recalled echo (GRE) (T1 in-phase): Metastases are darker to the liver. **C** Axial arterial phase image (ART): Metastases show faint irregular ring-shaped enhancement. **D** Axial delayed phase image (DEL): Metastases show peripheral washout with enhanced central parts. **E** Axial single shot TSE (SSTSE) with longer echo time (TE): The solid parts of the lesions become darker than on the T2 fatsat image. **F** Axial opposed-phase T1-w GRE image (T1 opposed-phase): The liver shows signs of moderate fatty infiltration. **G** Coronal SSTSE (SSTSE): The largest lesion is well visible (*arrow*). **H** Coronal delayed phase image (DEL): The largest lesion shows peripheral washout with enhanced central parts (*arrow*)

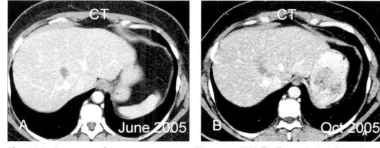
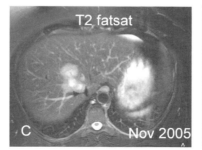
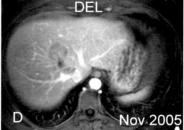

Fig. 24.3. Breast carcinoma metastases, CT versus MRI findings. A Axial CT image shows a hypodense lesion which was considered to indicate suspected metastasis. **B** Axial CT image (5 months later) shows approximately three lesions which were considered more likely to indicate suspected metastases. **C** Axial fat-sat TSE image (T2 fatsat) and **D** axial delayed phase image (DEL) show lesions with typical appearance of metastases, rendering the diagnosis with a much higher level of confidence

25 Kahler's Disease (Multiple Myeloma) Liver Metastases

Kahler's disease or multiple myeloma is a malignant proliferation of plasma cells usually located in the bone marrow. The extramedullary involvement occurs and is found in about 70% of autopsy cases. Hepatic involvement in multiple myeloma has not been proven to have major therapeutic consequences. Liver tests may be abnormal and the liver lesions may mimic metastatic disease. It can also be clinically and biologically silent. Ultrasound (US)-guided biopsy may facilitate diagnosis. MR imaging may have some advantage because of the high prevalence of benign lesions in the general population and a relatively low specificity of CT and US for liver lesions. MR imaging should be considered in patients with multiple myeloma with suspicion of hepatic spread.

MR Imaging Findings

At MR imaging the lesions are hyperintense on T2-weighted images and typically hypointense on T1-weighted images. After injection of gadolinium, in the arterial phase, the central parts of the lesion will show intense enhancement. In the delayed phase, the entire lesion will be enhanced, with persistent enhancement in the later phases. On the T1-w opposed-phase imaging, diffuse fatty infiltration may be present in combination with perifocal fatty sparing due to the parenchymal or vascular compression. Extrahepatic lesions, particularly with bones, may be present. Such lesions show similar arterial enhancement to the liver lesions (Figs. 25.1, 25.2). MR imaging can visualize the vascularity as well as the interval growth. US is non-specific and the lesions may even mimic cysts in the setting of steatosis with increased echogenicity of the background liver (Fig. 25.3).

Differential Diagnosis

The differential diagnosis may include other hypervascular liver metastases, such neuroendocrine types.

Management

MR imaging may facilitate the diagnosis or help to distinguish the solid versus the non-solid lesions and avoid unnecessary biopsy in the setting of multiple myeloma with suspicion of hepatic dissemination. Treatment may include surgery.

Literature

1. Chemlal K, Couvelard A, Grange MJ, et al. (1999) Nodular lesions of the liver revealing multiple myeloma. Leukemia Lymphoma 33:389–392
2. Nguyen BD, Dash N, Lupetin AR (1992) MR imaging of hepatic plasmacytoma: a case report. Clin Imag 16:98–101
3. Caturelli E, Squillante MM, Castalvetere M, et al. (1993) Myelomatous nodular lesions of the liver: diagnosis by ultrasound-guided fine needle biopsy. J Clin Ultras 21:133–137
4. Dohy H, Abe T, Takata N, et al. (1979) Successful hepatectomy for solitary plasmacytoma. N Engl J Med 300:1218–1219
5. Thiruvengadam R, Remedios BP, Goolsby HJ, et al. (1990) Multiple myeloma presenting as space-occupying lesions of the liver. Cancer 65:2784–2786

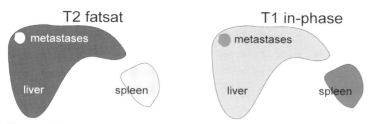

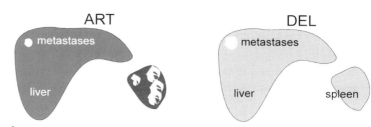

Fig. 25.1. Metastases, hypervascular Kahler liver and skeletal lesions, drawings. T2 fatsat: metastasis in the liver is very bright; **T1 in-phase**: metastasis is hypointense to the liver; **ART**: at least a part of the lesion shows intense enhancement; **DEL**: metastasis shows persistent enhancement of the entire lesion

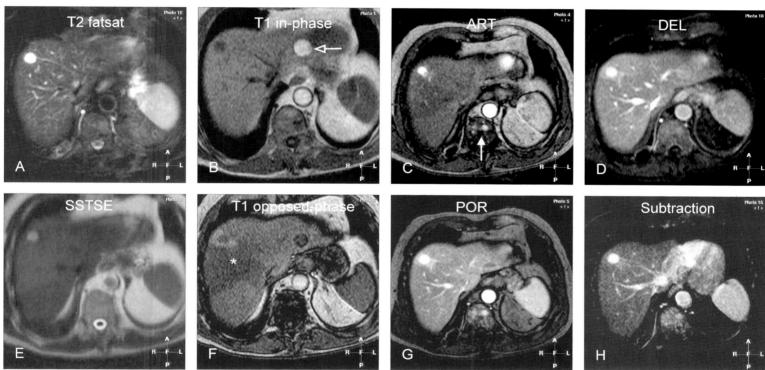

Fig. 25.2. Metastases, hypervascular Kahler liver and skeletal lesions, MRI findings. A Axial TSE image (T2 fatsat): Metastasis in the liver is very bright. **B** Axial in-phase image (T1 in-phase): Metastasis is hypointense to the liver. Ghost artifact from the aorta (*open arrow*). **C** Axial arterial phase image (ART): At least a part of the lesion shows intense enhancement. Note also the vertebral lesions (*arrow*). **D** Axial delayed phase image (DEL): Metastasis shows persistent enhancement of the entire lesion. **E** Axial SSTSE image (T2 fatsat): Metastasis is relatively bright to the liver. **F** Axial opposed-phase image (T1 opposed-phase) shows fatty infiltration in a part of the liver (*). Note the fatty sparing, especially around the liver lesion. **G** Axial portal phase image (POR) shows persistent and perilesional enhancement of the liver metastasis as well as the vertebral lesions. **H** Subtraction image shows the enhanced liver and vertebral lesions

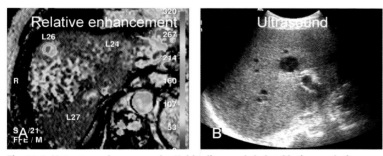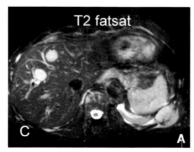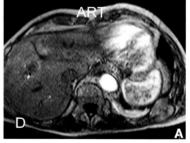

Fig. 25.3. Metastases, hypervascular Kahler liver and skeletal lesions, relative enhancement (computer-generated image); US and MRI findings (another patient). A Relative enhancement based on the arterial phase image shows most intense enhancement in the center of the lesion. **B–D** US and MRI show liver and skeletal metastases in another patient

26 Melanoma Liver Metastases I – Focal Type

Malignant melanoma of the uvea is the second most common type of primary malignant melanoma in humans and is remarkable for its purely hematogenous dissemination and its tendency to metastasize to the liver. Traditionally, hepatic metastases are initially present in 40–60 % of patients. Eventually, the liver is involved in up to 95 % of patients. Fifty percent of patients also have developed extrahepatic metastases which occur often in the lungs, bone, skin, and brain. Delayed dissemination is rather frequent, and the propensity for late hepatic metastasis of uveal melanoma has been designated one of the most unusual phenomena in tumor biology. There is no consensus about screening of patients who have uveal melanoma and have suspected hepatic metastases. US has a sensitivity of only 37 %; this is lower compared to CT. Particularly MR imaging is highly sensitive and specific for melanoma liver metastases.

MR Imaging Findings

MR imaging displays high signal intensity in the larger lesions on T2-weighted images. The smaller lesions may appear isointense. On T1-weighted images and especially on fat suppressed T1-weighted images, the melanin-containing metastases have high signal intensity. After injection of gadolinium in the arterial phase, melanoma metastases show intense enhancement. In the delayed phase, the lesions show wash-out and the larger lesions will become heterogeneous whereas smaller lesions may fade to isointensity. Ultrasound and CT are often non-specific (Figs. 26.1, 26.2). Melanoma metastases can show rapid interval growth (doubling time around 3 months). At laparoscopy and biopsy, the melanin typically appears dark.

Differential Diagnosis

Melanin-containing liver lesions (high signal on T1-weighted images) that show enhancement in the arterial phase after injection of gadolinium in a patient with an underlying uveal melanoma have no differential diagnosis. Other hypervascular liver lesions should be considered in the differential of non-melanotic liver metastases.

Literature

1. Eskelin S, Pyrhönen S, Summanen P, et al. (1999) Screening for metastatic malignant melanoma of the uvea revisited. Cancer 85:1151–1159
2. Middleton WD, Hiskes SK, Tefey SA, Vousher LD (1997) Small (1.5 cm or less) liver metastases: US-guided biopsy. Radiology 205:729–732
3. Hussain SM, Semelka RC (2005) Hepatic imaging: comparison of modalities. Radiol Clin N Am 43:929–947

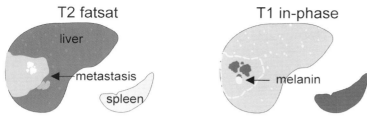
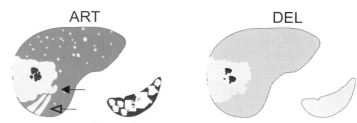

Fig. 26.1. Melanoma metastases, focal, drawings. T2 fatsat: a large lesion (*arrow*) with central necrosis is visible. The smaller lesions are difficult to see. **T1 in-phase:** a brighter area (*arrow*) indicates the presence of melanin; **ART:**

numerous smaller and larger lesions show intense enhancement. Note two lesions (*solid arrow*) with wedge-shaped enhancement (*open arrow*). **DEL:** most lesions show washout and become isointense

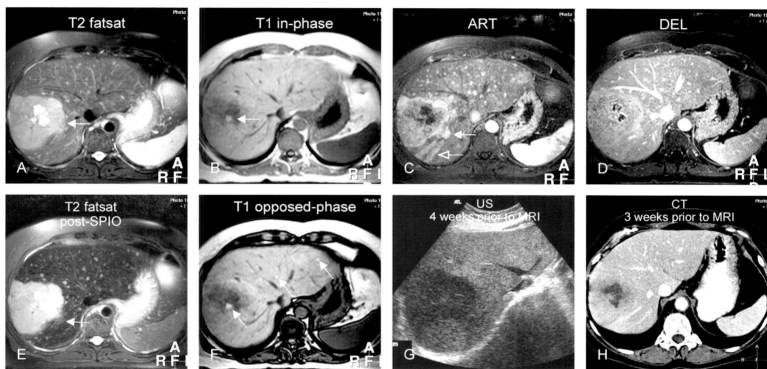

Fig. 26.2. Melanoma metastases, focal, melanotic, MRI findings. A Axial fatsat T2-w TSE image (T2 fatsat): Large melanoma metastasis (*arrow*) contains central necrosis. **B** Axial in-phase T1-w GRE (T1 in-phase): The large metastasis contains melanin with high signal (*arrow*). **C** Axial arterial phase image (ART): Larger metastasis shows intense irregular ring-shaped enhancement with multiple enhancing smaller metastases in the entire liver. Note also lesions (*solid arrow*) with wedge-shaped enhancement (*open arrow*). **D** Axial delayed phase image (DEL): Metastases become isointense and are difficult

to recognize. **E** Axial T2-w post-superparamagnetic iron oxide (SPIO) (T2 fatsat post-SPIO): Note the improved conspicuity of the larger as well as the smaller lesions (*arrow*). **F** Axial opposed-phase GRE image (T1 opposed-phase): The high signal of the metastases is caused by the paramagnetic effect of melanin (*arrows*). **G** Ultrasound shows only the larger lesion. **H** Computed tomography in the portal phase only shows the larger lesion. The findings are comparable to the delayed phase MR image in **D**

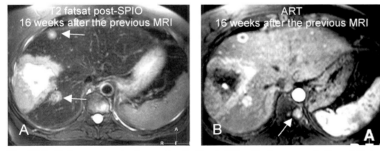
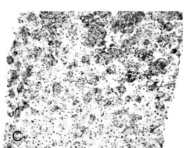
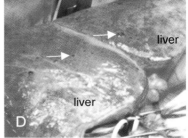

Fig. 26.3. Melanoma metastases, focal, direct MR pathology correlation. A Fat-suppressed T2-w TSE image after SPIO shows interval increase in size of the hepatic metastases (*arrows*). **B** Arterial phase image shows irregular ring-shaped and heterogeneous enhancement of the hepatic metastases as well as

a new bone metastasis (*arrow*). **C** Photomicrograph shows melanin-containing hepatocytes (parenchymal spread). H&E, × 100. **D** Laparoscopic photograph shows dark, melanin-containing capsular lesions (*arrows*)

27 Melanoma Liver Metastases II – Diffuse Type

Melanoma liver metastases can be diffused and may even be more difficult to recognize on ultrasound and CT. Diffuse metastases of liver may mimic subtle changes of vascularity and may have little to no contrast to the background and may appear as insignificant findings. In addition, techniques such as fluorodeoxyglucose-positron emission tomography (FDG-PET) may be negative in such cases. MR imaging can provide specific diagnosis by demonstrating the presence of melanin on T1-weighted images. In such cases, the extrahepatic disease may also be present, which can be evaluated with MR imaging as well. Therefore, MR imaging should be the modality of choice with suspected melanoma liver metastases.

MR Imaging Findings

MR imaging of melanoma metastases that present as diffused lesions show a heterogeneous and increased signal intensity of the entire liver on T2-weighted images. On T1-weighted images, the high signal intensity of diffuse melanoma metastases may be unremarkable because it may overlap with the normal high signal intensity of the liver, although after injection of gadolinium very intense heterogeneous enhancement of almost the entire liver will be present which may be persistent in the later phases. There may be some free fluid surrounding the liver. In such cases, CT and FDG-PET may be inconclusive. The findings may remain undetected or may be described as vascular abnormalities and the diagnosis may remain obscured (Figs. 27.1 – 27.3).

Management

Isolated hepatic perfusion particularly with tumor necrosis factor and melphalan appears to be an effective treatment for unresectable hepatic malignancies including melanoma metastases.

Literature

1. Eskelin S, Pyrhönen S, Summanen P, et al. (1999) Screening for metastatic malignant melanoma of the uvea revisited. Cancer 85:1151–1159
2. Alexander HR, Libutti SK, Pingpank JF, et al. (2003) Hyperthermic isolated hepatic perfusion with (IHP) using melphalan for patients with popular melanoma metastatic to liver. Clin Cancer Res 9:6343–6349
3. Grover A, Alexander HR (2004) The past decade of experience with isolated hepatic perfusion. Oncologist 9:653–664

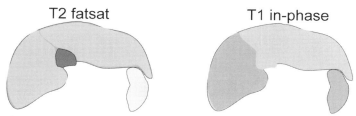

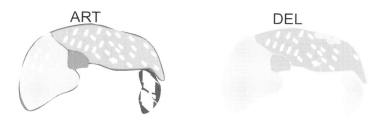

Fig. 27.1. Melanoma metastases, diffuse, drawings. T2 fatsat: melanoma metastases have caused a diffuse increased signal of the liver except in the caudate lobe; T1 in-phase: the right liver has abnormally decreased signal; ART: the liver shows diffuse and patchy abnormal enhancement in almost the entire liver; DEL: the left liver retains its patchy enhancement

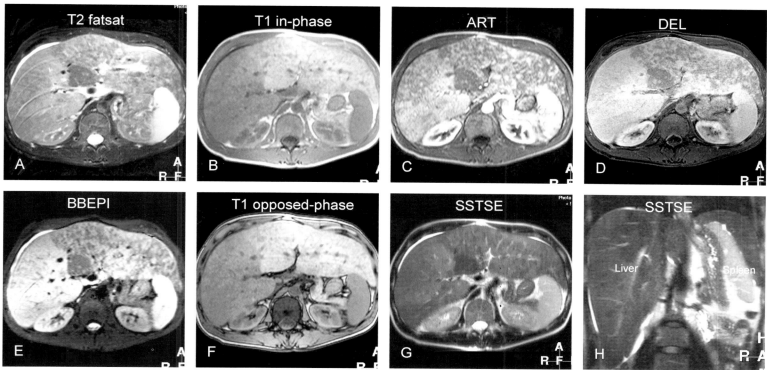

Fig. 27.2. Melanoma metastases, diffuse, MRI findings. A Axial fatsat T2-w TSE image (T2 fatsat): Melanoma metastases have caused a diffuse increased signal of the liver except in the caudate lobe. **B** Axial in-phase T1-w GRE (T1 in-phase): The liver shows abnormally decreased signal on the right side of the liver. **C** Axial arterial phase post-Gd 2D T1-w GRE image (ART): The liver shows diffuse and patchy abnormal enhancement in almost the entire liver. **D** Axial delayed post-Gd 3D GRE image (DEL): The left liver retains its patchy enhancement, whereas the right liver has abnormally increased enhancement. **E** Axial T2-w black-blood echoplanar image (BB-EPI): The right side of the liver has a higher signal than the left side. **F** Axial opposed-phase T1-w GRE image (T1 opposed-phase): The liver shows no signs of fatty infiltration. **G** Axial T2-w SSTSE image (SSTSE axial): The liver is surrounded by a small amount of ascites. **H** Coronal T2-w SSTSE image (SSTSE coronal): The liver is clearly enlarged and has an abnormally high signal

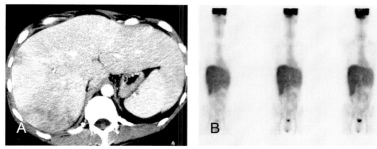

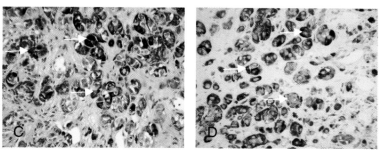

Fig. 27.3. Melanoma metastases, diffuse, CT, FDG-PET, and MR-pathology correlation. A Contrast-enhanced CT in portal phase (prior to MR) showed „vascular abnormalities". **B** FDG-PET (after CT and prior to MRI) showed normal activity in the liver without any evidence of metastases. **C** Photomicrograph of the liver biopsy shows diffuse sinusoidal infiltration of melanin-containing tumor cells (*arrows*). H&E, ×200. **D** Photomicrograph shows abundant specific immunohistochemical staining of the melanin-containing cells (*arrows*). Melan-A, ×200

28 Neuroendocrine Tumor I – Typical Liver Metastases

Neuroendocrine cells, which are present throughout the gastrointestinal (GI) tract, the pancreas, and the lungs, can give rise to a variety of tumors. Tumors that arise in the GI tract are called „neuroendocrine tumors" (NET) or „carcinoids" and tumors from the pancreas are called „islet cell tumors." The latter include insulinoma, gastrinoma, glucagonoma, vasoactive intestinal peptide-producing tumor (VIPoma), and somatostatinoma. The incidence of all NET has been estimated to be 2.0/100,000 for men and 2.4/100,000 for women. Etiology is unknown. Tumors may present with clinical symptoms and/or lymph node and liver metastases. The primary may be small and difficult to locate. The single most important predictor of poor survival in patients with neuroendocrine tumors is hepatic metastases. The extent of liver metastases correlates with the subsequent survival. For instance, patients without any liver metastases of gastrinomas have a 5-year survival of 95%, and with numerous bilobar metastases this figures drops to only 15%. Patients may present with liver metastases with an unknown primary.

MR Imaging Findings

At MR imaging, the liver metastases of neuroendocrine tumors are typically multiple (>5 lesions), relatively small (a few centimeters in diameter), similar in size with sharp margins to the liver, and predominantly very bright (with almost fluid-like signal intensity) on T2-weighted images. At T1-weighted images, the appearance is often unremarkable (low signal intensity compared to spleen). On gadolinium-enhanced images, the lesions show irregular ring-shaped or heterogeneous enhancement in the arterial phase and washout of contrast in the delayed phase images without any evidence of perilesional capsular enhancement (Figs. 28.1–28.3).

Differential Diagnosis

Other primary or secondary hypervascular liver lesions form the differential. To distinguish between NET and other types of liver metastases, an additional somatostatin-receptor scintigraphy (SRS) scan or a US-guided biopsy may be helpful.

Management

Management is often tailored and may include one or a combination of the following: surgical (curative or debulking), chemotherapy, and biotherapy (somatostatin analogues).

Literature

1. Capella C, Heitz PU, Hofler H, et al. (1995) Revised classification of neuroendocrine tumours of the lung, pancreas and gut. Virchows Arch 425:547–560
2. Hemminki K, Li X (2001) Incidence trends and risk factors of carcinoid tumors. A nationwide epidemiologic study from Sweden. Cancer 92:2204–2210
3. Kloppel G, Anlauf M (2005) Epidemiology, tumor biology and histopathological classification of neuroendocrine tumours of gastrointestinal tract. Clin Gastroenterol 19:507–517

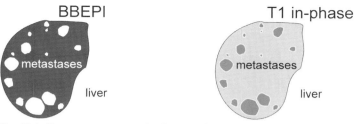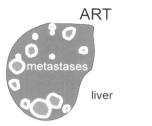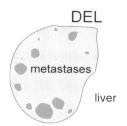

Fig. 28.1. Metastases, neuroendocrine, multiple, drawings. BBEPI: metastases are very bright to the liver; **T1 in-phase**: metastases are hypointense to the liver; **ART**: metastases show an intense irregular ring-shaped as well as peri- lesional enhancement; DEL: metastases show washout without any promi- nent capsular enhancement

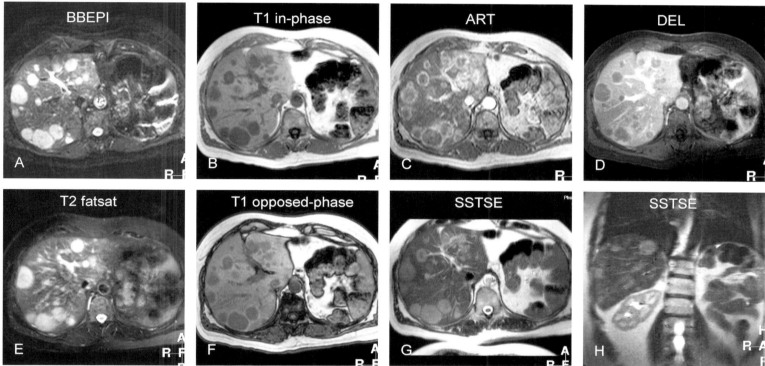

Fig. 28.2. Metastasis, neuroendocrine, multiple, MRI findings. A Axial black-blood echoplanar imaging (BBEPI) image: Metastases are very bright to the liver. **B** Axial in-phase T1-w GRE (T1 in-phase): Metastases are hypointense to the liver. **C** Axial arterial phase image (ART): Metastases show an intense irregular ring-shaped as well as a perilesional enhancement. **D** Axial delayed phase image (DEL): Metastases show washout of contrast, without any capsular enhancement. **E** Axial TSE image (T2 fatsat): Metastases are very bright to the liver, mimicking non-solid lesions such as cysts or hemangio- mas. **F** Axial opposed-phase image (T1 opposed-phase) shows slight signal drop in the liver indicating subtle steatosis. Note that metastases are surrounded by persistent high perifocal signal due to compressed liver. **G** Axial SSTSE image (SSTSE) shows the metastases as bright lesions, but much less brighter than fluid (e.g., in the spinal canal). **H** Coronal SSTSE image (SSTSE) with a longer TE shows that the metastases become darker, further indicating their solid nature

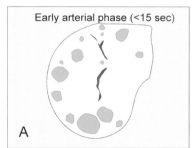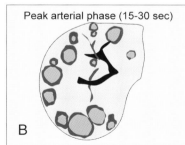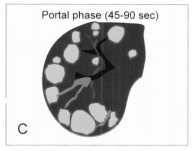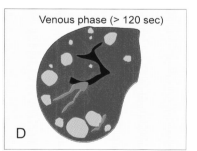

Fig. 28.3. Metastases, neuroendocrine, the enhancement pattern. A Early arterial phase: faint ring-shaped enhancement of metastases; no enhancement of the liver. **B** Peak arterial phase: Metastases show intense ring-shaped as well as perilesional enhancement; the liver shows 25–30% of the peak enhance- ment. **C** Portal phase: The liver shows the peak enhancement; the metastases show less perilesional enhancement. The liver veins are enhanced. **D** Venous phase: The lesions show washout without any capsular enhancement. Tissues show homogeneous enhancement

29 Neuroendocrine Tumor II – Pancreas Tumor Metastases

The tumors arising from the pancreas may comprise up to 45 % of all neuroendocrine tumors and about 40 % may be malignant with liver metastases. Of these, the majority are non-functioning tumors. Insulinomas are the most common pancreatic NET. They are usually small and solitary and 90 % are located within the pancreas; only 6 – 10 % of insulinomas are malignant. Multiple tumors present in 10 % of cases and may be associated with multiple endocrine neoplasia type 1 (MEN-1). In malignant tumors, all patients will have liver metastases.

MR Imaging Findings

At MR imaging, neuroendocrine tumor metastases from pancreas tumor are often small, and appear hyperintense on T2-weighted images and low signal intensity on T1 images. After injection of gadolinium, lesions show intense homogeneous or ring shaped enhancement with variable perifocal enhancement. In the delayed phase, the lesions show washout and become heterogeneous. At CT, the lesions may be less conspicuous because CT is performed as a single-phase study due to radiation issues. For this reason CT may not be a suitable technique for follow-up of such lesions (Figs. 29.1 – 29.3).

Management

Hepatic metastases treatment may include (1) primary tumor resection, (2) resection in combination with ablation, (3) transarterial chemoembolization, and (4) medical therapies including somatostatin analogues, radiation, and systemic chemotherapy. Surgical resection of neuroendocrine hepatic metastases is a proven treatment of symptoms related to systemic hormone release. Advances in operative techniques and equipment have made hepatic resections safer, especially in tertiary, high-volume centers. Although the neuroendocrine tumors are frequently characterized by an indolent course, historic controls with hepatic metastases without resection or ablation have a much-reduced 5-year survival, which varies from 20 % to 30 %. Recently, several groups have reported an improved 5-year survival of 50 – 70 % with resection of neuroendocrine hepatic metastases.

Literature

1. Capella C, Heitz PU, Hofler H, et al. (1995) Revised classification of neuroendocrine tumours of the lung, pancreas and gut. Virchows Arch 425:547 – 560
2. Kloppel G, Anlauf M (2005) Epidemiology, tumor biology and histopathological classification of neuroendocrine tumours of gastrointestinal tract. Clin Gastroenterol 19:507 – 517
3. Touzios JG, Kiely JN, Pitt SC, et al. (2005) Neuroendocrine hepatic metastases: does aggressive management improve survival? Ann Surg 241:776 – 785

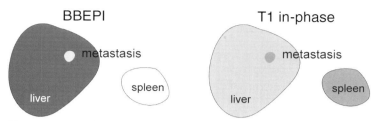
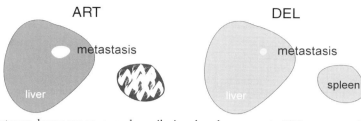

Fig. 29.1. Metastasis, neuroendocrine pancreas tumor metastasis, before octreotide treatment, drawings. BBEPI: metastasis is hyperintense to the liver; T1 in-phase: metastasis is hypointense to the liver; ART: metastasis shows intense homogeneous and perilesional enhancement; DEL: metastasis shows washout with some persistent enhancement

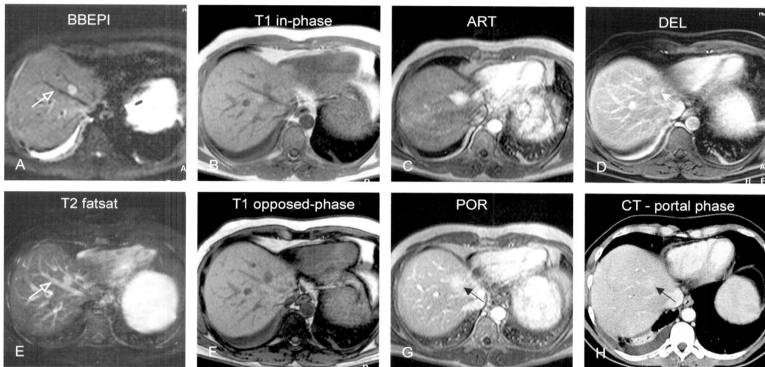

Fig. 29.2. Metastasis, neuroendocrine pancreas tumor metastasis, before octreotide treatment, MRI findings. A Axial BBEPI image (BBEPI): Metastasis is hyperintense to the liver. The conspicuity of the lesion is improved due to dark vessels (*open arrow*). **B** Axial in-phase image (T1 in-phase): Metastasis is hypointense to the liver. **C** Axial arterial phase image (ART): Metastasis shows intense homogeneous and perilesional enhancement, and therefore appears larger. **D** Axial delayed phase image (DEL): Metastasis shows washout with some persistent enhancement. **E** Axial TSE image (T2 fatsat): Metastasis has a similar appearance to some of the in-plane bright vessels (*open arrow*), and hence lesser conspicuity than on the BBEPI image. **F** Axial opposed-phase image (T1 opposed-phase) shows no steatosis. **G** Axial portal phase image (POR): The metastasis (*arrow*) is difficult to appreciate because of the washout of contrast. **H** Axial CT in portal phase: The metastasis (*arrow*) appears almost isodense to the liver and is difficult to appreciate

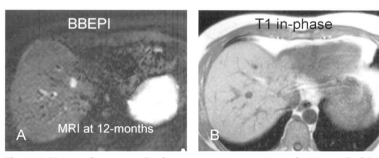
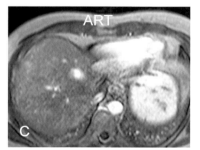
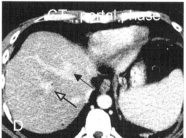

Fig. 29.3. Metastasis, neuroendocrine pancreas tumor metastasis, 12 months follow-up after octreotide treatment, MRI findings. A Axial BBEPI image (BBEPI): Metastasis has decreased in size. **B** Axial in-phase image (T1 in-phase): Metastasis is difficult to see due to its smaller size. **C** Axial arterial phase image (ART): Metastasis shows less intense enhancement compared to the previous MRI. **D** Axial CT in portal phase: Due to decreased size and vascularity, the metastasis is even more difficult to assess than the previous CT. Also it is difficult to distinguish from some of the vessels (*open arrow*)

30 Neuroendocrine Tumor III – Gastrinoma Liver Metastases

Gastrinomas can occur in the pancreas, stomach, duodenum, and proximal jejunum. About 90 % of these tumors are located within the „gastrinoma triangle," which is formed by the junction between the neck and body of the pancreas medially, the second and third portions of the duodenum inferiorly, and the junction of the cystic and common bile ducts superiorly. The tumors produce gastrin and can give rise to ulcers, diarrhea, and reflux (Zollinger-Ellison syndrome). Gastrinomas, relative to insulinomas, are more often extrapancreatic and multiple. They also tend to be even smaller and less vascular than insulinomas. These features make them even more difficult to localize than insulinomas. As many as 60 % of gastrinomas are malignant; 25 % of these tumors are associated with MEN-1, which is more common in the setting of multiple and extrapancreatic tumors. At the time of diagnosis, 30 % of pancreatic tumors and 10 % of duodenal tumors have metastasized. Metastases most commonly involve the lymph nodes and liver.

MR Imaging Findings

Gastrinoma liver metastases typically appear as multiple liver lesions with somewhat variable signal intensity and size. On T2-weighted imaging, most lesions have high signal intensity compared to the normal liver and comparable signal intensity to the spleen. On the T1-weighted images, the lesions have low signal intensity. After injection of gadolinium, small lesions have almost homogeneous enhancement with varied perifocal enhancement and the larger lesions may have ring-shaped or heterogeneous enhancement in the arterial phase. In the delayed phase, the smaller lesions show complete wash-out whereas the larger lesions may show persistent or even increased enhancement in the central part of the lesions. MR imaging can also show extrahepatic localization, such as nodal involvement. The involved nodes often have a similar appearance to the hepatic metastases (Fig. 30.1 – 30.3).

Literature

1. Kumbasar B, Kamel IR, Tekes A, et al. (2004) Imaging of neuroendocrine tumors: accuracy of helical CT versus SRS. Abdom Imaging 29:696 – 702
2. Noone TC, Hosey J, Firat Z, Semelka RC (2005) Imaging and localization of islet-cell tumours of pancreas on CT and MRI. Best Pract Res Clin Endocrinol Metab 19:195 – 211
3. Semelka RC, Custodio CM, Balci NC, Woosley JT (2000) Neuroendocrine tumors of the pancreas: spectrum of appearances on MRI. J Magn Reson Imaging 11:141 – 148

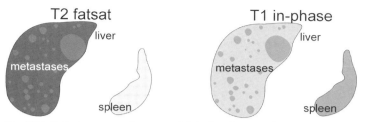
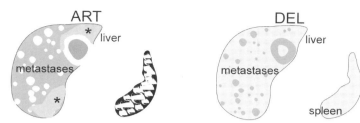

Fig. 30.1. Metastases, gastrinoma, multiple drawings. T2 fatsat: metastases are variable in size and slightly hyperintense to the liver; **T1 in-phase:** metastases are hypointense to the liver; **ART:** larger lesions show irregular ring-shaped and the smaller lesions homogeneous enhancement; note also the parenchymal enhancement (*); **DEL:** metastases show washout

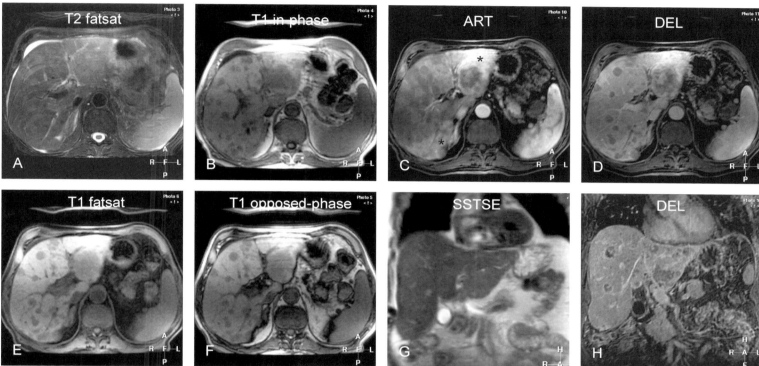

Fig. 30.2. Metastases, gastrinoma, multiple, MRI findings. A Axial TSE image (T2 fatsat): Metastases are variable in size and slightly hyperintense to the liver. Note also ascites. **B** Axial in-phase image (T1 in-phase): Metastases are hypointense to the liver. **C** Axial arterial phase image (ART): Larger lesions show irregular ring-shaped and the smaller lesions homogeneous enhancement; note also the parenchymal enhancement (*). **D** Axial delayed phase image (DEL): Metastases show washout. **E** Axial fat-suppressed GRE image (T1 fatsat): Metastases show better delineation to the liver due to improved liver-to-lesion contrast. **F** Axial opposed-phase image (T1 opposed-phase) shows no fatty infiltration. **G** Coronal SSTSE image (SSTSE) shows irregular contours of the liver suggesting capsular involvement. **H** Coronal delayed image (DEL) shows multiple metastases with washout and central persistent enhancement

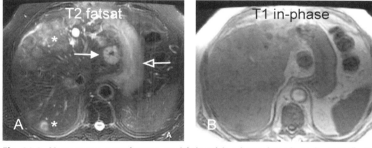
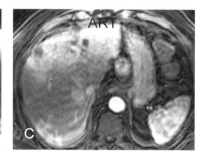
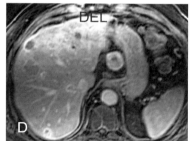

Fig. 30.3. Metastases, gastrinoma, multiple with a large lymph node, MRI findings. A Axial TSE image (T2 fatsat) shows multiple liver metastases (*), a large lymph node (*solid arrow*), and thickened stomach wall (*open arrow*). **B** Axial in-phase image (T1 in-phase): Metastases are hypointense to the liver. **C, D** Axial arterial and delayed phase images (ART/DEL): Metastases appear in similar fashion

31 Neuroendocrine Tumor IV – Carcinoid Tumor Liver Metastases

The term „carcinoid" is used for neuroendocrine tumors (NET) of extrapancreatic origin. Endocrine tumors of the gastrointestinal tract, which are known as carcinoids, originate from the diffuse neuroendocrine cell system. These cells are scattered throughout the mucosa of the GI tract and express neuroendocrine markers such as chromogranin A. Carcinoid tumors can produce serotonin and can cause flushing, diarrhea, and bronchial obstruction (carcinoid syndrome). There are 14 cell types which produce different hormones. Carcinoid tumors show a non-random distribution in the GI tract: stomach (2–3%; recent studies: 11–41%), duodenum and proximal jejunum (22%), distal jejunum and ileum (23–28%), appendix (19%), cecum and ascending colon (9%), and rectosigmoid (20%). The carcinoid type of tumors is found in up to 55% of patients with NET and up to 60% may be malignant with hepatic metastases.

MR Imaging Findings

Carcinoid tumor liver metastases may have a variable signal intensity on T1- and T2-weighted images. On T2-weighted images lesions may have low signal intensity areas, as well as high signal intensity areas. The low signal intensity areas correspondingly will have high signal intensity on T1-weighted images. These findings are consistent with the presence of hemorrhage or protein content within the lesions. After injection of gadolinium, the lesions show peripheral ring-shaped enhancement in the arterial phase and wash-out in the delayed phase. The lesions may be large in size. The presence of calcifications, which are better appreciated on CT, is a non-specific finding. Relatively large lesions may have cystic components centrally which may be filled with colloid or protein-rich fluid, appearing high on T1-weighted images. Larger tumors also tend to have solid peripheral components with persistent enhancement (Figs. 31.1–31.3).

Differential Diagnosis

Hemorrhage and other hemorrhagic tumors should be distinguished based on characteristic MR imaging findings.

Literature

1. Capella C, Heitz PU, Hofler H, et al. (1995) Revised classification of neuroendocrine tumours of the lung, pancreas and gut. Virchows Arch 425:547–560
2. Kloppel G, Anlauf M (2005) Epidemiology, tumor biology and histopathological classification of neuroendocrine tumours of gastrointestinal tract. Clin Gastroenterol 19:507–517
3. Touzios JG, Kiely JN, Pitt SC, et al. (2005) Neuroendocrine hepatic metastases: does aggressive management improve survival? Ann Surg 241:776–785
4. McGill DB, Rakela J, Zinsmeister AR, et al. (1990) A 21 year experience with major hemorrhage after percutaneous liver biopsy. Gastroenterology 99:1396–1400

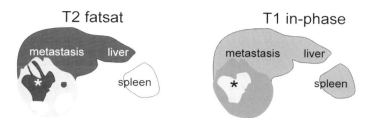

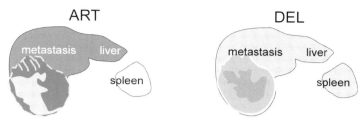

Fig. 31.1. Metastasis, carcinoid with hemorrhage, drawings. T2 fatsat: dark hematoma (*) is located in the center of the metastasis, which is predominantly hyperintense to the liver; **T1 in-phase:** hematoma shows high signal caused by methemoglobin (*); **ART:** parts of the metastasis show heterogeneous enhancement; **DEL:** peripheral parts of the metastasis show more enhancement than the central hemorrhagic part

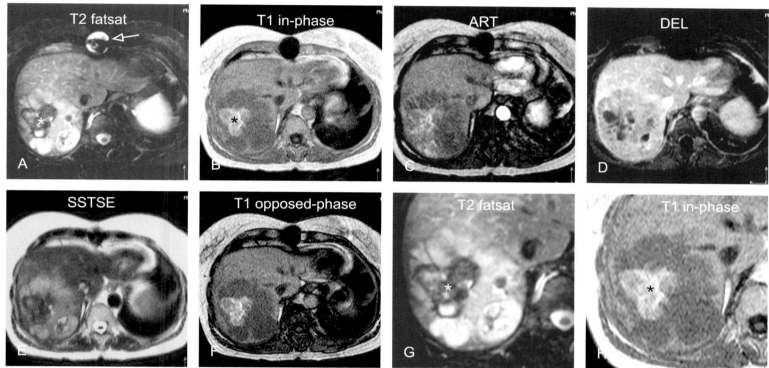

Fig. 31.2. Metastasis, carcinoid with hemorrhage, MR findings. A Axial fat-suppressed T2-w TSE image (T2 fatsat): Dark hematoma (*) is located in the center of the metastasis, which is predominantly hyperintense to the liver. Artifact caused by the metal wire after sternotomy (*open arrow*). **B** Axial in-phase image (T1 in-phase): Hematoma shows high signal caused by methemoglobin (*). **C** Axial GRE image in the arterial phase (ART): Parts of the metastasis show heterogeneous enhancement. **D** Axial delayed phase (DEL): The hematoma appears to remain unenhanced. **E** Axial SSTSE image (SSTSE) shows decreased signal in the solid parts of the metastasis. **F** Axial opposed-phase image (T1 opposed-phase) shows increased perilesional signal caused by steatotic liver (*arrow*). **G** A detailed view of fat-suppressed T2-weighted image (T2 fatsat) shows the central hematoma in more detail (*). **H** Axial in-phase image (T1 in-phase) shows the hemorrhage bright (*)

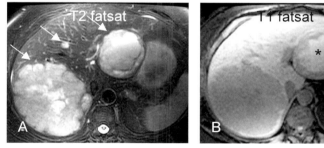

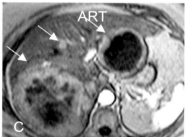

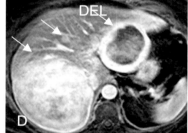

Fig. 31.3. Metastasis (another patient), carcinoid, protein-producing, MRI findings. A Axial TSE (T2 fatsat) shows three carcinoid metastases with variable solid component (*arrows*). **B** Axial fat-suppressed T1-w image (T1 fatsat): One of the lesions contains fluid with high signal (*), consistent with high protein content. **C** Axial arterial phase image (ART) shows enhancement of mainly the solid parts (*arrows*). **D** Axial delayed phase image (DEL) shows persistent enhancement of the solid parts (*arrows*)

32 Neuroendocrine Tumor V – Peritoneal Spread

Peritoneal carcinomatosis has been described in association with neuroendocrine tumors. Overall peritoneal spread from neuroendocrine tumors can occur in 10% of cases. Carcinoid tumors produce peritoneal spread in 27% and non-gastrinoma pancreatic tumors in 11% of cases. Peritoneal spread from gastrinoma is rare. In addition to the nature of the primary tumor, the size of the primary tumor of >5 cm is associated with the presence of peritoneal disease from pancreatic endocrine tumors. In patients with carcinoid tumors, an ileal primary tumor is more often associated with peritoneal spread than carcinoid tumor at other locations. Patients with peritoneal metastases can also have concurrent liver metastases. However, it should be kept in mind that capsular implants may show ingrowths and mimic liver lesions at imaging. Particularly, MR imaging can accurately detect peritoneal nodules, liver capsular nodules, ascites, and presence of soft tissue masses within the mesentery as well as in the greater omentum.

MR Imaging Findings

At MR imaging, the peritoneal carcinomatosis with capsular spread to the liver presents as high signal intensity on T2-weighted images with increased thickness of the peritoneal lining and irregularity of the liver capsule. Some lesions around the liver may become large and show ingrowths into the liver and may mimic liver lesions. At T1-weighted images the findings are non-specific. After injection of gadolinium, in the arterial phase, the nodular component and thickened peritoneal and capsular lining show increased enhancement which persists in the later phases. Based on the sequences with high soft tissue contrast and routine gadolinium-enhanced imaging, MR imaging provides more accurate information than other modalities including CT (Figs. 32.1–32.3). MR imaging can better distinguish ascites from solid components.

Differential Diagnosis

Peritoneal spread from other malignancies (ovarian, breast, colorectal). Correlation with clinical history and localization of the primary tumor may facilitate distinction.

Literature

1. Vasseur B, Cadiot G, Zins M, et al. (1996) Peritoneal carcinomatosis in patients with digestive endocrine tumors. Cancer 78:1686–92
2. Lebtahi R, Cadiot G, Sarda L, et al. (1997) Clinical impact of somatostatin receptor scintigraphy in the management of patients with neuroendocrine gastroenteropancreatic tumors. J Nucl Med 38:853–8
3. Krenning EP, Kwekkeboom DJ, Bakker WH, et al. (1993) Somatostatin receptor scintigraphy with [111In-DTPAD-Phe1]- and [123I-Tyr3]-octreotide: the Rotterdam experience with more than 1,000 patients. Eur J Nucl Med 20:716–31
4. Berger JF, Laissy JP, Limot O, et al. (1996) Differentiation between multiple liver hemangiomas and liver metastases of gastrinomas: value of enhanced MRI. JCAT 20:349–55

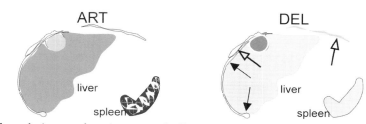

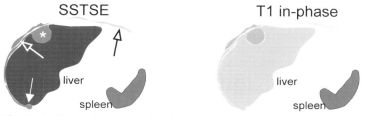

Fig. 32.1. Metastasis, neuroendocrine, peritoneal and capsular involvement, drawings. SSTSE: large (*) and a small capsular in growth (*solid arrow*) appear as hyperintense liver; peritoneal involvement (*open arrows*); T1 in-

phase: lesions are hypointense to the liver; **ART:** all lesions show enhancement; **DEL:** note the difference between the capsular (*solid arrows*) and the peritoneal enhancement (*open arrows*)

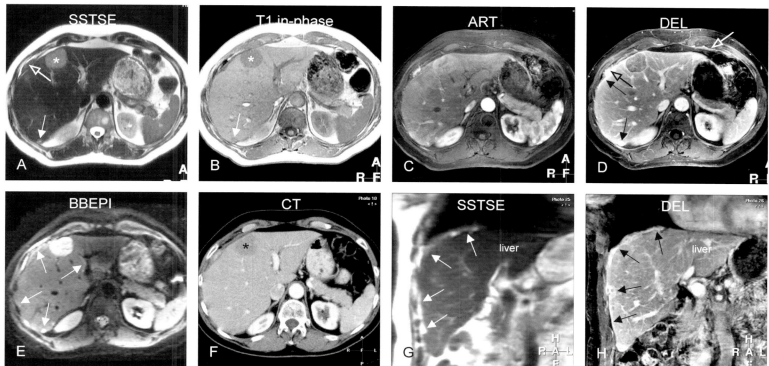

Fig. 32.2. Metastasis, neuroendocrine, peritoneal and capsular involvement, MRI findings at 3.0T. A Axial SSTSE image (SSTSE): Capsular thickening (*solid arrow*) and a large ingrowth (*) are hyperintense to the liver; the peritoneal thickening appears darker (*open arrow*). **B** Axial in-phase T1-w GRE (T1 in-phase): Similar appearance of the larger (*) and the smaller (*arrow*) capsular lesions suggests their common origin. **C** Axial arterial phase image (ART): The lesions show intense enhancement. **D** Axial delayed phase image (DEL): The capsular (*solid arrows*) and peritoneal (*open arrows*) lesions

show increased and persistent enhancement. **E** Axial BBEPI image (T2 fat-sat): Compared to SSTSE, the conspicuity of the capsular lesions (*arrows*) is improved. **F** Axial contrast-enhanced CT (CT) shows the largest lesion (*) well; the smaller capsular lesions are difficult to recognize. **G** Coronal SSTSE image (SSTSE) shows diffuse and irregular capsular thickening (*arrows*). **H** Coronal delayed phase image (DEL) shows abnormal capsular enhancement (*arrows*)

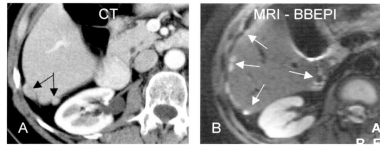

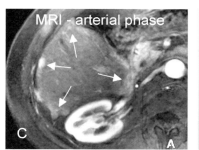

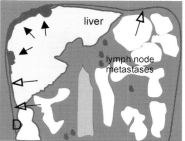

Fig. 32.3. Metastasis, neuroendocrine, peritoneal and capsular involvement, CT and MRI findings at a different anatomic level, drawing. A Axial enhanced (single phase) CT shows two capsular lesions (*arrows*). **B** Axial BBEPI image (MRI-BBEPI) shows multiple bright lesions (*arrows*). **C** Axial arterial phase

image (MRI – arterial phase) shows intense enhancement of the capsular lesions (*arrows*). **D** Drawing illustrates the capsular (*solid arrows*), peritoneal (*open arrow*) spread, and lymph node metastases

33 Ovarian Tumor Liver Metastases – Mimicking Giant Hemangioma

Ovarian cancer has the highest mortality rate of all gynecologic malignancies, in which about 70% of patients have peritoneal involvement at the time of diagnosis. The tumors have a tendency to show direct spread as well as intraperitoneal dissemination. The staging system is surgically based: *stage I,* disease being limited to one or both ovaries; *stage II,* extraovarian spread within the pelvis; *stage III,* diffuse peritoneal disease involving the upper abdomen; *stage IV,* distant metastases including hepatic lesions. Common sites of intraperitoneal seeding include the omentum, paracolic gutters, liver capsule, and diaphragm. Thickening, nodularity, and enhancement are all signs of peritoneal involvement. Microscopic peritoneal and liver capsular spread remain challenging to detect at imaging. Some investigators have shown that MR imaging is superior in visualization of small or equivocal peritoneal implants compared with CT.

MR Imaging Findings

At MR imaging, the intrahepatic, liver capsular and peritoneal carcinomatosis presents as high signal intensity on T2-weighted images. Liver lesions may grow diffusely and replace the entire hepatic parenchyma; capsular lesions may show ingrowths into the liver. The high signal of the liver lesions may show similarity with giant hemangiomas in the liver. On T1-weighted images the findings are non-specific. After injection of gadolinium, the liver lesions show heterogeneous enhancement in the arterial phase, which remains heterogeneous in the delayed phase due to washout of the contrast as opposed to giant hemangiomas, which typically show persistent enhancement in the delayed phase (Figs. 33.1, 33.2). Thickened peritoneum and omentum show high signal intensity on T2-weighted images with persistent delayed enhancement (Fig. 33.3). MR imaging facilitates better distinction between fluid and non-fluid components.

Differential Diagnosis

Clinical correlation is recommended to differentiate from other disseminated malignancies (breast, colorectal).

Management

Early ovarian cancer is treated with comprehensive staging laparotomy, whereas advanced but operable disease is treated with primary cytoreductive surgery (debulking) followed by adjuvant chemotherapy. Patients with unresectable disease may benefit from neoadjuvant (preoperative) chemotherapy before debulking.

Literature

1. Woodward PJ, Hosseinzadeh K, Saenger JS (2004) From the archives of the AFIP: radiologic staging of ovarian carcinoma with pathologic correlation. Radiographics 24:225–246
2. Low RN, Carter WD, Saleh F, et al. (1995) Ovarian cancer: comparison of findings with perfluorocarbon-enhanced MR imaging, In-111-CYT-103 immunoscintigraphy, and CT. Radiology 195:391–400
3. Low RN, Semelka RC, Worawattanakul S, et al. (1999) Extrahepatic abdominal imaging in patients with malignancy: comparison of MR imaging and helical CT, with subsequent surgical correlation. Radiology 210:625–632

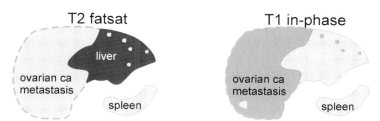 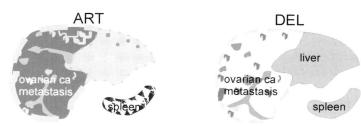

Fig. 33.1. Metastasis, ovarian carcinoma metastases, drawings. T2 fatsat: a large metastasis and several smaller lesions (left liver) are hyperintense to the liver; **T1 in-phase:** metastases are hypointense to the liver; **ART:** metastases show intense heterogeneous enhancement; **DEL:** metastases show persistent heterogeneous enhancement. Note that the liver capsule along the larger lesion is permeated

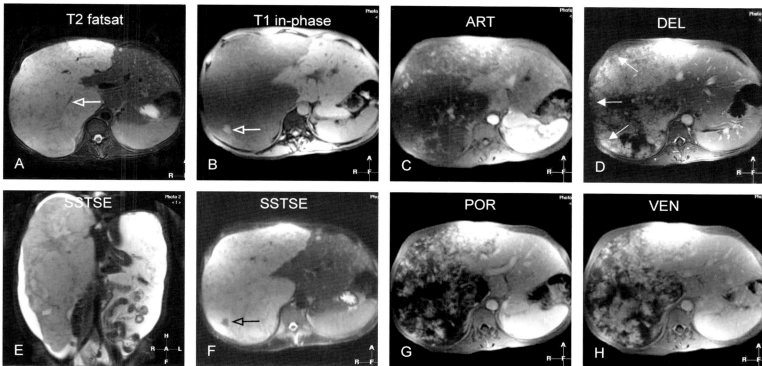

Fig. 33.2. Metastasis, ovarian carcinoma metastases, MRI findings. A Axial TSE image (T2 fatsat): A large metastasis and several smaller lesions (left liver) are hyperintense to the liver. Note that the larger lesions contain low signal intensity linear structures, including vessels (*open arrow*). **B** Axial in-phase image (T1 in-phase): Metastases are hypointense to the liver. The larger lesion contains an area of high signal intensity (*open arrow*), most likely mucin. **C** Axial arterial phase image (ART): Metastases show intense heterogeneous enhancement. **D** Axial delayed phase image (DEL): Metastasis shows persistent heterogeneous enhancement. Note that the liver capsule along the larger lesion is permeated and appears irregular (*arrows*). **E** Coronal SSTSE image (SSTSE) shows that the right liver is completely replaced by the tumor with abundant ascites, suggesting pseudomyxoma peritonei. **F** Axial SSTSE image (SSTSE) shows a small dark area with the large metastasis, consistent with mucin (*open arrow*). **G, H** Axial portal (POR) and venous (VEN) phase images show the progressive heterogeneous enhancement of the larger lesion

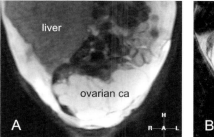 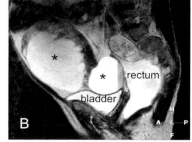 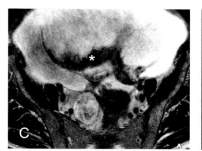 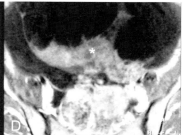

Fig. 33.3. Metastasis, ovarian carcinoma in the pelvis (primary tumor evaluation in the same patient), MRI findings. A Coronal TSE image through the pelvis shows the enlarged liver and the ovarian carcinoma with cystic and solid components. **B** Sagittal TSE image: Ovarian carcinoma consists of several cystic and solid components (*). **C, D** Axial TSE and gadolinium-enhanced delayed phase images show thickened wall of one of the cysts with enhancement (*)

34 Renal Cell Carcinoma Liver Metastasis

Renal cell carcinoma (RCC) is the 7th leading malignant condition among men and the 12th among women, accounting for 2.6% of all cancers. The aim of preoperative imaging in RCC is to adequately assess tumor size, localization and organ confinement, to identify lymph node and/or visceral metastases, and to reliably predict the presence and extent of any thrombus of the vena cava. In 25% of patients, advanced disease, including locally invasive or metastatic renal-cell carcinoma, is found at presentation. Moreover, a third of the patients who undergo resection of localized disease will have a recurrence. Median survival for patients with metastatic disease is about 13 months. Thus, there is a great need for more effective surgical and medical therapies. Nephrectomy may be warranted, even in the presence of metastatic disease. The detection of visceral metastases appears to be crucial since it has been shown that even patients with metastatic disease might benefit from radical nephrectomy followed by systemic immunotherapy. MR imaging provides more comprehensive locoregional evaluation of the primary lesion(s) including the distinction from concurrent (complicated) renal cysts, vascular invasion, and liver metastases.

MR Imaging Findings

At MR imaging, renal cell carcinoma liver metastases appear low signal intensity on T1-weighted images and moderately high signal intensity on T2-weighted images with fat suppression. After administration of gadolinium, renal cell carcinoma liver metastases may show variable enhancement patterns including an intense homogeneous to heterogeneous enhancement in the arterial phase. In the portal and delayed phase the metastases often show washout and may become more heterogeneous (Figs. 34.1, 34.2).

Differential Diagnosis

Other hypervascular liver lesions including primary tumors as well as secondary tumors from other sources such as pancreas may have very similar appearance and need clinical correlation or US-guided biopsy for confirmation of proper diagnosis (Fig. 34.3).

Management

Surgical excision of a solitary metastasis in patients with advanced RCC is recommended in many cases, but this approach has not yet been proved to be effective in prolonging survival.

Literature

1. Semelka RC, Shoenut JP, Magro CM, et al. (1993) Renal cancer staging: comparison of contrast-enhanced CT and gadolinium-enhanced fat-suppressed spin-echo and gradient-echo MR imaging. JMRI 3:597–602
2. Heidenreich A, Ravery V (2004) European Society of Oncological Urology: preoperative imaging in renal cell cancer. World J Urol 22:307–15
3. Mickisch GH, Garin A, van Poppel H, et al. (2001) Radical nephrectomy plus interferon-alfa-based immunotherapy compared with interferon alfa alone in metastatic renal-cell carcinoma: a randomized trial. Lancet 358:966–70
4. Figlin RA (1999) Renal cell carcinoma: management of advanced disease. J Urol 161:381–6

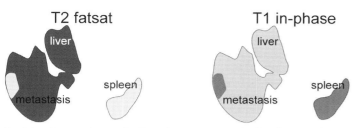 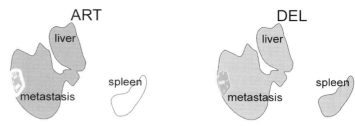

Fig. 34.1. Metastasis, renal cell carcinoma metastasis, drawings. T2 fatsat: Metastasis is hyperintense to the liver; **T1 in-phase:** metastasis is hypointense to the liver; **ART:** metastasis shows intense heterogeneous enhancement; **DEL:** metastasis shows some washout with persistent heterogeneous enhancement

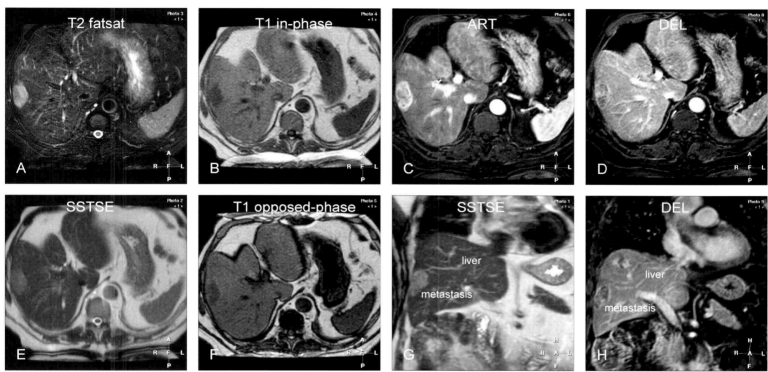

Fig. 34.2. Metastasis, renal cell carcinoma metastasis, MRI findings. A Axial TSE image (T2 fatsat): Metastasis is hyperintense to the liver. **B** Axial in-phase image (T1 in-phase): Metastasis is hypointense to the liver. **C** Axial arterial phase image (ART): Metastasis shows heterogeneous enhancement. **D** Axial delayed phase image (DEL): Metastasis shows some washout with persistent heterogeneous enhancement. **E** Axial SSTSE image (SSTSE): Metastasis is slightly hyperintense. **F** Axial opposed-phase image (T1 opposed-phase) shows slight signal drop in the liver indicating subtle steatosis. Note that metastases are surrounded by persistent high perifocal signal due to compressed liver. **G** Coronal SSTSE image (SSTSE) shows the metastasis as a relatively bright lesion. **H** Coronal delayed image (DEL) shows the metastasis with persistent heterogeneous enhancement

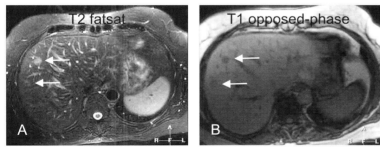 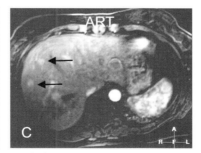 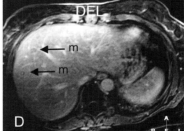

Fig. 34.3. Metastases, pancreas carcinoma metastases (another patient), MRI findings. A Axial TSE image (T2 fatsat) shows two metastases that are slightly hyperintense to the liver (*arrows*). **B** Axial opposed-phase image (T1 opposed-phase): metastases are hypointense to the liver (*arrows*). **C** Axial arterial phase image (ART): metastases show faint, homogenous enhancement (*arrows*). **D** Axial delayed phase image (DEL) shows washout within lesions (m).

Primary Solid Liver Lesions in Cirrhotic Liver

IIC

35 Cirrhosis I – Liver Morphology

Damage to the liver, which often leads to fibrosis and cirrhosis, can be caused by several factors, including toxic agents, metabolic disorders, obesity, alcoholism, and viral infections. Aflatoxin is considered an important cause of cirrhosis in endemic areas, such as Africa and Asia. Metabolic and genetic disorders, including hemochromatosis, can lead to cirrhosis as well. Alcohol may directly damage the liver cells but it also impairs the uptake as well as the oxidation of fatty acids in the hepatocellular mitochondria. Excess dietary fat and carbohydrates are stored as fatty acids and triglycerides in the hepatocytes. In addition, damaged liver cells lose their ability to efficiently remove triglycerides from the liver. Therefore, obesity, diabetes (type II) as well as alcoholism can lead to fatty liver. Long-standing steatosis can lead to steatohepatitis, which may progress to fibrosis, and eventually to cirrhosis. Viral hepatitis is currently the most important etiologic factor leading to liver fibrosis and cirrhosis in North America.

MR Imaging Findings

Cirrhosis induces several intra- and extrahepatic changes including enlargement of the caudate lobe and the left lateral segment of the liver, atrophy of the right hepatic lobe and the left medial segment, nodularity of the liver surface, coarse liver architecture, ascites, splenomegaly, and the development of collaterals. At MR imaging, cirrhotic liver shows changed morphology which may include irregular contours, atrophy of certain segments (usually segment IV), central atrophy, and hypertrophy of some segments. Cirrhotic livers contain regenerative nodules which may develop into dysplastic nodules and hepatocellular carcinomas over time (Figs. 35.1 – 35.3).

Literature

1. Hussain SM, Zondervan PE, et al. (2002) Benign versus malignant hepatic nodules: MR imaging findings with pathologic correlation. Radiographics 22:1023 – 36
2. Ito K, Mitchell DG, Gabata T, Hussain SM (1999) Expanded gallbladder fossa: simple MR imaging sign of cirrhosis. Radiology 211:723 – 726
3. Ito K, Mitchell DG, Siegelman ES (2002) Cirrhosis: MR imaging features. Magn Reson Imaging Clin N Am 10:75 – 92
4. Nonomura A, Enomoto Y, Takeda M, et al. (2005) Clinical and pathological features of non-alcoholic steatohepatitis. Hepatol Res 33:116 – 121

T1 fatsat 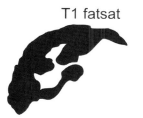 SSTSE 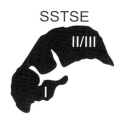 T1 opposed-phase 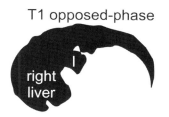 SSTSE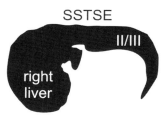

Fig. 35.1. Cirrhosis, morphology of the liver, drawings. T1 fatsat: multiple regenerative nodules cause irregular contours of the liver; **SSTSE:** hypertrophy of segments I, II and III with right-sided atrophy; note also irregular

contours; **T1 opposed-phase:** Segment I and right-sided hypertrophy; note also irregular contours; **SSTSE:** Segments II and II with right-sided hypertrophy.

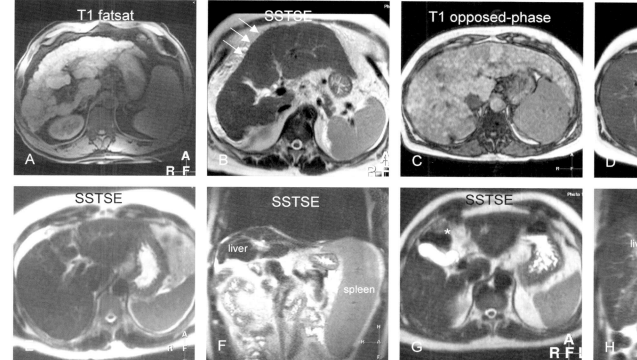

Fig. 35.2. Cirrhosis, morphology of the liver, MRI findings from six different patients. A Axial fat-suppressed T1-w gradient recalled echo (GRE) image (T1 fatsat): Multiple bright nodules and septa cause irregular contours of the liver. **B** Axial single shot turbo spin echo (SSTSE) image (SSTSE): Segment I, II, and III hypertrophy with right-sided atrophy is present. Note the fine irregularity of the liver contours due to intrahepatic nodules (*arrows*). **C** Axial opposed-phase image (T1-opposed-phase): Multiple bright nodules with predominant right-sided and segment I hypertrophy are present. **D** Axial SSTSE

image (SSTSE): Prominent left- and right-sided hypertrophy (i.e., segmental regenerative). **E** Axial SSTSE image (SSTSE) shows segment IV atrophy. **F** Coronal SSTSE image (SSTSE) shows atrophy of the liver and splenomegaly. **G** Axial SSTSE image (SSTSE) shows absence of segment IV due to complete atrophy. Note the interposition of the bowel loops with the empty gallbladder fossa (*). **H** Coronal SSTSE image (SSTSE) shows hypertrophy of the right and the left lateral segment of the liver

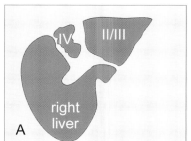 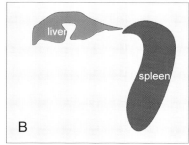 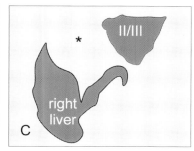 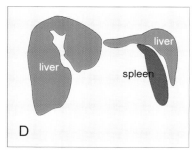

Fig. 35.3. Cirrhosis, morphology of the liver, drawings. A Atrophy of segment IV, with relative hypertrophy of the right liver and segments II/III. **B** Atrophy of

the liver with splenomegaly. **C** Complete disappearance of segment IV with empty gallbladder fossa (*). **D** Hypertrophy of the right and the left liver

36 Cirrhosis II – Regenerative Nodules and Confluent Fibrosis

Cirrhosis is mainly composed of regenerative nodules (RNs) that are surrounded by fibrous septa. In addition to the nodules, cirrhotic livers may have areas of increased segmental fibrosis which may mimic malignancy particularly on ultrasound (US) and computed tomography (CT) because these modalities lack the inherent tissue contrast and routine use of dynamic contrast-enhanced imaging. Also the RNs may be challenging to distinguish from malignancy on these modalities. MR imaging is highly sensitive and specific for diffuse liver lesions including cirrhosis and related abnormalities.

MR Imaging Findings

At MR imaging, RNs show variable signal intensity on T1-weighted sequences (low, iso, high). By definition, RNs show low signal intensity on T2-weighted sequences and do not show any detectable enhancement in the arterial phase after injection of gadolinium. In the later phase, cirrhotic livers often show septal enhancement with some enhancement of the RNs. Unlike previous reports, MR imaging facilitates the distinction between confluent fibrosis and segmental or diffuse hepatocellular carcinoma. Confluent fibrosis typically has slightly increased signal on T2-weighted images but lacks arterial enhancement or washout in the delayed phases. Instead, confluence fibrosis shows persistent enhancement in the delayed phases due to the presence of fibrosis (Figs. 36.1, 36.2).

Pathology

RNs result from a localized proliferation of hepatocytes and their supporting stroma. RNs include monoacinar RNs, multiacinar RNs, cirrhotic nodules, lobar or segmental hyperplasia, and focal nodular hyperplasia. RN is a well-defined region of parenchyma that has enlarged in response to necrosis, altered circulation, or other stimuli. The diameter varies between less than a millimeter to a few centimeters. Macronodular cirrhosis contains nodules >3 mm. Cirrhotic nodules are RNs that are largely or completely surrounded by fibrous septa (Fig. 36.3).

Literature

1. International Working Party (1995) Terminology of nodular hepatocellular lesions. Hepatology 22:983–993
2. Hussain SM, Zondervan PE, et al. (2002) Benign versus malignant hepatic nodules: MR imaging findings with pathologic correlation. Radiographics 22:1023–36
3. Ohtomo K, Baron RL, Dodd GD III, et al. (1993) Confluent hepatic fibrosis in advanced cirrhosis: evaluation with MR imaging. Radiology 189:871–874

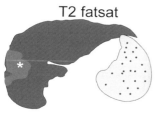
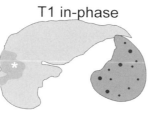
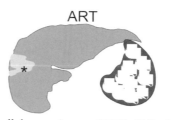
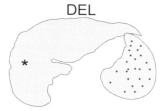

Fig. 36.1. Cirrhosis, confluent fibrosis. T2 fatsat: the right liver shows atrophy with slightly increased signal (*). **T1 in-phase:** the same part has a decreased signal (*). The spleen contains Gamna Gandy bodies. **ART:** the suspected part (*) shows slightly increased enhancement which may suggest an hepa-tocellular carcinoma (HCC); **DEL:** the suspected part of the liver (*) becomes almost isointense due to persistent enhancement, compatible with confluent fibrosis

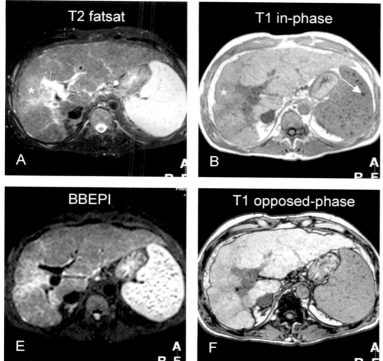
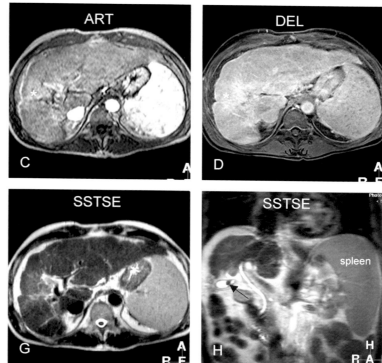

Fig. 36.2. Cirrhosis, confluent fibrosis, MRI findings. A Axial fat-suppressed T2-w TSE image (T2 fatsat): The liver shows irregular contours with multiple nodules and atrophy of the right liver with slightly increased signal (*). **B** Axial T1-w in-phase GRE image (T1 in-phase): A part of the right liver has decreased signal (*). The enlarged spleen shows Gamna Gandy bodies as a sign of portal hypertension. **C** Axial arterial phase image (ART): A part of the right liver shows some increased enhancement (*). **D** Axial delayed phase image (DEL): The enhanced liver (*) does not lose its contrast (no washout), compatible with confluent fibrosis. **E** Axial T2-w black-blood echoplanar imaging (BBEPI) image: Due to lack of refocusing pulses, the (iron containing) Gamna Gandy bodies appear larger. **F** Axial T1-w opposed-phase image (T1 opposed-phase) shows the liver with multiple regenerative nodules. **G** Axial SSTSE (SSTSE) shows the liver with irregular contours. **H** Coronal SSTSE (SSTSE) shows the atrophy of the right liver with enlarged spleen. Note a small stone in the gallbladder (*arrow*)

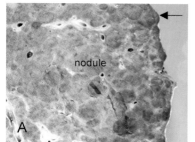
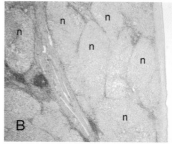
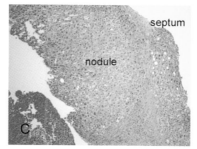
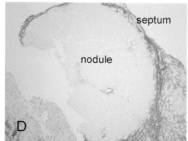

Fig. 36.3. Cirrhosis, histopathology based on the material from other patients. A Photograph of part of an explant cirrhotic liver with multiple nodules surrounded with septa. The contours of the liver are very irregular (*arrow*). **B** Photomicrograph shows multiple regenerative nodules (*n*) surrounded by septa consistent with cirrhosis. H&E, × 40. **C** Photomicrograph shows a nodule in more detail surrounded by a septum. H&E, × 100. **D** Photomicrograph shows the nodule in **C** with better demarcation due to specific staining of the fibrotic septum. Sirius red stain, × 100

37 Cirrhosis III – Dysplastic Nodules

Cirrhotic livers may contain various types of nodules including regenerative nodules, dysplastic nodules, and hepatocellular carcinoma (HCC). These nodules are part of the stepwise carcinogenesis of HCC, which is based on increasing cellularity and size of the liver lesion. In 1995, an International Working Party of Gastroenterology proposed a terminology in which dysplastic features of the hepatic nodule were expressed. The currently accepted nomenclature in stepwise carcinogenesis of HCC is regenerative nodule → low grade dysplastic nodule → high grade dysplastic nodule → small HCC → large HCC. Dysplastic lesions are composed of hepatocytes which show histologic characteristics of abnormal growth caused by presumed or proved genetic alteration. Dysplastic nodules include dysplastic focus and dysplastic nodule. Dysplastic focus is defined as a cluster of hepatocytes less than 1 mm in diameter with dysplasia but without definite histologic criteria of malignancy. Dysplasia indicates the presence of nuclear and cytoplasmic changes, such as minimal to severe nuclear atypia and increased amounts of cytoplasmic fat or glycogen, within the cluster of cells that compose the focus. Dysplastic foci are common in cirrhosis.

MR Imaging Findings

At MR imaging, the signal intensity and enhancement characteristics of the dysplastic nodules are not yet well established. Due to a gradual stepwise transition from a regenerative nodule into a low-grade dysplastic nodule, a high-grade dysplastic nodule, and eventually into a small and a large HCC, the hepatocytes within hepatic nodules undergo numerous changes that might not be reflected in their signal intensity or vascularity. So, current MRI sequences might not be able to distinguish regenerative nodules from dysplastic nodules with certainty. A majority of high-grade dysplastic lesions and well-differentiated small HCC may have high signal intensity on T1-weighted images. Other findings associated with dysplastic nodules may be fat accumulation, gradual increase in size, increased signal intensity, and increased enhancement (Figs. 37.1 – 37.3).

Management

In a cirrhotic liver, any nodule with increased size, changed signal intensity, and increased enhancement warrants clinical correlation with alpha-fetoprotein and follow-up with MR imaging.

Literature

1. International Working Party (1995) Terminology of nodular hepatocellular lesions. Hepatology 22:983 – 993
2. Hussain SM, Zondervan PE, et al. (2002) Benign versus malignant hepatic nodules: MR imaging findings with pathologic correlation. Radiographics 22:1023 – 36
3. Van den Bos IC, Hussain SM, Terkivatan T, et al. (2006) Step-wise carcinogenesis of hepatocellular carcinoma in the cirrhotic liver: demonstration on serial MR imaging. JMRI (in press)

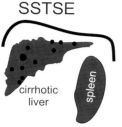
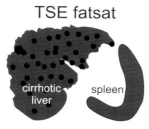
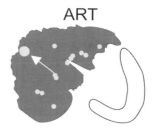
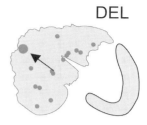

Fig. 37.1. Dysplastic nodules, cirrhotic liver, drawings. Coronal SSTSE: multiple low signal intensity nodules are visible in a cirrhotic liver with ascites. **TSE fatsat:** all nodules have low signal intensity; **ART:** the largest nodule (*arrow*) shows increased enhancement; other nodules show variable enhancement; **DEL:** the largest (*arrow*) as well as other nodules do not show any tumor capsule

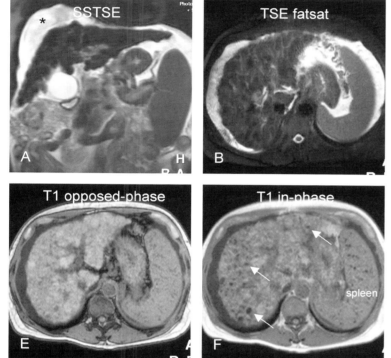
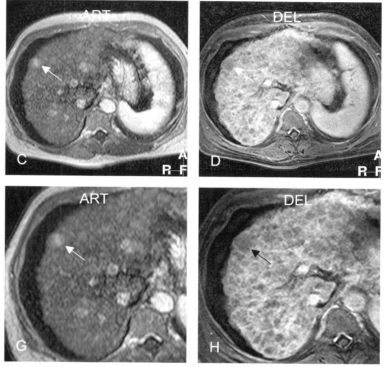

Fig. 37.2. Dysplastic nodules, cirrhotic liver, MRI findings. A Coronal SSTSE image (SSTSE): Multiple low signal intensity nodules are present with a cirrhotic liver with splenomegaly and ascites (*). **B** Axial fat-suppressed TSE image (TSE fatsat): All nodules show low signal intensity. **C** Axial arterial phase image (ART): The largest nodule shows increased enhancement (*arrow*); other lesions show variable enhancement. **D** Axial delayed phase image (DEL): The largest nodule (*arrow*) does not show any enhancing tumor capsule. **E** Axial opposed-phase image (T1 opposed-phase): Most hepatic nodules are bright. **F** Axial in-phase image (T1 in-phase): Several nodules lose their signal due to iron accumulation, i.e. siderotic nodules (*arrows*); note also the dark Gamna-Gandy bodies in the spleen. **G** Detailed view of the arterial phase (ART): The largest nodule clearly shows enhancement (*arrow*). **H** Detailed view of the delayed phase (DEL): The largest nodule does not show a tumor capsule (*arrow*)

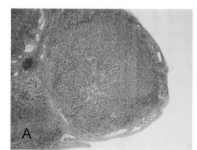
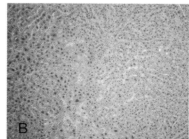
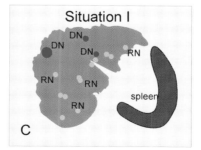
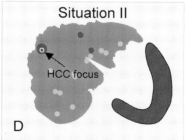

Fig. 37.3. Dysplastic nodules, histopathology, drawings. A Photomicrograph shows a large nodule surrounded by fibrous septa. H&E stain, ×20. **B** A detailed photomicrograph shows increased cellularity with variable size of the nuclei indicating at least dysplastic changes. H&E stain, ×100. **C** Situation I shows the presence of several dysplastic (DN) and regenerative (RN) nodules in a cirrhotic liver. **D** Situation II shows the presence of a focus of HCC with the largest DN (*arrow*)

38 Cirrhosis IV – Dysplastic Nodules – HCC Transition

Developing hepatocellular carcinoma (HCC) in cirrhosis can be demonstrated on serial MR imaging. State-of-the-art MR imaging may show a spectrum of findings in the initial detection of developing HCC, including (1) localized fatty infiltration within a developing dysplastic nodule that gradually evolves into HCC in combination with a slowly increasing alpha-fetoprotein (AFP); (2) development of a focus of HCC with high signal intensity on T2-weighted imaging within a dysplastic nodule; and (3) prominent neovasculature. These findings confirm the stepwise carcinogenesis of HCC is regenerative nodule → low grade dysplastic nodule → high grade dysplastic nodule → small HCC → large HCC. MR imaging should be the modality of choice for the evaluation and follow-up of patients with cirrhosis.

MR Imaging Findings

At MR imaging, developing HCC may be associated with fat accumulation (visible on in- and opposed-phase imaging), gradual increase in size, increased signal intensity on T2-weighted images with a nodule-in-nodule appearance, and increased enhancement in the arterial phase, and washout with enhancement of a tumor capsule in the delayed phase imaging of the dynamic gadolinium-enhanced imaging. These observations can only be made optimally if the MR imaging protocol includes a number of important sequences such as chemical shift imaging, T2-weighted imaging with and without fat suppression, and dynamic gadolinium-enhanced imaging (Figs. 38.1–38.3).

Differential Diagnosis

The differential diagnosis of small enhancing lesions within livers with hepatitis or cirrhosis includes dysplastic nodule, small HCC, arterioportal shunt, and pseudolesions (i.e., areas with non-specific transient increased enhancement). Follow-up MR imaging facilitates differentiation.

Literature

1. Van den Bos IC, Hussain SM, Terkivatan T, et al. (2006) Step-wise carcinogenesis of hepatocellular carcinoma in the cirrhotic liver: demonstration on serial MR imaging. JMRI (in press)
2. Sakamoto M, Hirohashi S, Shimosato Y (1991) Early stages of multistep hepatocarcinogenesis: adenomatous hyperplasia and early hepatocellular carcinoma. Hum Pathol 22:172–178
3. Mitchell DG, Rubin R, Siegelman ES, et al. (1991) Hepatocellular carcinoma within siderotic regenerative nodules: appearance as a nodule within a nodule on MR images. Radiology 178:101–103
4. Ito K, Fujita T, Shimizu A, et al. (2004) Multiarterial phase dynamic MRI of small early enhancing hepatic lesions in cirrhosis or chronic hepatitis: differentiating between hypervascular hepatocellular carcinomas and pseudolesions AJR 183:699–705

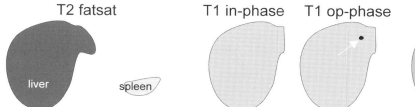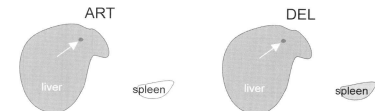

Fig. 38.1. Dysplastic nodules (DN)-HCC transition in a patient with hepatitis C for >20 years. T2 fatsat: no lesions are visible; T1 in- and op-phase: a small focus of fatty infiltration suggests a nodule with fat (*arrow*); ART: the nodule is hypointense due to fat suppression (*arrow*); no apparent enhancement is visible; DEL: the nodule remains hypointense (*arrow*)

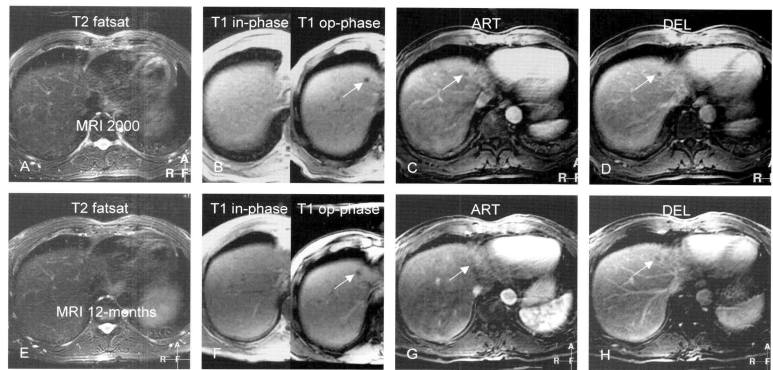

Fig. 38.2. DN-HCC transition in a patient with hepatitis C for >20 years, MRI findings. A Axial fat-suppressed T2-w TSE image (T2 fatsat): No lesions are visible. B Axial T1-in- and opposed-phase images (T1-in and op): A small focus of decreased signal (*arrow*) suggests a nodule with fatty infiltration. C Axial arterial phase image (ART): The nodule appears hypointense due to fat suppression; no apparent enhancement is present. D Axial delayed phase image (DEL): The nodule (*arrow*) remains hypointense. E (Patient refused a follow-up MRI at 3 months and came back after 1 year.) Axial fat-suppressed TSE image (T2 fatsat): no lesions are visible. F Axial T1-in- and opposed-phase images (T1-in and op): The nodule has increased in size on the opposed phase image (*arrow*). G Axial arterial phase image (ART): The nodule shows some enhancement (*arrow*). H Axial delayed phase image (DEL): The nodule (*arrow*) may have some washout. The findings suggest at least a dysplastic nodule with a focus of HCC (patient refused liver transplantation or resection)

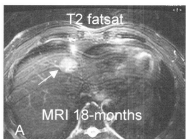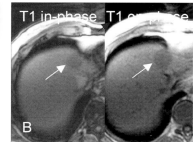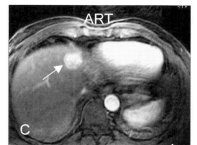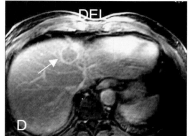

Fig. 38.3. DN-HCC transition, follow-up MRI. A Axial fat-suppressed TSE image (T2 fatsat): a large hyperintense lesion (*arrow*). B Axial T1-in- and opposed-phase images (T1-in and op): No signs of fatty infiltration are present in the large lesion (*arrows*). C Axial arterial phase image (ART): The nodule shows intense (almost) homogeneous enhancement (*arrow*). D Axial delayed phase image (DEL): The nodule is surrounded by a tumor capsule (*arrow*). The findings are consistent with an HCC

39 Cirrhosis V – Cyst in a Cirrhotic Liver

Hepatic cysts are common lesions (they may occur in up to 20% of the general population). Most hepatic cysts are considered to be developmental in origin. Currently, most hepatic cysts are discovered as incidental findings at cross-sectional imaging. Smaller cysts (< 10 mm) at US and CT may be difficult to distinguish from solid lesions, and may cause diagnostic problems especially in patients with an underlying liver disease such as cirrhosis. On imaging studies, small cysts may mimic hepatocellular carcinomas (HCC) in cirrhotic livers. MR imaging is highly reliable for the detection and characterization of cysts even in the presence of underlying parenchymal liver disease.

MR Imaging Findings

At MR imaging, cysts are typically low in signal intensity on T1-weighted images, high in signal intensity on T2-weighted images, and retain signal intensity on longer echo time (e.g., > 120 ms) T2-weighted images. After injection of contrast, cysts do not show any enhancement. On delayed post-gadolinium images (up to 5 min) cysts remain unenhanced. MRI is particularly valuable when lesions are small (Figs. 39.1, 39.2). The cysts differ from small HCC based on the signal intensity and enhancement. As opposed to cysts, small HCC may vary from low to moderately high signal intensity on T2-weighted images, and often show increased arterial enhancement.

Differential Diagnosis

Small cysts in the setting of cirrhosis may mimic small HCC on US and CT. MR imaging can reliably distinguish these entities. Hepatic cysts concurrent with cirrhosis are most likely present before the onset of the underlying parenchymal liver disease which leads to cirrhosis (Fig. 39.3).

Literature

1. Murakami T, Imai A, Nakamura H, et al. (1996) Ciliated foregut cyst in cirrhotic liver. J Gastroenterol 31:446–449
2. Hussain SM, Semelka RC, Mitchell DG (2002) MR imaging of hepatocellular carcinoma. Magn Reson Imaging Clin N Am 10:31–52
3. Mortele KJ, Ros PR (2001) Cystic focal liver lesions in the adult: differential CT and MR imaging features. Radiographics 21:895–910
4. Hussain SM, Semelka RC (2005) Liver masses. Magn Reson Imaging Clin N Am 13:255–275

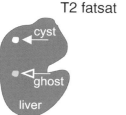
T2 fatsat

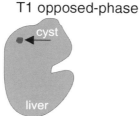
T1 opposed-phase

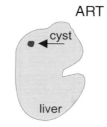
ART

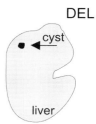
DEL

Fig. 39.1. Cyst in a cirrhotic liver, drawings. T2 fatsat: cyst is very bright (fluid-like) compared to the liver with smooth and sharp margins (*solid arrow*); note the slightly undulating contours of the liver and a ghost artifact of the cyst (*open arrow*); **T1 opposed-phase:** cyst is hypointense to the liver; **ART:** cyst shows no enhancement; **DEL:** cyst remains unenhanced

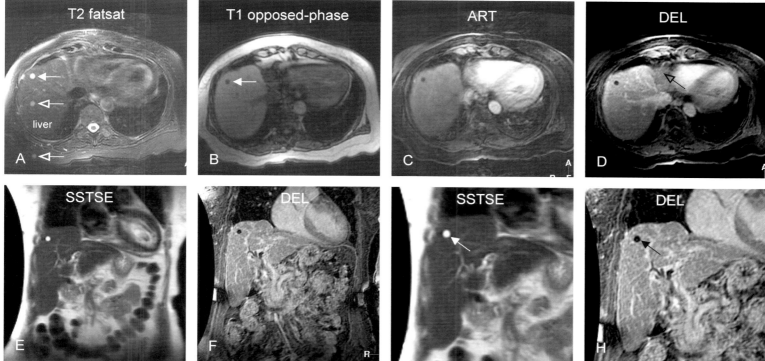

Fig. 39.2. Cyst (solitary) in a cirrhotic liver, MRI findings. A Axial fat-suppressed T2-w TSE image (T2 fatsat) shows a small sharply marginated bright cyst (*solid arrow*) with ghost artifacts (*open arrows*). **B** Axial opposed-phase image (T1 in-phase): The cyst has low signal intensity. The liver contours are somewhat undulating. **C** Axial gadolinium-enhanced 3D GRE image in the arterial phase (ART): The cyst shows no enhancement. **D** Axial delayed phase (DEL): The cyst remains unenhanced. **E** Coronal T2-w SSTSE image with longer echo time (TE) of 120 ms (SSTSE): The cyst (*arrow*) retains its high signal intensity due to high fluid content (typical sign of non-solid liver lesions). **F** Coronal delayed phase (DEL): The cyst remains unenhanced. **G** A detailed view of the coronal T2-w SSTSE image shows the bright cyst (*arrow*). **H** A detailed view of the coronal delayed phase (DEL) shows the liver with typical cirrhotic morphology (irregular contours and enhanced septa), and the unenhanced cyst (*arrow*)

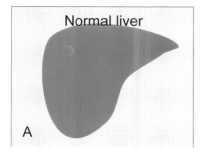
Normal liver

Liver with fibrosis

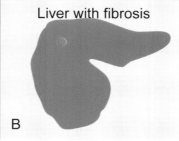
Liver with cirrhosis

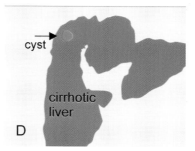

Fig. 39.3. Cyst in a cirrhotic liver, schematic drawings explaining the coincidental cyst and cirrhosis. A–C Normal liver with cyst should have been present prior to the development of fibrosis and cirrhosis. **D** A detail view of the drawing shows the irregular contours of the cirrhotic liver containing a simple cyst

40 Cirrhosis VI – Multiple Cysts in a Cirrhotic Liver

As cysts are common in the liver, multiple small cysts may concur with cirrhosis. Such lesions may have overlapping features with small HCC at imaging. Proper diagnosis is important to avoid unnecessary follow-up and liver biopsy.

MR Imaging Findings

At MR imaging, cysts are typically low in signal intensity on T1-weighted images, high in signal intensity on T2-weighted images, and retain signal intensity on longer echo time (e.g., > 120 ms) T2-weighted images. After injection of contrast, cysts do not show any enhancement. On delayed post-gadolinium images (up to 5 min) cysts remain unenhanced. MRI is particularly valuable when lesions are small. Flow-sensitive MR imaging sequences can be used to reliably distinguish between small cysts from small intrahepatic vessels (Figs. 40.1, 40.2). It is critical to perform multiphasic dynamic gadolinium-enhanced imaging in the setting of multiple cysts. Particularly, based on these sequences cysts may reliably be distinguished from small HCCs. As opposed to multiple cysts, small HCCs show early arterial enhancement.

Differential Diagnosis

Multiple small cysts in the setting of cirrhosis may mimic multiple small HCCs. US may be reliable for cysts that are uncomplicated and located superficially in a cirrhotic liver (Fig. 40.3). At CT, it may be challenging to characterize small lesions in the setting of cirrhosis. If MR imaging shows multiple peribiliary cysts, an underlying congenital biliary disease should be considered within the differential diagnosis of patients with multiple liver cysts and cirrhosis.

Literature

1. Murakami T, Imai A, Nakamura H, et al. (1996) Ciliated foregut cyst in cirrhotic liver. J Gastroenterol 31:446–449
2. Hussain SM, Semelka RC, Mitchell DG (2002) MR imaging of hepatocellular carcinoma. Magn Reson Imaging Clin N Am 10:31–52
3. Hussain SM, Semelka RC (2005) Liver masses. Magn Reson Imaging Clin N Am 13:255–275

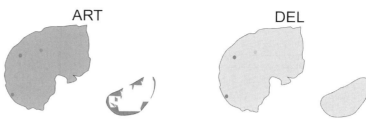

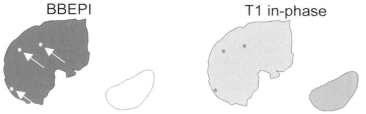

Fig. 40.1. Cyst (multiple) in a cirrhotic liver, drawings. BBEPI: Cysts (*arrows*) are very bright (fluid-like) compared to the liver with smooth and sharp margins; note the slightly undulating contours of the liver, indicating the presence of cirrhosis; **T1 in-phase**: Cysts are hypointense to the liver; **ART**: Cysts show no enhancement; **DEL**: Cysts remain unenhanced

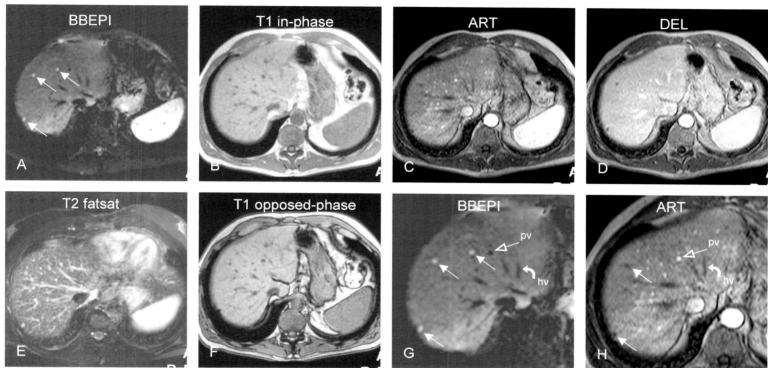

Fig. 40.2. Cysts in a cirrhotic liver, MRI findings. A Axial black-blood echo planar imaging (BBEPI) shows three hyperintense small lesions (*arrows*), which in the setting of cirrhosis may mimic foci of hepatocellular carcinoma. **B** Axial in-phase image (T1 in-phase): The cysts are hardly visible. **C** Axial gadolinium-enhanced GRE image in the arterial phase (ART): The cysts show no enhancement. **D** Axial delayed phase (DEL): Two cysts are visible as unenhanced lesion, whereas the third is not quite recognizable. **E** Axial T2-weighted fat-suppressed TSE (T2-w fatsat): Small cysts and small vessels are difficult to distinguish due to high signal. **F** Axial opposed-phase image (T1 opposed-phase): The cysts are hardly visible. **G** A detailed view of the BBEPI image shows the portal vein (*open arrow*) and hepatic vein (*curved arrow*) with signal void due to flow, whereas the cysts (*solid arrows*) appear bright. **H** A detailed view of the axial arterial phase (ART) shows enhancement of the portal vein (*open arrow*) and no enhancement of the hepatic veins (*curved arrow*) and cysts (*solid arrows*)

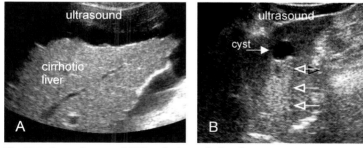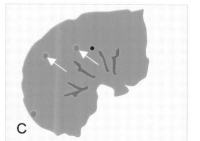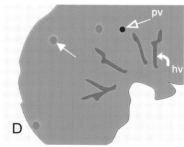

Fig. 40.3. Cysts, ultrasound (US) and schematic drawings. A US shows typical appearance of cirrhotic liver with irregular contours, which is surrounded by ascites. **B** US shows typical appearance of a simple hepatic cyst (*solid arrow*) with increased sound transmission (*open arrows*). **C** Drawing based on BBE-PI shows multiple cysts within a cirrhotic liver (*arrows*). **D** A detailed view of the drawing shows that the portal vein (*open arrow*) and hepatic vein (*curved arrow*) can be distinguished from the cyst (*solid arrow*) based on the presence of flow and anatomic orientation

41 Cirrhosis VII – Hemangioma in a Cirrhotic Liver

Hepatocellular carcinoma may occur in up to 22% of patients with long-standing cirrhosis. Hemangiomas can occur in up to 20% of the general population. In the setting of cirrhosis, however, the incidence of hemangiomas (about 2%) is lower than expected. The events leading to cirrhosis may obliterate and change the appearance and vascularity of particularly small hemangiomas. MR imaging is likely to offer some advantages over CT in this challenging setting. In general, contrast enhancement of the cirrhotic liver at CT is often suboptimal. Because of its greater sensitivity to small differences in intrinsic tissue contrast as well as gadolinium enhancement, MR imaging is likely to perform better than CT for the detection and characterization of liver lesions especially in the setting of cirrhosis.

MR Imaging Findings

At MR imaging, small and medium-sized hemangiomas have a characteristic appearance with moderately high signal intensity on T2-weighted sequences and peripheral nodular enhancement in the arterial phase and persistent enhancement in the delayed phase (Figs. 41.1, 41.2). This characteristic appearance of hemangioma may however change due to gradual parenchymal changes that lead to cirrhosis (Fig. 41.3). The signal intensity as well as the enhancement pattern may become unreliable even on state-of-the-art MR imaging. Therefore, atypical small, and fibrotic or hyalinized hemangiomas may be difficult to diagnose. In such cases, clinical correlation with alpha-fetoprotein and follow-up studies are preferred to US-guided biopsy, which may be undesirable in the setting of cirrhosis.

Differential Diagnosis

Small HCCs can show moderately high signal intensity on T2-weighted images but the signal intensity is typically much lower than for the hemangiomas and the signal may decrease on heavily T2-weighted sequences due to their solid nature. In addition, HCCs usually do not show any persistent enhancement in the delayed phase.

Literature

1. Brancatelli G, Federle MP, Blachar A, et al. (2001) Hemangioma in the cirrhotic liver: diagnosis and natural history. Radiology 219:69–74
2. Dodd GD III, Baron RL, Oliver JH III, et al. (1999) Spectrum of imaging findings of the liver in end stage cirrhosis. II. Focal abnormalities. AJR 173:1185–1192
3. De Caralt TM, Ayuso JR, Ayuso C, et al. (1999) Distortion of subcapsular hepatic hemangioma by hepatic cirrhosis. Can Assoc Radiol J 50:137–138
4. Hussain SM, Semelka RC (2005) Liver masses. Magn Reson Imaging Clin N Am 13:255–275

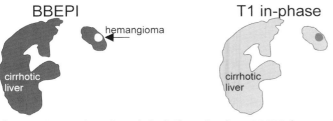

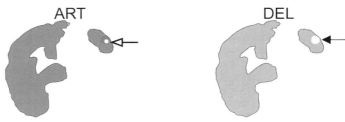

Fig. 41.1. Hemangioma in a cirrhotic liver, drawings. BBEPI: hemangioma is markedly hyperintense to the cirrhotic liver (*solid arrow*); **T1 in-phase**: hemangioma is hypointense to the cirrhotic liver; **ART**: hemangioma typi-cally shows a peripheral nodular enhancement (*open arrow*); DEL: hemangioma becomes completely enhanced and retains its contrast (*solid arrow*)

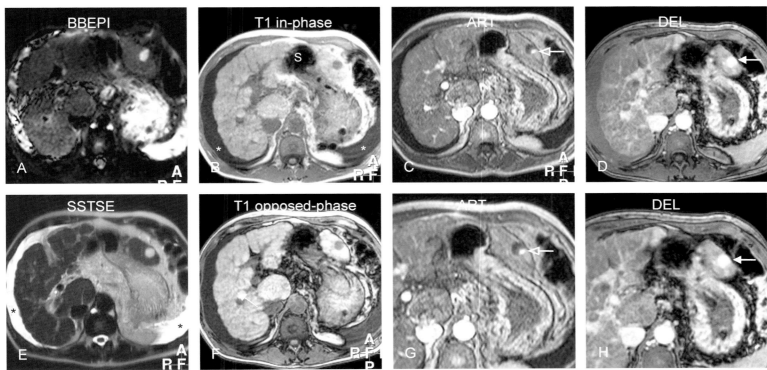

Fig. 41.2. Hemangioma in a cirrhotic liver, MRI findings. A Axial T2-weighted black-blood echo planar imaging (BBEPI): Hemangioma is hyperintense to the liver (*arrow*). **B** Axial in-phase (T1 in-phase): Hemangioma is hypointense to the cirrhotic liver (irregular contours, multiple regenerative nodules, and ascites). Note the ascites (*) and the interposition of the stomach (S) due to liver atrophy. **C** Axial arterial phase image (ART): Hemangioma shows typical peripheral nodular enhancement (*open arrow*). **D** Axial delayed phase (DEL): Hemangioma is completely enhanced and retains its contrast (*arrow*). **E** Axial T2-w SSTSE image with TE of 120 ms (SSTSE): Hemangioma retains its high signal indicating its non-solid nature. Ascites (*). **F** Axial opposed-phase image (T1 opposed-phase): Hemangioma is hypointense to the liver. **G** A detailed view of the arterial phase shows more clearly the peripheral nodular enhancement (*open arrow*). **H** A detailed view of the delayed phase shows the homogeneously enhanced hemangioma (*arrow*)

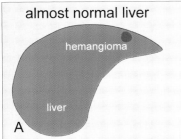
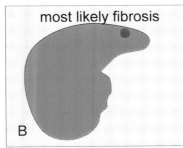
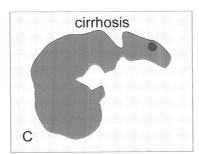
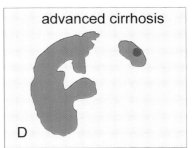

Fig. 41.3. Preexisting hemangioma in cirrhotic liver, temporal changes, drawings. A Drawing shows almost normal contours and morphology of the liver. **B** Drawing shows signs of fibrosis (enlargement of the right liver; rounded edges). **C** Drawing shows signs of cirrhosis (irregular contours with nodules, atrophy, and left-sided hypertrophy. **D** Drawing shows signs of advanced cirrhosis such as complete atrophy of the area around the falciform ligament with interposition of stomach

42 HCC in Cirrhosis I – Typical Small with Pathologic Correlation

Hepatocellular carcinoma (HCC) is a malignant neoplasm composed of cells with hepatocellular differentiation. Small HCC is defined as measuring ≤2 cm in diameter. The criteria used to distinguish HCC from high-grade dysplastic nodules are not clearly defined. At histology, criteria in favor of malignancy include prominent nuclear atypia, high nuclear-cytoplasmic ratio with nuclear density twice normal, plates three or more cells thick, numerous unaccompanied arteries, mitoses in moderate numbers, and invasion of stroma or portal tracts. Most small HCC cannot be distinguished histologically from dysplastic nodules with certainty. By understanding the events of the stepwise carcinogenesis of HCC and taking advantage of the abundant neovascularity of HCC, one can more easily make sense of the complex nodularity depicted in cirrhotic livers on multiple MRI pulse sequences.

MR Imaging Findings

At MR imaging, small HCCs are often detected on the arterial phase as early enhancing lesions. On T2-weighted images, such lesions may have slightly increased signal compared to the surrounding parenchyma but may appear as isointense or even low in signal intensity areas. Classically, an early enhancing nodule of ≤2 cm with moderately increased signal intensity on T2-weighted images should be considered a small HCC (Figs. 42.1, 42.2). The appearance on T1-weighted sequences may vary and often does not play a role in the diagnosis unless a nodule shows evidence of fatty infiltration on chemical shift imaging. Fatty infiltration as well as increased vascularity are recognized signs of small HCC.

Pathology

At pathology, multiple regenerative nodules surrounded by fibrous septa may be present in cirrhotic livers. At gross pathology, HCC may appear as a dominant yellowish nodule (Fig. 42.3). At histology, small HCCs are usually well differentiated. Increased cellularity, loss of normal reticulin structure, and plates of more than three cells thick are features of HCC. Also, invasion of stroma or portal tracts is highly suggestive of malignancy.

Literature

1. International Working Party (1995) Terminology of nodular hepatocellular lesions. Hepatology 22:983 – 993
2. Hussain SM, Zondervan PE, et al. (2002) Benign versus malignant hepatic nodules: MR imaging findings with pathologic correlation. Radiographics 22:1023 – 36
3. Hussain SM, Semelka RC, Mitchell DG (2002) MR imaging of hepatocellular carcinoma. Magn Reson Imaging Clin N Am 10:31 – 52
4. Van den Bos IC, Hussain SM, Terkivatan T, et al. (2006) Step-wise carcinogenesis of hepatocellular carcinoma in the cirrhotic liver: demonstration on serial MR imaging. JMRI (in press)

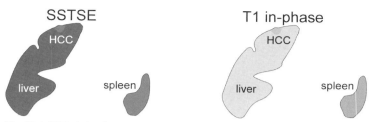
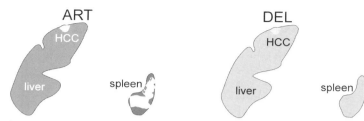

Fig. 42.1. HCC, cirrhosis, small, drawings. SSTSE: HCC is only minimally hyperintense to the cirrhotic liver; **T1 in-phase:** HCC is almost isointense to the liver; **ART:** HCC shows intense and homogeneous enhancement with slight bulging of the liver contour; **DEL:** HCC shows some washout and becomes somewhat heterogeneous

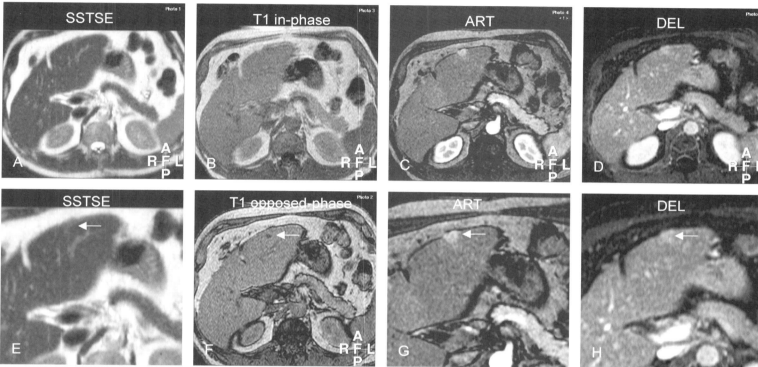

Fig. 42.2. HCC, cirrhosis, small, typical MRI findings. A Axial SSTSE image (SSTSE): HCC is minimally hyperintense to the cirrhotic liver, with rounded edges and peripheral atrophy. **B** Axial in-phase image (T1 in-phase): HCC is isointense compared to the liver. **C** Axial arterial phase image (ART): HCC shows intense homogeneous enhancement with some bulging of the liver contour. **D** Axial delayed phase image (DEL): HCC shows some washout and becomes heterogeneous. **E** A detailed view of the axial SSTSE image (SSTSE): HCC is minimally hyperintense compared to the liver (*arrow*). **F** Axial opposed-phase image (T1 opposed-phase): HCC is predominantly isointense to the liver, though a small area within the lesion shows decreased signal due to fatty infiltration (*arrow*). **G** A detailed view of the axial arterial phase image (ART): HCC shows intense homogeneous enhancement with some bulging of the liver contour (*arrow*). **H** A detailed view of the axial delayed phase image (DEL): HCC shows some washout and becomes heterogeneous (*arrow*)

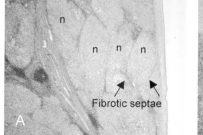
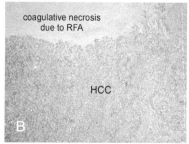
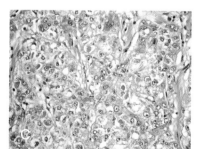
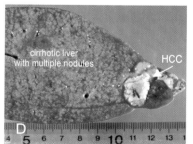

Fig. 42.3. HCC, cirrhosis, small, direct MR-pathology correlation. A Photomicrograph of the liver shows multiple nodules (*n*) surrounded by fibrous septa, compatible with cirrhosis. H&E, ×40. **B** Photomicrograph shows typical aspect of HCC with coagulative necrosis after local treatment with radiofrequency ablation (RFA) therapy. H&E, ×100. **C** Photomicrograph shows poorly differentiated HCC. H&E, ×400. **D** Photograph of the explant (3 months after MRI above) shows a small HCC containing two RFA needle marks (*arrow*)

43 HCC in Cirrhosis II – Small With and Without a Tumor Capsule

Small (≤2 cm) hepatocellular carcinoma (HCC) may not show a tumor capsule at imaging. True tumor capsule, however, is a specific sign of mainly the larger HCC, and histologically is composed of fibrous tissue with relatively large extracellular space. In contrast, pseudocapsule is a term used for non-specific tissue changes that may be present around hepatic lesions. Pseudocapsules may be composed of compressed liver parenchyma, inflammatory infiltrates, compressed vessels, and non-steatosis. MR imaging facilitates differentiation between true capsule and pseudocapsule.

MR Imaging Findings

At MR imaging, very small HCC may show low signal on T1-weighted images, high signal on T2-weighted images, intense homogeneous enhancement in the arterial phase, and washout with heterogeneity in the delayed phase. Relatively larger lesions may show a true tumor capsule with increasing thickness. The true capsule has low signal intensity on T1- as well as T2-weighted images and shows enhancement in the delayed phase (Figs. 43.1–43.3). Pseudocapsules display high signal on T2-weighted images.

Management

A diagnostic biopsy of an HCC with a capsule may cause rupture with increased probability of dissemination. Currently, treatments for HCC include liver transplantation (LTX), resection, and minimally invasive treatment (MIT). LTX can cure both the tumor and the underlying cirrhosis. *LTX* is effective in patients with a single tumor (≤5 cm) or no more than three tumors, each 3 cm or less in diameter. If LTX is not possible and the liver has sufficient functional reserve, *resection* may be an option. *MIT* has become an alternative to (1) resection, (2) a means for local control while patients may be waiting for LTX, and (3) a method for palliation. MIT includes laser therapy, cryotherapy, thermal ablation, ethanol or acetic acid injection, and arterial chemoembolization.

Literature

1. Hussain SM, Zondervan PE, et al. (2002) Benign versus malignant hepatic nodules: MR imaging findings with pathologic correlation. Radiographics 22:1023–36
2. Hussain SM, Semelka RC, Mitchell DG (2002) MR imaging of hepatocellular carcinoma. Magn Reson Imaging Clin N Am 10:31–52
3. Mazzaferro V, Regalia E, Doci R, et al. (1996) Liver transplantation for the treatment of small hepatocellular carcinomas in patients with cirrhosis. N Engl J Med 334:693–699

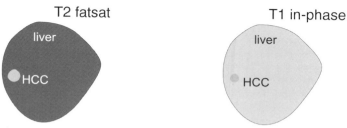 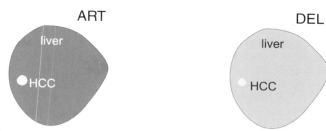

Fig. 43.1. HCC, cirrhosis, small, drawings. T2 fatsat: HCC is hyperintense to the liver; **T1 in-phase:** HCC is slightly hypointense to the liver; **ART:** HCC shows intense homogeneous enhancement; **DEL:** HCC shows washout with some residual enhancement but no tumor capsule

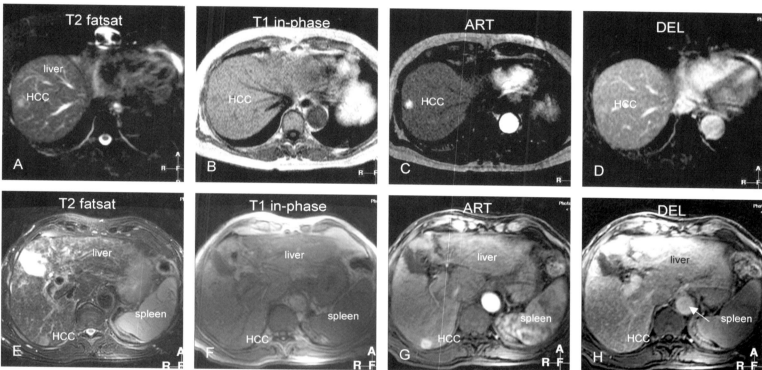

Fig. 43.2. HCC, cirrhosis, small HCC without a capsule, slightly larger HCC with a tumor capsule, MRI findings. A Axial fat suppressed T2-w TSE image (T2 fatsat): HCC is hyperintense to the liver. **B** Axial in-phase image (T1 in-phase): HCC is slightly hypointense to the liver. **C** Axial arterial phase image (ART): HCC shows intense homogeneous enhancement. **D** Axial delayed phase image (DEL): HCC shows washout with some residual enhancement but no tumor capsule. **E** Axial TSE image (T2 fatsat) in a different patient: HCC is hyperintense to the liver. **F** Axial in-phase image (T1 in-phase): HCC is slightly hypointense to the liver. **G** Axial arterial phase image (ART): HCC shows intense homogeneous enhancement. **H** Axial delayed phase image (DEL): HCC shows washout with an enhanced tumor capsule

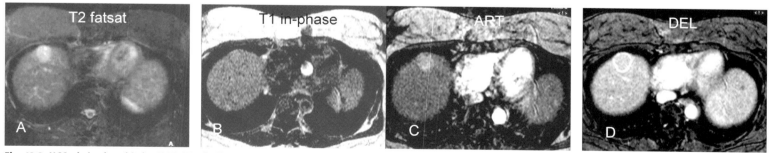

Fig. 43.3. HCC, cirrhosis, mid-size HCC, MRI findings. A Axial TSE image (T2 fatsat): HCC is hyperintense to the liver, containing two smaller brighter nodules. **B** Axial in-phase image (T1 in-phase): HCC is surrounded by a dark capsule. **C** Axial arterial phase image (ART): HCC shows almost homogeneous enhancement. **D** Axial delayed phase image (DEL): HCC shows washout with enhanced capsule

44 HCC in Cirrhosis III – Nodule-in-Nodule Appearance

High-grade dysplastic nodules and small hepatocellular carcinoma (HCC) (≤2 cm) may have a nodule-in-nodule appearance on MR images, especially if a focus of HCC originates within a siderotic regenerative nodule. Such a lesion in fact is a developing HCC and can be considered as a transition between low-grade dysplastic nodule and a small HCC. State-of-the-art MR imaging displays a spectrum of findings in the initial detection of developing HCCs, including (1) localized fatty infiltration within a developing dysplastic nodule that gradually evolves into HCC, maybe in combination with increasing alpha-fetoprotein; (2) development of a focus of HCC with high signal intensity on T2-weighted imaging in a dysplastic nodule; and (3) prominent neovasculature as the initial sign of developing HCC. These findings may represent various genetic pathways of developing HCC.

MR Imaging Findings

At MR imaging, the appearance of a developing or small HCC may consist of low intensity of a large nodule, with one or more internal foci of higher signal intensity on T2-weighted images. On T1-weighted chemical shift imaging, such lesions may show signal loss due to fatty infiltration. In the arterial phase, the central nodule may show more enhancement, indicating the development of increased tumor neovascularity (Figs. 44.1 – 44.3).

Management

The recognition of developing HCC is important because the average doubling time for volume of such HCCs may be less than 3 months. In addition, early detection of HCC provides more options for patient management.

Literature

1. Mitchell DG, Rubin R, Siegelman ES, et al. (1991) Hepatocellular carcinoma within siderotic regenerative nodules: appearance as a nodule within a nodule on MR images. Radiology 178:101 – 103
2. Sadek AG, Mitchell DG, Siegelman ES, et al. (1995) Early hepatocellular carcinoma that develops within macroregenerative nodules: growth rate depicted at serial MR imaging. Radiology 195:753 – 756
3. Van den Bos IC, Hussain SM, Terkivatan T, et al. (2006) Step-wise carcinogenesis of hepatocellular carcinoma in the cirrhotic liver: demonstration on serial MR imaging. JMRI (in press)
4. Kanai T, Hirohashi S, Upton MP, et al. (1987) Pathology of small hepatocellular carcinoma: a proposal for a new gross classification. Cancer 60:810 – 819

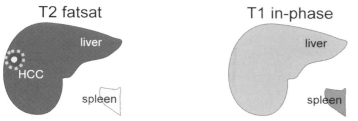

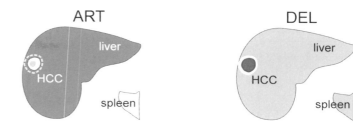

Fig. 44.1. HCC, cirrhosis, nodule-in-nodule, drawings. T2 fatsat: HCC shows a hyperintense smaller nodule within a larger darker lesion; **T1 in-phase:** HCC is isointense to the liver; **ART:** HCC shows intense (almost) homoge-neous enhancement (the inner nodule is surrounded by more enhance-ment); **DEL:** HCC shows washout with enhancement of a thick fibrous tu-mor capsule

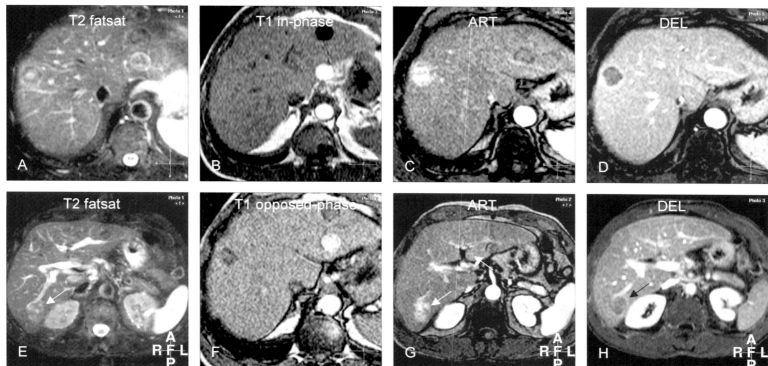

Fig. 44.2. HCC, cirrhotic liver, nodule-in-nodule, MRI findings. A Axial fat sup-pressed T2-w TSE image (T2 fatsat): HCC shows a nodule-in-nodule appear-ance (a bright nodule within a darker nodule). **B** Axial in-phase image (T1 in-phase): HCC is isointense to the liver. **C** Axial arterial phase image (ART): HCC shows intense (almost) homogeneous enhancement with more enhancement around the inner nodule. **D** Axial delayed phase image (DEL): HCC shows washout with an enhancing thick tumor capsule, a specific sign of HCC. **E** Axial fat suppressed T2-w TSE image at a lower anatomic level (T2 fatsat) shows a second HCC with predominantly high signal (*arrow*). **F** Axial opposed-phase T1-w GRE image (T1 opposed-phase): HCC shows loss of signal due to fatty infiltration. **G** Axial arterial phase image at a lower ana-tomic level (ART) shows heterogeneous enhancement of the second HCC (*arrow*). **H** Axial delayed phase image at a lower anatomic level (DEL): HCC shows washout with an enhancing tumor capsule that partially surrounds the HCC (*arrow*)

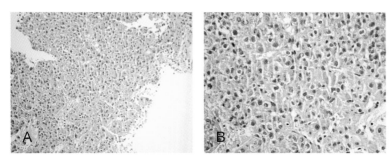

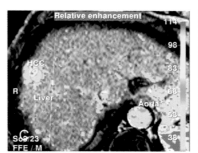

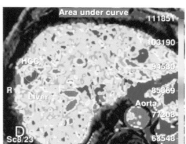

Fig. 44.3. HCC, MR biopsy correlation. A Photomicrograph from a subcutane-ous metastasis of one of the lesions in the liver (shown above) shows a lesion of hepatocellular origin. H&E, × 200. **B** A detailed view shows the abnormal hepatocytes arranged in thickened cell plates (more than two). H&E, × 400. **C** Pixelwise presentation of the relative enhancement (based on the dynamic imaging) shows the presence of tumor vessels (*red areas*). **D** Pixelwise pre-sentation of the area-under-the-curve shows the enhancement of the tumor capsule

45 HCC in Cirrhosis IV – Mosaic Pattern with Pathologic Correlation

Hepatocellular carcinoma (HCC) is the most common primary cancer of the liver. The overall 5-year survival rate without any treatment is less than 5%. HCC is more frequent in the East and Southeast Asia. The incidence of HCC, however, is rising in Europe and North America. In a recent study, the incidence of HCC in the United States increased from 1.4 per 100,000 between 1976 and 1980, to 2.4 per 100,000 between 1991 and 1995. Men are affected three times as often as women and blacks twice as often as whites. The age-specific incidence of HCC has progressively shifted toward a younger population, reaching a peak at about 80–84 years of age between 1981 and 1985, and dropping to 75–79 years of age between 1991 and 1995. Large (>2 cm) HCC may have a number of characteristic features, such as mosaic pattern, tumor capsule, extracapsular extension with the formation of satellite nodule(s), vascular invasion, and extrahepatic dissemination, including lymph node and distant metastases.

MR Imaging Findings

The mosaic pattern is present in 88% of the lesions larger than 2 cm. On T1- and T2-weighted MR images, the mosaic pattern appears as areas of variable signal intensities, whereas on gadolinium-enhanced images, the lesions enhance in a heterogeneous fashion during the arterial and later phases (Figs. 45.1, 45.2). Tumor capsule, a characteristic sign of HCC, is present in 60–82% of large HCCs. The tumor capsule is hypointense on both T1- and T2-weighted images. Vascular invasion occurs in 24% of large HCCs. Extrahepatic dissemination of large HCCs occurs in up to 48% with lung metastases, lymph node metastases, bone metastases, etc.

Pathology

At gross pathology, large HCC appears as a dominant nodule among a myriad of regenerative nodules of the cirrhotic liver. The nodule may be composed of several smaller nodules (mosaic) contained within a grossly visible true fibrous capsule. At histology, the tumor may show increased cellularity, abnormal hepatocytes, thickened cell plates, and hemorrhage (Fig. 45.3).

Literature

1. Hussain SM, Semelka RC, Mitchell DG (2002) MR imaging of hepatocellular carcinoma. Magn Reson Imaging Clin N Am 10:31–52
2. El-Serag HB, Mason AC (1999) Rising incidence of hepatocellular carcinoma in the United States. N Engl J Med 340:745–750
3. Kadoya M, Matsui O, Takashima T, et al. (1992) Hepatocellular carcinoma: correlation of MR imaging and histopathologic findings. Radiology 183:819–825

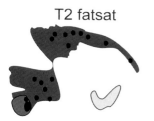
T2 fatsat

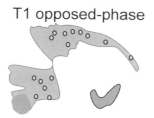
T1 opposed-phase

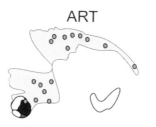
ART

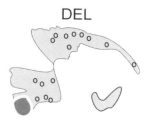
DEL

Fig. 45.1. HCC, cirrhotic liver, mosaic pattern. T2 fatsat: HCC appears as a nodule with areas of variable signal intensity (mosaic pattern) within a cirrhotic liver. **T1 opposed-phase:** HCC is almost isointense to the liver. **ART:** HCC shows enhancement in some and negligible enhancement in other areas; **DEL:** HCC shows washout in the enhancing parts of the tumor with the enhancement of the tumor capsule

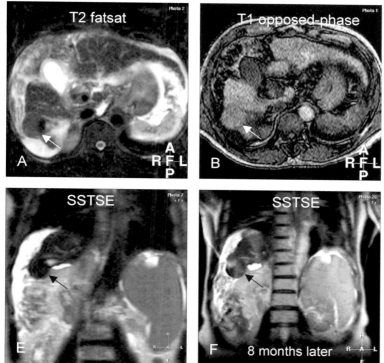

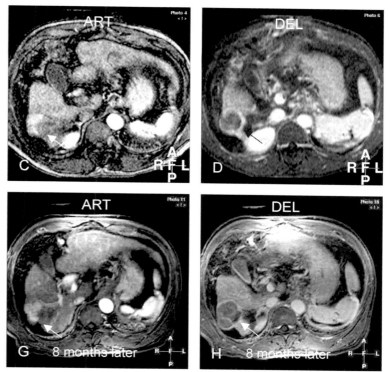

Fig. 45.2. HCC, cirrhotic liver, mosaic pattern, MRI findings. A Axial fat-suppressed T2-w TSE image (T2 fatsat): HCC nodule has areas with higher and lower (mosaic) than the cirrhotic liver (*arrow*). **B** Axial T1-w opposed-phase GRE image (T1 opposed-phase): HCC is isointense to the cirrhotic liver (*arrow*). **C** Axial arterial phase post-Gd T1-w GRE image (ART): HCC shows more enhancement in some parts and less in other parts, indicating the mosaic pattern (*arrow*). **D** Axial delayed post-Gd T1-w GRE image (DEL): HCC shows washout in the enhanced areas with enhancement of the tumor capsule (*arrow*). **E** Coronal T2-w SSTSE image with a TE of 120 ms (SSTSE): HCC is isointense to the cirrhotic liver (*arrow*). **F** Coronal T2-w SSTSE image (SSTSE) 8 months later: HCC has increased in size (*arrow*). **G** Axial arterial phase post-Gd T1-w GRE image 8 months later (ART): HCC is larger in size with a mosaic enhancement pattern (*arrow*). **H** Axial delayed phase post-Gd T1-w GRE image 8 months later (DEL): HCC shows the enhanced tumor capsule and septa within a larger lesion (*arrow*)

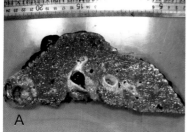

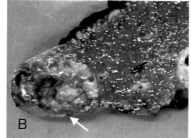

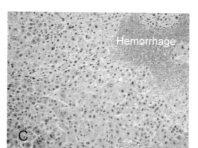

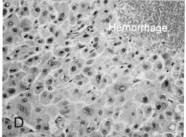

Fig. 45.3. HCC with mosaic pattern, cirrhosis, direct MR-explant correlation. A Photograph of the entire explant provides an overview of the cirrhotic liver and a large HCC. **B** A detailed photograph of the area with HCC (*arrow*) that correlates well with the T2 coronal image. **C** Photomicrograph of the HCC shows thickened cell plates with abnormal hepatocytes and an area with hemorrhage. H&E, ×200. **D** Photomicrograph shows in detail the hepatocytes composed of abnormal nuclei and cytoplasm compatible with HCC. H&E, ×400

46 HCC in Cirrhosis V – Typical Large with Mosaic and Capsule

Edmondson et al. divided HCCs into nodular (81%), massive (23%), and diffuse (3%). In 1987, Kanai et al. proposed a new gross classification: (1) Type 1: single nodular type; (2) Type 2: single nodular type with extranodular growth; (3) Type 3: contiguous multinodular type; (4) Type 4: poorly demarcated nodular type; and (5) early HCC (< 12 mm): a lesion that does not destroy the underlying liver structure. Type 1 and 2 lesions are said to be more likely to show an expanding growth. Type 3 and 4, as well as small HCC, may predominantly display a replacing growth. Type 1 lesions show a remarkable response to minimally invasive treatment, such as transcatheter arterial embolization. The lesions with mosaic pattern may be considered as Type 3 lesions. Such lesions are a configuration of confluent small nodules separated by thin septa.

MR Imaging Findings

At T1-weighted images, large HCCs with a mosaic pattern may predominantly have a high signal intensity compared to the surrounding liver. These lesions may be surrounded by a low signal intensity fibrous capsule. The individual nodules within such HCCs may have a slightly variable signal, hence giving rise to the characteristic mosaic appearance. The high signal intensity on T1 may be caused by high copper protein content. On contrast-enhanced imaging, some nodules may enhance more than others, again expressing the mosaic pattern based on vascularity. On delayed contrast-enhanced images, the individual nodules as well as the lesion may be contained within capsules (Figs. 46.1, 46.2). The possibility of fatty infiltration of the lesion can be excluded on chemical shift imaging.

Pathology

High signal intensity on T1-weighted images may be associated with well-differentiated HCC (Fig. 46.3A, B). MR imaging is well able to show HCC without tumor capsule with the suggestion of infiltrating growth pattern (Fig. 46.3C, D).

Literature

1. Edmondson HA, Steiner PE (1954) Primary carcinoma of the liver: a study of 100 cases among 18,900 necropsies. Cancer 7:462–503
2. Kanai T, Hirohashi S, Upton MP, et al. (1987) Pathology of small hepatocellular carcinoma: a proposal for a new gross classification. Cancer 60:810–819
3. Ebara M, Fukuda H, Kojima Y, et al. (1999) Small hepatocellular carcinoma: relationship of signal intensity to histopathologic findings and metal content of the tumor and surrounding hepatic parenchyma. Radiology 210:81–88
4. Muramatsu Y, Nawano S, Takayasu K, et al. (1991) Early hepatocellular carcinoma: MR imaging. Radiology 181:209–213

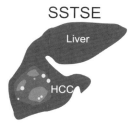

SSTSE

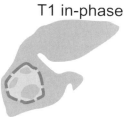

T1 in-phase

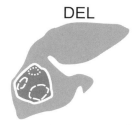

ART

DEL

Fig. 46.1. HCC, cirrhosis, large, mosaic, drawings. SSTSE: HCC contains several nodules with variable signal intensity indicating a mosaic pattern; **T1 in-phase:** HCC is predominantly hyperintense to the liver with a darker tumor capsule; **ART:** HCC shows more and intense enhancement in some areas of the tumor; **DEL:** HCC shows washout in the enhanced areas with an enhanced thick tumor capsule

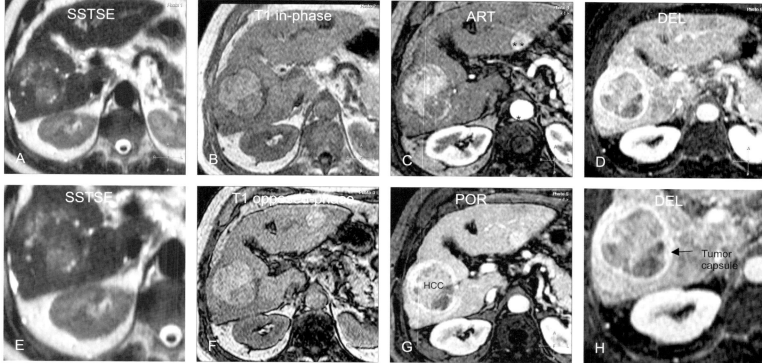

Fig. 46.2. HCC, cirrhotic liver, large, mosaic pattern, typical MRI findings. A Axial SSTSE image (SSTSE): HCC is predominantly hyperintense to the liver. The tumor capsule is hypointense and not visible. **B** Axial in-phase image (T1 in-phase): HCC is predominantly hyperintense to the cirrhotic liver with a darker tumor capsule. **C** Axial arterial phase image (ART): HCC shows intense enhancement in some areas, indicating the mosaic pattern. **D** Axial delayed phase image (DEL): HCC shows washout with enhanced thick tumor capsule. **E** A detailed view of the SSTSE image (SSTSE): HCC shows areas with high and low signal indicating the mosaic pattern. **F** Axial opposed-phase T1-w GRE image (T1 opposed-phase): HCC as well as the cirrhotic liver show no signs of fatty infiltration. **G** Axial portal phase image (POR): HCC shows washout with enhanced thick tumor capsule. **H** A detailed view of the axial delayed phase 2D T1-w GRE image (DEL): HCC is surrounded by an enhanced thick tumor capsule (*arrow*)

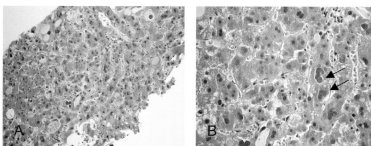

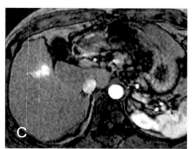

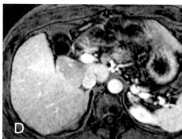

Fig. 46.3. HCC, direct MR-biopsy correlation in A and B. A Photomicrograph of a US-guided biopsy from the tumor (shown above) shows thickened cell plates with abnormal nuclei, compatible with HCC. H&E, × 200. **B** Photomicrograph shows enlarged atypical nuclei (*arrows*) with abnormal cytoplasm of the hepatocytes. H&E, × 400. **C, D** Arterial and delayed phase images, respectively, from another patient show an HCC with diffuse, infiltrating growth without a tumor capsule

47 HCC in Cirrhosis VI – Mosaic Pattern with Fatty Infiltration

Hepatocellular carcinomas (HCCs) may present as T1-bright lesions. The recent literature indicates that high signal intensity on T1-weighted images is correlated with the presence of an increased amount of copper protein in the lesion. Fatty change is generally present in approximately 10% of HCCs. Fatty accumulation within cirrhotic nodules may be an indication of ongoing dysplastic changes. Dysplasia indicates the presence of nuclear and cytoplasmic changes, such as minimal to severe nuclear atypia and an increased amount of cytoplasmic fat or glycogen. In fact, a nodule with fatty infiltration may be the initial presentation of a developing HCC. Chemical shift (in- and opposed-phase) imaging is a simple and highly sensitive and specific method for demonstrating fatty infiltration in tissues including liver lesions.

MR Imaging Findings

At T1-weighted opposed-phase imaging, fat-containing HCCs show signal loss compared to the in-phase imaging. HCCs may be composed of various smaller nodules with a variable amount of fat and variation in the signal intensity on T1-weighted images (mosaic pattern). In addition, the lesion may be surrounded by a tumor capsule (Figs. 47.1, 47.2). These are the characteristic diagnostic features of mainly a large fat-containing HCC.

Pathology

At pathology, nodules may have a variable amount of dysplastic changes which include small cell and large cell dysplasia (Fig. 47.3A, B). Fat accumulation can also be considered as part of the ongoing dysplastic changes within cirrhotic nodules and HCC. Fibrous capsule may surround fatty areas within HCCs, which appear bright at histology (Fig. 47.3C, D).

Differential Diagnosis

Hepatocellular adenomas contain fat in up to 70% of cases but tumor morphology and enhancement differ from those in fatty HCCs. Hepatic angiomyolipoma and lipoma are rare fatty tumors.

Literature

1. Ebara M, Fukuda H, Kojima Y, et al. (1999) Small hepatocellular carcinoma: relationship of signal intensity to histopathologic findings and metal content of the tumor and surrounding hepatic parenchyma. Radiology 210:81–88
2. Hussain SM, Semelka RC, Mitchell DG (2002) MR imaging of hepatocellular carcinoma. Magn Reson Imaging Clin N Am 10:31–52
3. Van den Bos IC, Hussain SM, Terkivatan T, et al. (2006) Step-wise carcinogenesis of hepatocellular carcinoma in the cirrhotic liver: demonstration on serial MR imaging. JMRI (in press)
4. Hussain SM, Van den Bos IC, Dwarkasing S, et al. (2006) Hepatocellular adenoma: findings at state-of-the-art magnetic resonance imaging, ultrasound, computed tomography and pathologic analysis. Eur Radiol 16:1873–1886

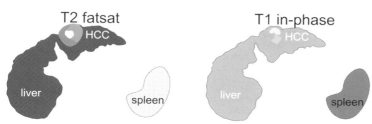
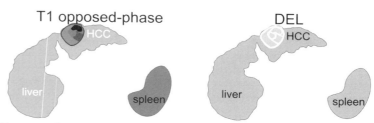

Fig. 47.1. HCC, cirrhotic liver, mosaic pattern with fatty lesion, drawings. T2 fat-sat: HCC appears as dominant nodule that is slightly hyperintense to the liver with a brighter center; **T1 in-phase:** HCC is almost isointense to the liver.

T1 opposed-phase: parts of HCC shows moderate to marked signal loss due to variable amount of fatty infiltration; **DEL:** HCC shows washout with enhanced septae and a tumor capsule

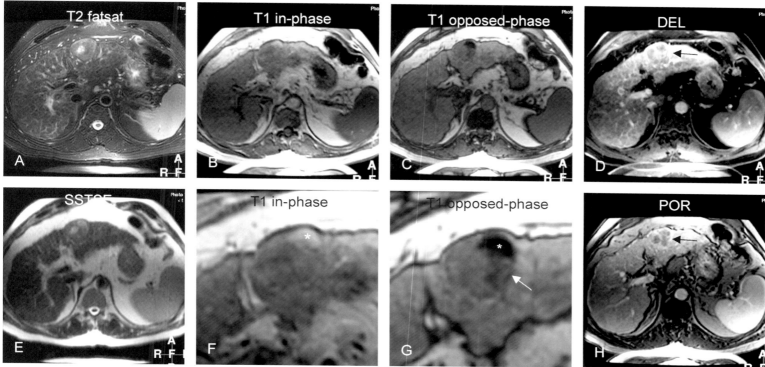

Fig. 47.2. HCC, cirrhotic liver, mosaic pattern with fatty lesion, MRI findings. A Axial TSE image (T2 fatsat): HCC appears as a dominant nodule that is slightly hyperintense to the liver with a brighter center. **B** Axial in-phase image (T1 in-phase): HCC is almost isointense to the liver. **C** Axial opposed-phase image (T1 opposed-phase): parts of HCC show moderate to marked signal loss due to the variable amount of fatty infiltration. **D** Axial delayed phase image (DEL): HCC shows washout with enhanced septa and a tumor capsule (*arrow*). **E** Axial SSTSE image (SSTSE): HCC is predominantly

hyperintense to the liver. **F** A detailed view of the in-phase image (T1 in-phase): one part of the HCC is much brighter (*). **G** A detailed view of the opposed-phase image (T1 opposed-phase): one part of the HCC shows marked signal loss, whereas another part shows moderate signal loss (*arrow*), which is related to the amount of fatty infiltration. **H** Axial portal phase image (POR): HCC shows washout with enhanced septa and a tumor capsule (*arrow*)

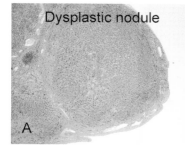
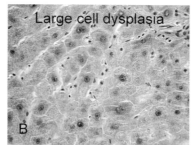
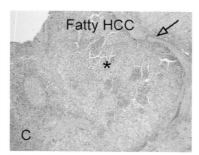
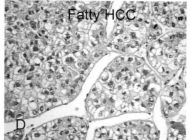

Fig. 47.3. HCC, direct MR-biopsy correlation. A Photomicrograph shows a dysplastic nodule surrounded by fibrous septa. H&E, ×40. **B** Photomicrograph shows typical large cell dysplasia with large abnormal hepatocytes with thickened plates. H&E, ×400. **C** Photomicrograph shows the HCC (shown

above) with the most fatty part (*) surrounded by a fibrous tumor capsule (*open arrow*). H&E, ×100. **D** Photomicrograph shows in detail the hepatocytes composed of abnormal nuclei and cytoplasm with fat, consistent with the fatty HCC shown above. H&E, ×200

48 HCC in Cirrhosis VII – Large Growing Lesion with Portal Invasion

Large hepatocellular carcinomas (HCCs) have a number of characteristic features, including vascular invasion with or without extracapsular extension with the formation of satellite nodule(s). Vascular invasion in fact is also a hallmark of diffuse HCC. Both the portal as well as the hepatic veins may be affected. In a recent study, 15.5 % of cases showed macroscopic and 59.0 % microscopic venous invasion proved at histopathology. In this study, the lesions with vascular invasion were associated with a larger tumor size, a higher α-fetoprotein level, and less frequent encapsulation. In a meta-analysis of 7 reports with 1497 patients, portal vein invasion was found in 24 % of the cases with HCC.

MR Imaging Findings

Vascular invasion is visible as a lack of signal void on multislice T1-weighted gradient echo and flow-compensated T2-weighted fast spin-echo images. The signal in vessels may however vary on such sequences depending on the cardiac cycle and flow rate. On black-blood T2-weighted echoplanar MR imaging, flow within vessels is actively dephased by applying low diffusion gradients. On this sequence, normal vessels are visible with signal void whereas thrombosed vessels appear bright. On gadolinium-enhanced MR images, the tumor thrombus from HCC typically shows early enhancement on images acquired during the arterial phase and a filling defect on images acquired during later phases. A combination of various T2-weighted, T1-weighted, and dynamic gadolinium-enhanced sequences is critical in the detection of large HCC as well as small satellite nodules with vascular invasion (Figs. 48.1, 48.2). With the interval growth, the lesions may change their signal intensity and become more apparent (Fig. 48.3).

Differential Diagnosis

Rarely other liver lesions such as metastases and cholangiocarcinomas may show vascular invasion. Bland thrombosis of the hepatic vessels may be caused by underlying Budd-Chiari syndrome. Bland thrombosis however does not show any arterial enhancement. In the presence of unexplained portal vein thrombosis, any concealed diffuse HCC should be excluded.

Literature

1. Hussain SM, Semelka RC, Mitchell DG (2002) MR imaging of hepatocellular carcinoma. Magn Reson Imaging Clin N Am 10:31–52
2. Tsai T-J, Chau G-Y, Lui W-Y, et al. (2000) Clinical significance of microscopic tumor venous invasion in patients with resectable hepatocellular carcinoma. Surgery 127:603–608
3. Lee YT, Geer DA (1987) Primary liver cancer: pattern of metastasis. J Surg Oncol 36:26–31
4. Hussain SM, De Becker J, Hop WCJ, et al. (2005) Can a single-shot black-blood T2-weighted spin-echo echo-planar imaging sequence with sensitivity encoding replace the respiratory-triggered turbo spin-echo sequence for the liver? – An optimization and a feasibility study. JMRI 21:219–229

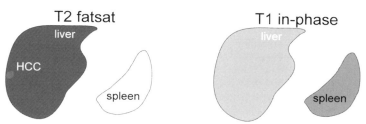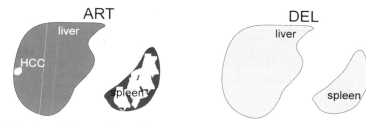

Fig. 48.1. HCC, cirrhosis, multiple. T2 fatsat: HCC is only slightly brighter to the cirrhotic liver; **T1 in-phase:** HCC is isointense to the cirrhotic liver; **ART:** HCC shows intense almost homogeneous enhancement; **DEL:** HCC becomes isointense to the liver

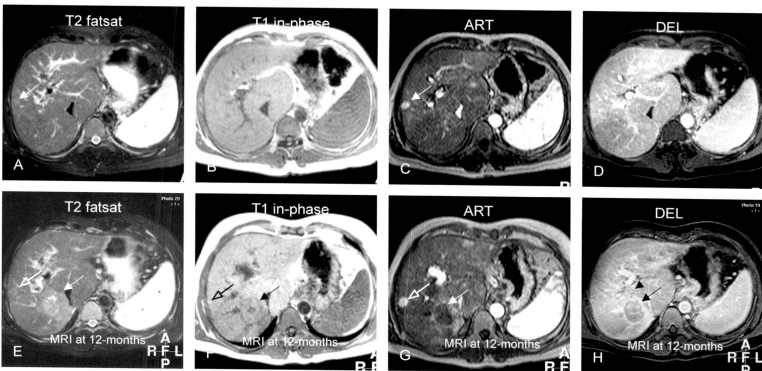

Fig. 48.2. HCC, cirrhosis, multiple growing lesions, MRI findings. A Axial TSE image (T2 fatsat): HCC is only slightly brighter to the cirrhotic liver (*arrow*). **B** Axial in-phase image (T1 in-phase): HCC is isointense to the cirrhotic liver. **C** Axial arterial phase image (ART): HCC shows intense almost homogeneous enhancement. **D** Axial delayed phase image (DEL): HCC becomes isointense to the liver. **E** Axial TSE image (T2 fatsat) at 12 months: smaller HCC is increased in size (*open arrow*). An additional larger HCC (*solid arrow*) has emerged with predominantly high signal to the liver. **F** Axial in-phase image (T1 in-phase): HCCs have predominantly low signal to the liver; note a bright nodule at the site of the smaller HCC (*open arrow*). Larger HCC is surrounded by a capsule (*solid arrow*). **G** Axial arterial phase image (ART): small HCC shows similar enhancement; the larger lesion shows heterogeneous enhancement. **H** Axial delayed phase image (DEL): small HCC becomes isointense to the liver. The larger lesion shows washout with enhancement of septa (*arrow*), and probably also suspicion of portal invasion (*arrowhead*)

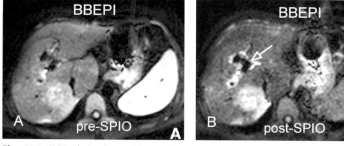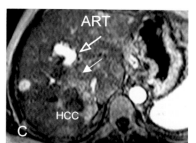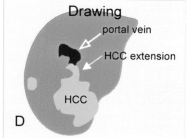

Fig. 48.3. HCC, cirrhosis, multiple lesions, additional MRI findings at 6 months. A Axial BBEPI image before uptake of SPIO: Both HCCs are hyperintense to the liver. **B** Axial BBEPI image after uptake of SPIO shows improved delineation of the HCC with abruptly ending right portal vein (*open arrow*). **C** A detailed view of the arterial phase image indeed shows a faint enhancing extension of the larger HCC (*solid arrow*) into the portal vein (*open arrow*). **D** Drawing presents the findings schematically

49 HCC in Cirrhosis VIII – Segmental Diffuse with Portal Vein Thrombosis

Diffuse hepatocellular carcinoma (HCC) is present in 4–13% of patients with HCC. The tumor can spread throughout most of the liver, and may be segmental in location. Typically, diffuse HCC is accompanied by extensive portal venous tumor thrombosis and a substantial elevation of serum alpha-fetoprotein (AFP) value. Serum AFP values may be elevated in up to 78% of patients. Diffuse HCC is often difficult to detect on imaging studies because of its permeative appearance and heterogeneity of background chronic liver disease. Portal venous tumor thrombosis may be an important clue to the diagnosis. Fibrous capsule and septa are often absent in diffuse HCC. Detection of portal venous thrombosis is crucial in the diagnosis of diffuse HCC on imaging.

MR Imaging Findings

At MR imaging, the affected segment(s) have subtle to markedly increased signal intensity on T2-weighted images. On heavily T2-weighted images, segmental dilatation of the bile ducts may also be present. On T1-weighted images, subtle hypointensity may be present. On gadolinium-enhanced images, the affected area may show only faint heterogeneous or patchy enhancement in the arterial phase. However, the lesion may show markedly heterogeneous enhancement in the delayed phase, likely due to a combined effect of washout and ongoing persistent enhancement (Figs. 49.1, 49.2). In some cases, portal vein thrombosis may be masked by the presence of the tumor. If necessary, maximum intensity projections may facilitate evaluation of the extent of the portal vein thrombosis (Fig. 49.3). Ascites may surround the liver. Hepatic veins are often unaffected.

Differential Diagnosis

Confluent fibrosis may be a challenge to distinguish from diffuse HCC on CT. MR imaging provides more characteristic imaging information.

Literature

1. Kanematsu M, Semelka RC, Leonardou P, et al. (2003) Hepatocellular carcinoma of diffuse type: MR imaging findings and clinical manifestations. JMRI 18:189–195
2. Okuda K, Noguchi T, Kubo Y, et al. (1981) A clinical and pathological study of diffuse type hepatocellular carcinoma. Liver 1:280–289
3. Tublin ME, Dodd 3rd GD, Baron RL (1997) Benign and malignant portal vein thrombosis: differentiation by CT characteristics. AJR 168:719–723
4. Kelekis NL, Semelka RC, Worawattanakul S, et al. (1998) Hepatocellular carcinoma in North America: a multiinstitutional study of appearance on T1-weighted, T2-weighted, and serial gadolinium-enhanced gradient-echo images. AJR 170:1005–13

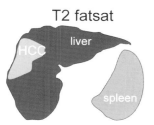
T2 fatsat

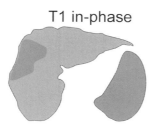
T1 in-phase

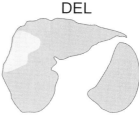
ART

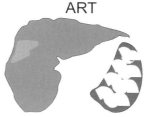
DEL

Fig. 49.1. HCC, cirrhotic diffuse HCC, portal invasion, iron deposition. T2 fatsat: HCC is much brighter than the dark liver due to mild iron deposition; the spleen has also a lower signal; **T1 in-phase:** HCC is slightly hypointense to the cirrhotic liver (irregular contours and splenomegaly); **ART:** a part of HCC shows faint heterogeneous enhancement; **DEL:** HCC shows some washout and becomes more heterogeneous

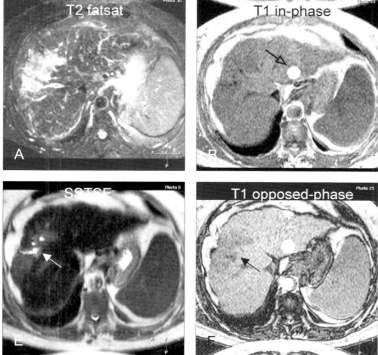
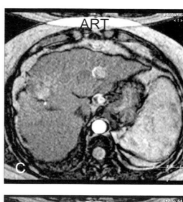
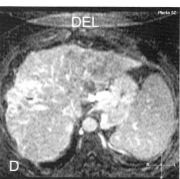
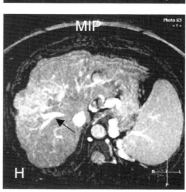

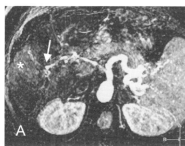
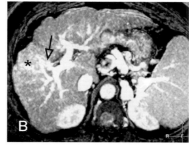
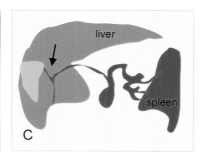
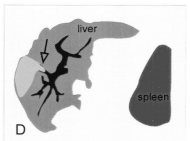

Fig. 49.2. HCC, cirrhotic liver, diffuse HCC, portal invasion, iron deposition, MRI findings. A Axial fat-suppressed TSE image (T2 fatsat): HCC is much brighter than the dark liver and the spleen due to iron deposition. **B** Axial in-phase GRE image (T1 opposed-phase): HCC is slightly hypointense compared to a slightly darker liver and spleen [liver and spleen have become darker compared to opposed-phase (shorter TE) image in **F**]. Pulsation artifact of the aorta (*open arrow*). **C** Axial arterial phase image (ART): HCC shows faint heterogeneous enhancement. **D** Axial delayed phase image (DEL): HCC shows some washout and becomes more heterogeneous. **E** Axial SSTSE image (SSTSE): HCC contains dilated bile ducts (*arrow*).The liver and the spleen are too dark due to iron deposition. **F** Axial opposed-phase image (T1 opposed-phase): HCC (*arrow*) is more hypointense in a brighter liver due to shorter TE. **G** Axial portal phase image (POR): HCC appears somewhat heterogeneous (*arrow*). **H** Maximum intensity projection (MIP): HCC shows no invasion of the right hepatic vein (*arrow*)

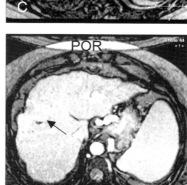

Fig. 49.3. HCC, diffuse in cirrhosis with portal invasion, MIPs and drawings. A A MIP of the arterial phase: The hypertrophic hepatic artery (*solid arrow*) feeds the tumor (*). **B** MIP of the portal phase: Note the disruption of the portal branch to segment VIII (*open arrow*), due to invasion (*). **C** Drawing shows the hypertrophic hepatic artery caused by the presence of cirrhosis and HCC (*solid arrow*). **D** Drawing illustrates the tumor invasion of the portal branch to segment VIII (*open arrow*)

50 HCC in Cirrhosis IX – Multiple Lesions Growing on Follow-up

In a large multi-institutional study of 354 hepatocellular carcinomas (HCCs), 56% were solitary, 40% multiple and 4% diffuse. Multiplicity of HCC may be based on transhepatic hematogenous spread, multifocal origin, or a combination of both. In general, the differential diagnosis of hypervascular liver lesions is wide-ranging. However, in the setting of cirrhosis the differential diagnosis can be practically narrowed down to HCC unless proven otherwise. Therefore, it is crucial to know the patient's history (e.g., viral and alpha-fetoprotein status) and to determine any morphological changes that suggest fibrosis or cirrhosis on imaging. These include (1) irregular or rounded liver contours; (2) abnormally large or small liver segments; (3) presence of nodules; (4) splenomegaly; (5) collaterals; and (6) ascites. Recognition of cirrhosis is particularly important if a patient presents with multiple hypervascular lesions.

MR Imaging Findings

At MR imaging, the combination of hypointensity on T1-weighted images, hyperintensity on T2-weighted images, and diffuse heterogeneous enhancement is the most common appearance of HCC on MR images. Small HCCs (2 cm) are frequently isointense on both T1-weighted and T2-weighted images and may be detected on immediate gadolinium-enhanced images only (Figs. 50.1. 50.2). Follow-up may be considered in patients with suspicion of multiple HCC (Fig. 50.3).

Differential Diagnosis

In the setting of cirrhosis, high-grade dysplastic nodules, vascular shunts, and pseudolesions may have some overlap with small and developing HCC. Without any clinical evidence of liver disease and the lack of imaging signs of cirrhosis, focal nodular hyperplasia syndrome, hepatocellular adenomas, and multiple metastases should be considered.

Literature

1. Kelekis NL, Semelka RC, Worawattanakul S, et al. (1998) Hepatocellular carcinoma in North America: a multiinstitutional study of appearance on T1-weighted, T2-weighted, and serial gadolinium-enhanced gradient-echo images. AJR 170:1005–1013
2. Ito K, Fujita T, Shimizu A, et al. (2004) Multiarterial phase dynamic MRI of small early enhancing hepatic lesions in cirrhosis or chronic hepatitis: differentiating between hypervascular hepatocellular carcinomas and pseudolesions. AJR 183:699–705
3. Hussain SM, Zondervan PE, et al. (2002) Benign versus malignant hepatic nodules: MR imaging findings with pathologic correlation. Radiographics 22:1023–1036

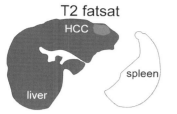
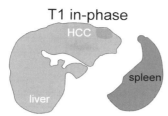
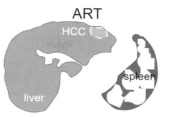
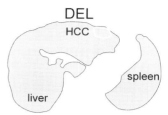

Fig. 50.1. HCC, cirrhosis, multiple. T2 fatsat: HCC is only slightly brighter than the cirrhotic liver; **T1 in-phase**: HCC is only slightly darker than the cirrhot- ic liver; **ART**: HCC shows faint heterogeneous enhancement; **DEL**: HCC shows washout with capsular enhancement

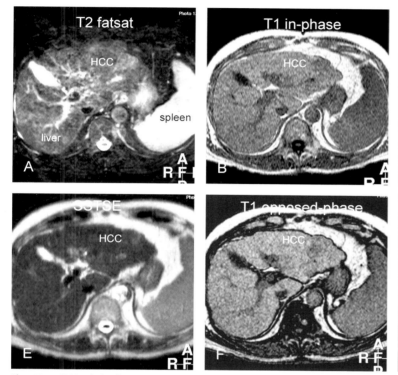
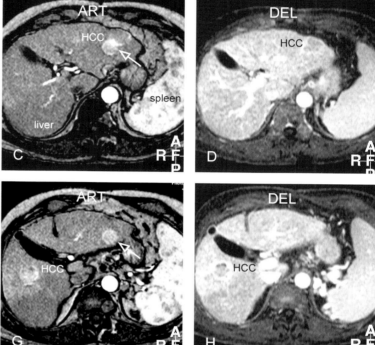

Fig. 50.2. HCC, cirrhosis, multiple lesions, MRI findings. A Axial TSE image (T2 fatsat): HCC is only slightly brighter than the cirrhotic liver and difficult to recognize, also because of ghost artifacts. **B** Axial in-phase image (T1 in-phase): HCC is only slightly darker than the cirrhotic liver. **C** Axial arterial phase image (ART): HCC shows faint heterogeneous enhancement. Ghost artifact of the aorta (*open arrow*). **D** Axial delayed phase image (DEL): HCC shows washout with capsular enhancement. **E** Axial SSTSE image (SSTSE): HCC is hardly visible within a cirrhotic liver with irregular contours. **F** Axial opposed-phase image (T1 opposed-phase): No fatty infiltration is present. **G** Axial arterial phase image (ART) at lower anatomic level shows a second HCC. Ghost artifact of the aorta (*open arrow*). **H** Axial delayed phase image (DEL): The second HCC also shows washout with capsular enhancement

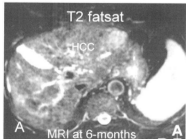
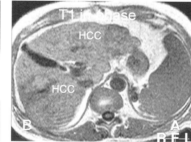
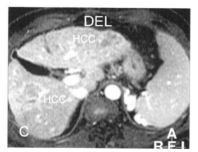
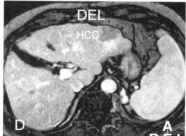

Fig. 50.3. HCC, cirrhosis, multiple lesions, MRI findings at 6 months. A Axial TSE image (T2 fatsat): HCC has become brighter and larger in size. **B** Axial in-phase image (T1 in-phase): HCC in the left liver is hypointense and HCC in the right liver is hyperintense to the liver. **C** Axial delayed phase image (DEL): HCC in the right liver is larger with washout and capsular enhance- ment. **D** Axial delayed phase image (DEL): HCC in the left liver shows more washout

51 HCC in Cirrhosis X – Capsular Retraction and Suspected Diaphragm Invasion

Hepatic capsular retraction adjacent to hepatic tumor is rare, although this finding has been described in a variety of malignant tumors [intrahepatic cholangiocarcinoma, hepatocellular carcinoma (HCC), and colorectal metastases] and benign entities (confluent fibrosis and hemangioma). Although retraction of the liver capsule adjacent to a hepatic tumor was first described in epithelioid hemangioendothelioma, many radiologists consider this sign to be associated with cholangiocarcinoma. Rarely, HCC may present with this sign and in combination with other imaging findings such as high signal intensity on T2-weighted images, and subtle cirrhotic morphology may hamper the diagnosis. In addition, if subcapsular location coincides with the subphrenic location of HCC, the possibility of diaphragm invasion may be raised.

MR Imaging Findings

At MR imaging, subcapsular HCC may show retraction of the liver capsule. The signal intensity of such HCC may be exceptionally high on T2-weighted images and mimic cholangiocarcinoma. The high signal intensity strongly suggests high fluid content and may be related to the cholangiocellular differentiation or a mixed type of HCC at histology. On T1-weighted images the findings may be unremarkable. The lesions may show only subtle enhancement in the arterial phase. The enhancement of a tumor capsule in the delayed phase and subtle cirrhotic morphology of the liver may facilitate the correct diagnosis. Small recurrences of such HCCs may also display high signal on T2-weighted images and may be successfully removed at surgery (Figs. 51.1 – 51.3).

Differential Diagnosis

Large, single, intrahepatic lesions with high signal intensity on T2-weighted images and capsular retraction may mimic intrahepatic cholangiocarcinoma. In such cases, it is crucial to assess any capsular enhancement in the delayed phase, search for any subtle signs of cirrhosis at imaging, and look for the clinical indicators of parenchymal liver disease.

Literature

1. Miller WJ, Dodd GD III, Federle MP, Baron RL (1992) Epithelioid hemangioendothelioma of the liver: imaging findings with pathologic correlation. AJR 159:53 – 57
2. Outwater E (1993) Capsular retraction in hepatic tumors [letter]. AJR 160:422
3. Yang DM, Kim HS, Cho SW, et al. (2002) Various causes of hepatic capsular retraction: CT and MR findings. Br J Radiol 75:994 – 1002
4. Verhoef C, Holman FA, Hussain SM, et al. (2005) Resection of extrahepatic hepatocellular carcinoma metastasis can result in long-term survival. Acta Chir Belg 105:533 – 536

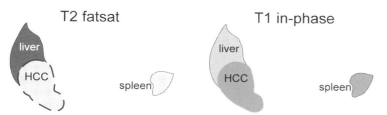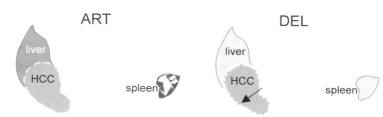

Fig. 51.1. HCC, cirrhosis, large, drawings. T2 fatsat: HCC is hyperintense to the liver and surrounded by a (ruptured) tumor capsule; **T1 in-phase:** HCC is hyperintense to the liver; **ART:** HCC shows faint enhancement predomi-

nantly in the periphery of the lesion; **DEL:** HCC shows washout with enhancement of the tumor capsule, which appears to be discontinuous at the subcapsular region (*arrow*)

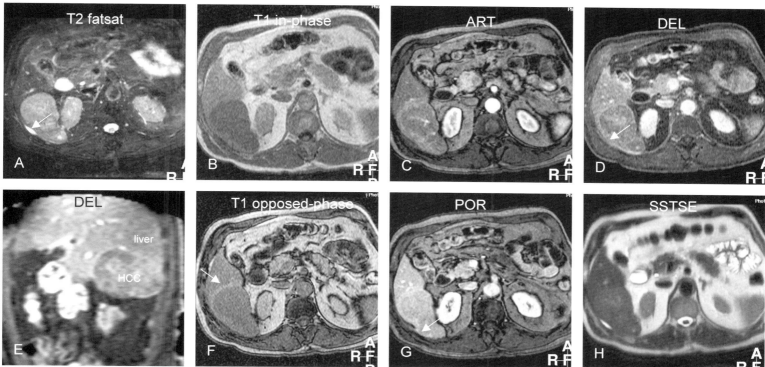

Fig. 51.2. HCC, cirrhosis, large, MRI findings. A Axial TSE image (T2 fatsat): HCC is hyperintense to the liver, which is surrounded by a discontinuous dark tumor capsule; note also a subtle umbilication (*arrow*). **B** Axial in-phase image (T1 in-phase): HCC is hypointense to the cirrhotic liver. **C** Axial arterial phase image (ART): HCC shows faint enhancement mainly in the periphery of the tumor. **D** Axial delayed phase image (DEL): HCC shows washout with enhanced capsule that particularly appears to be ruptured in

the subcapsular region (*arrow*). **E** Sagittal delayed phase image (DEL): Fatty liver has become darker with persistent perilesional high signal (*arrow*). **F** Axial opposed-phase image (T1 opposed-phase): Note the peri-lesional compressed bright liver parenchyma (*arrow*). **G** Axial portal phase image (POR): a part of the HCC appears to be attached to the diaphragm, suspicious of extrahepatic tumor extension (*arrow*). **H** Axial SSTSE image (SSTSE): HCC is slightly brighter in the central part (*arrow*)

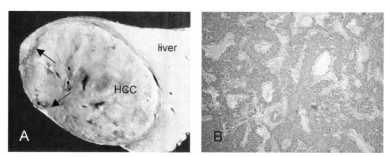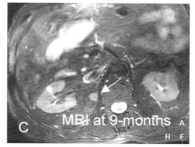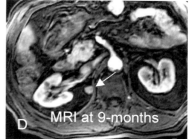

Fig. 51.3. HCC, cirrhosis, large, direct MR-pathology correlation. A Photograph of the resected specimen shows the HCC with a fibrous tumor capsule that is discontinuous at least at two places (*arrow*). The resection surfaces were considered to be free of tumor at pathology. **B** Photomicrograph shows large

glands within plates of abnormal hepatocytes that indicate a cholangiolar type of HCC. H&E, ×100. **C, D** Axial TSE and arterial phase images at 9 months follow-up show a recurrence at the diaphragm that was resected successfully (*arrow*)

52 HCC in Cirrhosis XI – Diffuse Within the Entire Liver with Portal Vein Thrombosis

Diffuse hepatocellular carcinoma (HCC) is present in up to 13 % of patients with HCC. The tumor can spread throughout the liver, and in some cases may replace almost the entire liver parenchyma by a permeative or extensive micronodular growth pattern. Extensive portal venous tumor thrombosis is a hallmark of such extensive diffuse HCC and the serum alpha-fetoprotein value is elevated in up to 78 % of patients. In addition, lymph node, bone, and lung metastases may be present. Diffuse HCC that infiltrates and replaces the entire liver may remain undetected on CT and US, mainly because of insufficient intrinsic soft tissue contrast in these modalities. The presence of portal venous tumor thrombosis is an important clue to the diagnosis.

MR Imaging Findings

At MR imaging, the entire liver shows heterogeneous increased signal intensity on T2-weighted images with irregular contours and ascites (spleen, if normal, may be used as a reference). On T1-weighted images, the liver may also appear heterogeneous with the presence of abnormally high signal at the level of the portal vein. Due to the presence of tumor thrombus, the portal vein is often expanded. On gadolinium-enhanced images, the entire liver shows marked heterogeneous or patchy enhancement in the arterial phase. The enhancement becomes more permeative or miliary in the delayed phase (Figs. 52.1, 52.2). US and CT may remain inconclusive in such cases (Fig. 52.3).

Differential Diagnosis

Hepatic vascular abnormalities such as bland portal vein thrombosis and Budd-Chiari syndrome may show some overlap on imaging with diffuse HCC, but the clinical settings and the relationship with the tumor markers differ considerably. Increased arterial enhancement of the liver due to altered vascularity is often a transient phenomenon, does not persist into the delayed phase and is often unaccompanied by tissue changes.

Literature

1. Kanematsu M, Semelka RC, Leonardou P, et al. (2003) Hepatocellular carcinoma of diffuse type: MR imaging findings and clinical manifestations. JMRI 18:189–195
2. Okuda K, Noguchi T, Kubo Y, et al. (1981) A clinical and pathological study of diffuse type hepatocellular carcinoma. Liver 1:280–289
3. Tublin ME, Dodd 3rd GD, Baron RL (1997) Benign and malignant portal vein thrombosis: differentiation by CT characteristics. AJR 168:719–723
4. Hussain SM, Semelka RC (2005) Hepatic imaging: Comparison of modalities. Radiol Clin N Am 43:929–947

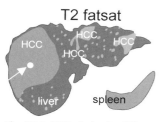 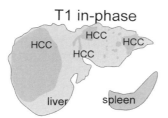 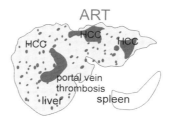 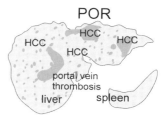

Fig. 52.1. HCC, cirrhosis, diffuse HCC with portal invasion, drawings. T2 fatsat: HCC is diffuse and hyperintense to the liver; note also the cirrhotic liver, a bright cyst (*arrow*) and ascites; **T1 in-phase:** HCC is hypointense to the liver;

ART: HCC shows heterogeneous permeative enhancement with enhancement of the portal vein tumor thrombosis; **DEL:** the entire liver remains strongly heterogeneous

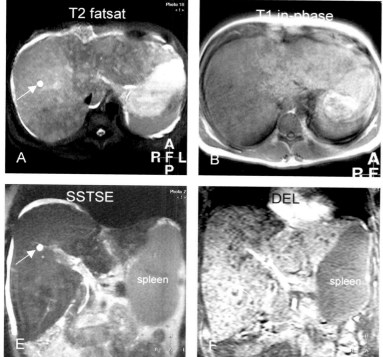 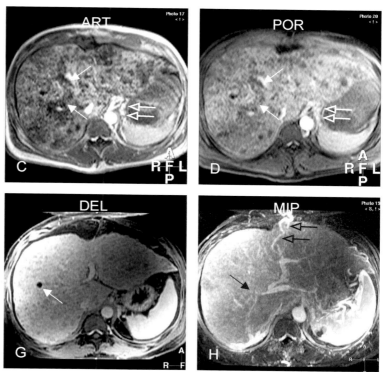

Fig. 52.2. HCC, cirrhosis, diffuse HCC with portal invasion, MRI findings. A Axial TSE image (T2 fatsat): HCC is diffuse and hyperintense to the liver; note also the cirrhotic liver, a bright cyst (*arrow*) and ascites. **B** Axial in-phase image (T1 in-phase): HCC is hypointense to the liver. **C** Axial arterial phase image (ART): HCC shows heterogeneous permeative enhancement with the portal vein tumor thrombosis (*solid arrows*) and esophageal varices (*open arrows*). **D** Axial portal phase image (POR): The liver remains heterogeneous with portal vein thrombosis (*solid arrows*) and varices (*open arrows*). **E** Coronal

SSTSE image (SSTSE): Note the cirrhotic liver with diffuse HCC, a cyst, ascites, and enlarged spleen. **F** Coronal delayed phase image (POR): The liver shows strong heterogeneous enhancement due to the diffuse HCC. **G** Axial delayed phase image (POR) at another level shows the cyst (*arrow*) and the liver with septal enhancement. **H** MIP of the delayed phase image shows the recanalization of the ligament falciform (*open arrows*) and thrombosed right portal vein (*solid arrow*)

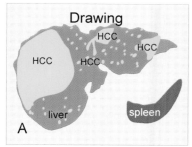 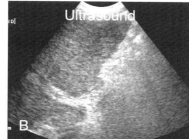 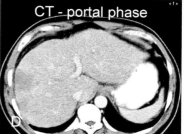 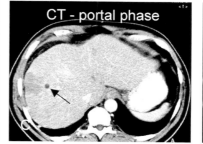

Fig. 52.3. HCC, cirrhosis, diffuse HCC with portal invasion, drawing and inconclusive US and CT prior to MRI. A Drawing shows the diffuse HCC within the cirrhotic liver. **B** Ultrasound was performed because of acute esophageal hemorrhage. No cause was found and the cirrhosis was not recognized. **C** and **D**

CT (following US) at two different anatomic levels showed a cyst (*arrow*) and "circulation changes". No cause of bleeding was found and MRI was requested which is shown above

53 HCC in Cirrhosis XII – With Intrahepatic Bile Duct Dilatation

Hepatocellular carcinomas (HCCs) rarely may show invasion with dilatation of the bile ducts and cause jaundice mimicking an intrahepatic cholangiocarcinoma. The treatment options and prognosis may differ. Therefore, early distinction is important. Intraductal cholangiocarcinoma is frequently limited to the mucosa but can invade the ductal wall at a late stage. It usually follows a relatively benign course, and long-term survival can usually be expected after complete surgical resection. In contrast, the bile duct invasion is a late and rare presentation in HCC with a relatively poor prognosis. Definitive surgical intervention is often not feasible because of tumor extension and associated advanced liver cirrhosis.

MR Imaging Findings

At MR imaging, segmental dilatation of the bile ducts in combination with a liver mass may suggest the presence of a cholangiocarcinoma. However, the history of parenchymal liver disease with cirrhosis may strongly indicate the presence of an underlying HCC. Also the mosaic pattern, tumor capsular enhancement, and portal vein thrombosis are indicators of HCC. In rare cases, several intrahepatic confluent nodules of HCC may be present that may also show intrahepatic bile duct dilatation. Such HCCs may be unusually bright on T2-weighted images and show intense arterial enhancement (Figs. 53.1 – 53.3).

Differential Diagnosis

The differential diagnosis should include (1) cholangiocarcinoma, (2) primary sclerosing cholangitis with a cholangiocarcinoma, and (3) liver metastases of a hepatoid type of stomach or gallbladder tumor, which often have an elevated alpha-fetoprotein value and clinically mimic HCC.

Management

Percutaneous biliary drainage and transarterial chemoembolization may be used for palliation.

Literature

1. Jung AY, Lee JM, Choi SH, et al. (2006) Computed tomography features of an intraductal polypoid mass differentiation between hepatocellular carcinoma with bile duct tumor invasion and intraductal papillary cholangiocarcinoma. JCAT 30:18 – 24
2. Kojiro M, Kawabata K, Kawano Y, et al. (1982) Hepatocellular carcinoma presenting as intrabile duct tumor growth: a clinicopathologic study of 24 cases. Cancer 49:2144 – 2147
3. Tamada K, Isoa N, Wada S, et al. (2001) Intraductal ultrasonography for hepatocellular carcinoma with tumor thrombi in the bile duct; comparison with polypoid cholangiocarcinoma. J Gastroenterol Hepatol 16:801 – 805
4. Lauffer JM, Mai G, Berchtold D, et al. (1999) Multidisciplinary approach to palliation of obstructive jaundice caused by a central hepatocellular carcinoma. Dig Surg 16:531 – 536

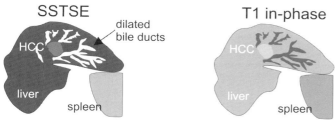 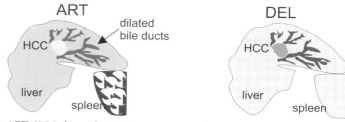

Fig. 53.1. HCC, with dilated bile ducts in a cirrhotic liver, drawings. SSTSE: HCC is slightly hyperintense to the liver and causes compression, encasement, and dilatation of the bile ducts; **T1 in-phase:** HCC is almost isointense to the liver; **ART:** HCC shows faint heterogeneous enhancement; **DEL:** HCC shows washout without a tumor capsule

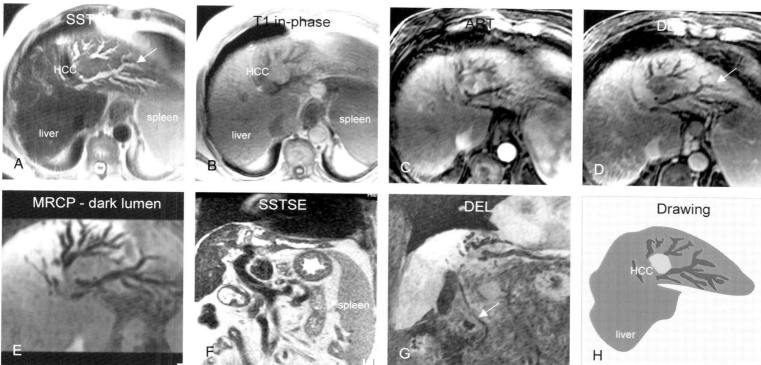

Fig. 53.2. HCC, dilated bile ducts in a cirrhotic liver, MRI findings. A Axial SSTSE image (SSTSE): HCC is slightly hyperintense and causes compression, encasement, and dilatation of the bile ducts (*arrow*). **B** Axial in-phase image (T1 in-phase): HCC is isointense to the liver. **C** Axial arterial phase image (ART): HCC shows faint heterogeneous enhancement. **D** Axial delayed phase image (DEL): HCC shows washout without any enhancing tumor cap-sule. **E** Coronal reformat based on the axial delayed phase image (MRCP – dark lumen) shows dark, dilated bile ducts in an enhanced liver. **F** Coronal SSTSE image (SSTSE) shows the enlarged spleen indicating portal hypertension. **G** Coronal delayed phase image (DEL) shows unenhanced dilated bile ducts in the left liver with normal common bile duct (*arrow*). **H** Drawing shows HCC with dilated bile ducts

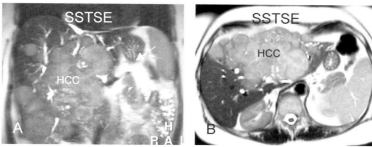 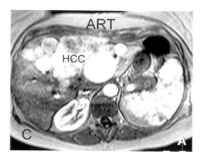 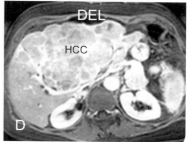

Fig. 53.3. HCC, dilated bile ducts, MRI findings in another patient with increased alpha-fetoprotein. A Coronal SSTSE image (SSTSE) shows a large multifocal HCC with interspersed dilated bile ducts. **B** Axial SSTSE image (SSTSE) of the massive HCC with dilated bile ducts. **C** Axial arterial phase image (ART) shows intense enhancement of the nodules within HCC. **D** Axial delayed phase image (DEL) shows washout with septa enhancement

Primary Solid Liver Lesions in Non-Cirrhotic Liver

54 Focal Nodular Hyperplasia I – Typical with Large Central Scar and Septa

Edmondson introduced the term focal nodular hyperplasia (FNH) in 1958. Currently, FNH is considered a benign, regenerative lesion. FNH is the second most common benign liver tumor after hemangioma and has a reported prevalence of 0.9 %. FNH occurs predominantly in women during their reproductive years. Approximately 20 % of patients have multiple FNHs, which often concur with other benign lesions such as hemangiomas and cysts.

MR Imaging Findings

Typically, FNH is iso- or hypointense on T1- (94 – 100 %), slightly hyper- or isointense on T2- (94 – 100 %) and with a bright central scar on T2-weighted images (84 %). FNH shows intense homogeneous enhancement in the arterial phase with enhanced central scar and septa in the later phases of the gadolinium-enhanced images (Figs. 54.1, 54.2). FNHs do not have a true tumor capsule, though the pseudocapsule surrounding some of the FNHs may be quite prominent. The central scar is well formed, typically high in signal intensity on T2-weighted images and shows enhancement on delayed contrast-enhanced images. After uptake of Kupffer cell-specific contrast media, central scar and septa may show improved conspicuity (Fig. 54.3A–C).

Pathology

The gross pathology of FNH is characterized by a network of central scar and septa that contain multiple nodules (macroscopically it resembles „focal cirrhosis") (Fig. 54.3D).

Management

Asymptomatic FNH does not need any treatment or follow-up.

Literature

1. Hussain SM, Terkivatan T, Zondervan PE, et al. (2004) Focal nodular hyperplasia: a spectrum of findings at state-of-the-art MR imaging, ultrasound, CT and pathology. Radiographics 24:3 – 19
2. Hussain SM, Zondervan PE, Ijzermans JN, et al. (2002) Benign versus malignant hepatic nodules: MR imaging findings with pathologic correlation. Radiographics 22:1023 – 36
3. Terkivatan T, Van den Bos IC, Hussain SM, et al. (2006) Focal nodular hyperplasia: lesion characteristics on state-of-the-art MRI including dynamic gadolinium-enhanced and superparamagnetic iron-oxide-uptake sequences in a prospective study. JMRI 24:864 – 872

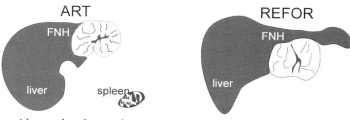
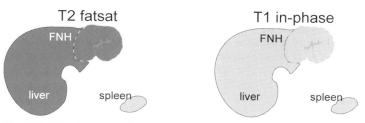

Fig. 54.1. FNH, drawings. T2 fatsat: FNH is isointense to the liver but visible due to the mass effect; **T1 in-phase:** FNH is isointense to the liver with faintly darker central scar; **ART:** FNH shows a very intense homogeneous enhance-ment with septal and central scar sparing; **REFOR:** coronal reconstruction of the arterial phase image shows the relationship of FNH to liver in a different anatomic orientation

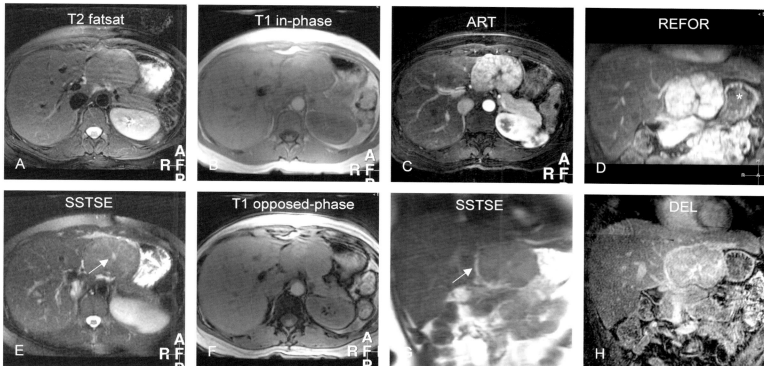

Fig. 54.2. FNH, large typical MRI findings at 3.0T. A Axial fat-suppressed turbo spin echo (TSE) image (T2 fatsat): FNH is isointense to the liver but visible due to the mass effect. **B** Axial in-phase image (T1 in-phase): FNH is isointense to the liver with a faintly darker central scar. **C** Axial arterial phase image (ART) with high resolution: FNH shows a very intense and homogeneous enhancement with septal and central scar sparing. **D** Coronal reformat based on the arterial phase image (REFOR): Almost the entire FNH is exophytic and causes compression of the stomach (*). **E** Axial single-shot TSE image (SSTSE) shows the bright central scar (*arrow*) better than on the T2 fatsat image. **F** Axial opposed-phase image (T1 opposed-phase): FNH shows no fatty infiltration. **G** Coronal T2-w SSTSE image (SSTSE): FNH is in part surrounded by a bright pseudocapsule (*arrow*). **H** Coronal delayed phase image (DEL): The central scar and the septa are enhanced

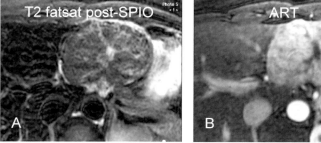
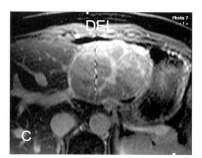
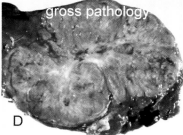

Fig. 54.3. FNH (same patient as shown above) and gross pathology (another patient). A Axial fat-suppressed TSE image (T2 fatsat) after uptake of superparamagnetic iron oxide (SPIO) shows signal loss in the liver as well as FNH with improved conspicuity of the septa and the central scar. **B** Axial arterial phase image (ART) shows the intratumoral enhanced nodules. **C** Axial de-layed phase image (DEL) shows the enhanced septa and the central scar in detail. **D** Photograph of a resected specimen shows nodules interspersed by the central scar and septa. Note the striking similarity with the lesion shown at MRI

55 Focal Nodular Hyperplasia II – Typical with Pathologic Correlation

Focal nodular hyperplasia is often discovered as an incidental finding on cross-sectional imaging. At ultrasound (US), the lesions may be difficult to characterize. Most radiologists recommend a computed tomography (CT) scan after the initial ultrasound. Despite the recent spectacular technical developments in CT and the introduction of multi-row detector ultra-fast CT, most centers still perform a single phase (usually portal phase) examination after injection of iodine contrast media. On such CTs, hypervascular lesions, such as FNH, cannot be characterized with certainty. Further evaluation is needed either with biopsy or MR imaging.

MR Imaging Findings

Typical FNH may not be well visible on T1-weighted or T2-weighted images because of its similarity with the surrounding liver tissue. The only components that may have distinct signal intensity are the central scar and the septa. Particularly, the central scar may be well visible on fat-suppressed T2-weighted images. If the central scar and the septa are not very prominent, FNH shows intense homogeneous enhancement in the arterial phase. The central scar and septa show delayed persistent enhancement (Figs. 55.1, 55.2). The combination of the signal intensity and typical enhancement pattern allow the visualization of the internal tumor anatomy. This allows very accurate diagnosis at MR imaging. Ultrasound lacks the intrinsic soft tissue contrast and therefore often remains inconclusive (Fig. 55.3A).

Pathology

At biopsy, it may be a challenge to diagnose FNH, which is a benign nodule that occurs in a liver that is otherwise histologically normal or nearly normal. Classic FNH is characterized by the presence of (a) abnormal nodular architecture, (b) malformed appearing vessels, and (c) cholangiolar proliferation. Specific stains may be needed to identify various components of FNH at biopsy (Fig. 55.3B – D). The non-classic FNH lacks one of the following classic features – nodular abnormal architecture or malformed vessels – but always shows bile ductular proliferation.

Management

Typical and asymptomatic FNH do not need any treatment or follow-up.

Literature

1. Nguyen BN, Flejou JF, Terris B, et al. (1999) Focal nodular hyperplasia of the liver. A comprehensive pathologic study of 305 lesions and recognition of new histologic forms. Am J Surg Pathol 23:1441 – 54
2. Hussain SM, Terkivatan T, Zondervan PE, et al. (2004) Focal nodular hyperplasia: a spectrum of findings at state-of-the-art MR imaging, ultrasound, CT and pathology. Radiographics 24:3 – 19
3. Hussain SM, Semelka RC (2005) Hepatic imaging: comparison of modalities. Radiol Clin N Am 43:929 – 947

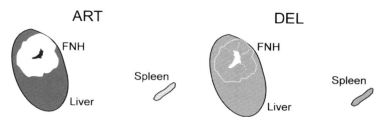
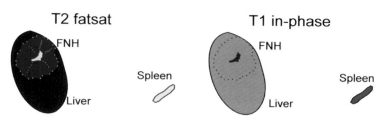

Fig. 55.1. FNH, drawings. T2 fatsat: FNH is slightly hyperintense to the liver with a brighter central scar and septa; **T1 in-phase:** FNH is isointense to the liver with a darker central scar; **ART:** FNH shows a very intense homoge-neous enhancement of the entire lesion, except the central scar; **DEL:** FNH becomes isointense with enhanced central scar, septa, and a pseudocapsule

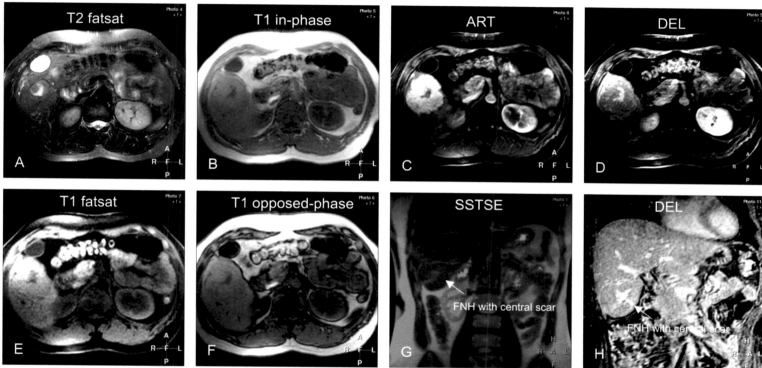

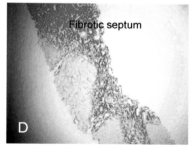

Fig. 55.2. FNH, typical MRI findings. A Axial fat-saturated T2-w TSE image (T2 fatsat): FNH is isointense to the liver with a brighter central scar. **B** Axial in-phase T1-w gradient recalled echo (GRE) (T1 in-phase): FNH is isointense to the liver with a darker central scar and a thin pseudocapsule. **C** Axial fat-suppressed arterial phase post-Gd 3D T1-w GRE image (ART): FNH shows very intense and homogeneous enhancement, except the central scar. **D** Axial delayed phase post-Gd 3D T1-w GRE image (DEL): FNH becomes isoin-tense with enhancement of the central scar and the septa. **E** Axial 2D T1-w GRE image (T1 fatsat) shows the central scar and the pseudocapsule better. **F** Axial opposed-phase 2D T1-w GRE image (T1 opposed-phase) shows no fatty infiltration either within the liver or in the FNH. **G** Coronal T2-w SSTSE (SSTSE) shows the FNH with a brighter central scar (*arrow*). **H** Coronal de-layed phase post-Gd 3D T1-w GRE image (DEL) with high spatial resolution clearly shows the enhanced central scar, the septa, and the pseudocapsule

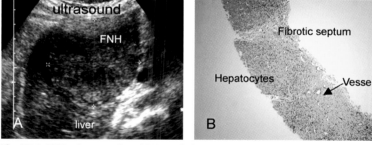
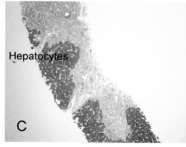

Fig. 55.3. FNH, ultrasound and MR pathology correlation. A Ultrasound (same patient) shows FNH with similar echogenicity as the liver, without revealing intratumoral morphology. **B** Photomicrograph of a biopsy shows nodules of FNH surrounded by a septum that contains vessels and inflammatory infil-trate. H&E, × 100. **C** Photomicrograph shows the stained hepatocytes within well-defined nodules. PAS stain, × 100. **D** Photomicrograph shows the stained fibrotic septa. SR stain, × 100

56 Focal Nodular Hyperplasia III – Typical with Follow-up Examination

The pathogenesis of focal nodular hyperplasia (FNH) is not well understood. Vascular malformation and vascular injury have been suggested as the underlying mechanism. The association with steroids has been denied more recently. FNH is the second most common benign liver tumor after hemangioma and has a reported prevalence of 0.9%. The male to female ratio is 1:8 and the tumors occur in relatively young patients. In principle, all benign liver lesions including FNH may show some growth over time. There are only sporadic cases of either increased or deceased size of FNH. We have not observed any FNH with major change in size on state-of-the-art MR imaging during the past 10 years. With any major change in diameter of a presumed FNH, the diagnosis should be doubted.

MR Imaging Findings
At MR imaging, the hallmarks of FNH are (1) T2-bright, large, well-formed central scar and septa; (2) near isointensity on T1- as well as T2-weighted images; (3) intense enhancement in the arterial phase; (4) fading to isointensity in the delayed phase with enhancement of the central scar and septa; and (5) no significant change in the size of the lesion over time (Figs. 56.1–56.3).

Gross Pathology
The *classic FNH* consists of lobulated contours and parenchyma that is composed of nodules surrounded by radiating fibrous septa originating from a central scar. The central scar contains malformed vascular structures. Among the classic FNHs, one or more macroscopic central scars are present in a majority of cases. The gross appearance of *non-classic FNH* is heterogeneous and globally resembles adenomas in most cases with vaguely lobulated contours and the lack of a macroscopic central scar in almost all cases.

Literature
1. Wanless IR, Mawdsley C, Adams R (1995) On the pathogenesis of focal nodular hyperplasia of the liver. Hepatology 5:1194–1200
2. Mathieu D, Kobeiter H, Maison P, et al. (2000) Oral contraceptive use and focal nodular hyperplasia of the liver. Gastroenterology 118:560–564
3. Nguyen BN, Flejou JF, Terris B, et al. (1999) Focal nodular hyperplasia of the liver. A comprehensive pathologic study of 305 lesions and recognition of new histologic forms. Am J Surg Pathol 23:1441–1454

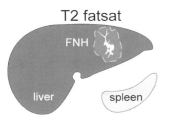
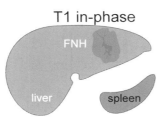
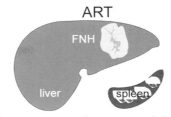
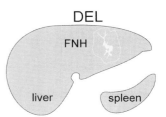

Fig. 56.1. FNH, drawings. T2 fatsat: FNH is slightly hyperintense to the liver with a brighter central scar and septa; **T1 in-phase:** FNH is slightly hypointense to the liver with a darker central scar; **ART:** FNH shows a very intense homogeneous enhancement of the entire lesion, except the central scar; **DEL:** FNH becomes isointense with enhanced central scar, septa, and a pseudocapsule

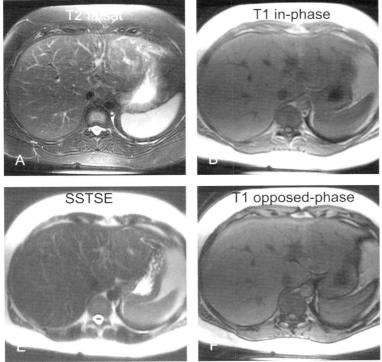
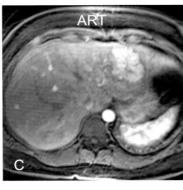
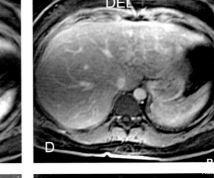
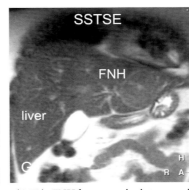
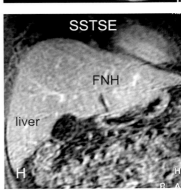

Fig. 56.2. FNH, typical MRI findings. A Axial fat-suppressed TSE image (T2 fatsat): FNH is slightly hyperintense to the liver with a brighter central scar, septa, and pseudo-capsule. **B** Axial in-phase image (T1 in-phase): FNH is slightly hypointense to the liver with a darker central scar. **C** Axial arterial phase image (ART): FNH shows very intense and homogeneous enhancement, except the central scar and the septa. **D** Axial delayed phase image (DEL): FNH becomes isointense with enhancement of the central scar and septa. **E** Axial SSTSE image (SSTSE) shows the bright central scar in the lesion. **F** Axial opposed-phase image (T1 opposed-phase) shows no fatty infiltration. **G** Coronal SSTSE (SSTSE) shows the FNH with a brighter central scar (*arrow*). **H** Coronal delayed phase image (DEL) shows the enhanced central scar

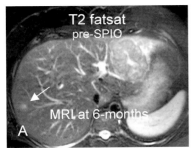
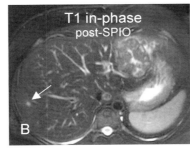
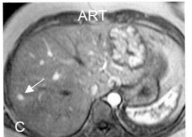
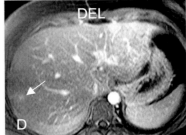

Fig. 56.3. FNH, 6 months follow-up MRI findings. A Axial TSE image (T2 fatsat) prior to SPIO uptake: FNH is unchanged. Note an additional smaller lesion (*arrow*). **B** Axial TSE image (T2 fatsat) after SPIO uptake: FNH, the liver, the spleen, and the small lesion (*arrow*) show decreased signal and hence contain Kupffer cells. **C** Axial arterial phase image (ART): FNH and the small lesion (*arrow*) show similar enhancement. **D** Axial delayed phase image (DEL) shows no change. In retrospect, the smaller lesion (*arrow*) was also present on the previous MRI

57 Focal Nodular Hyperplasia IV – Multiple FNH Syndrome

Multiple focal nodular hyperplasia (FNH) occurs in approximately 20–25% of patients with FNH. Multiple FNH syndrome consists of at least two FNH lesions and one or more of the following associated lesions: liver hemangioma, central nervous system vascular malformation, meningioma and astrocytoma. An incomplete expression is considered if FNH is seen with only one of the mentioned associated lesions. These patients may be symptomatic and frequently show abnormal liver function tests. Differentiation from multiple hepatocellular adenomas (HCAs) and multifocal hepatocellular carcinomas (HCCs) may be challenging. FNH may have a pseudocapsule composed of compressed parenchyma, perilesional vessels and inflammation. True fibrotic tumor capsule is a characteristic sign of HCC and is present in 60–80% of cases. The enhancement of HCA overlaps with FNH, but HCAs do not have a central scar and the majority of them contain fat.

MR Imaging Findings

At MR imaging, FNH should have (1) near isointensity on T1- and T2-weighted images, (2) intense enhancement in the arterial phase, and (3) fading to isointensity with enhancement of the central scar and septa in the delayed phase. In fatty liver, the pseudocapsule may be composed of a compressed non-fatty rim of hepatic parenchyma on opposed-phase images. The amount of scar tissue and the size of the central scar within FNH may vary. The central scar is typically high in signal intensity on T2-weighted and low in signal intensity on T1-weighted images. Multiple lesions often have concurrent hemangiomas and cysts (Figs. 57.1, 57.2).

Pathology

Multiple FNHs are histologically identical to the solitary type. At histology, FNH is composed of small nodules of normal hepatocytes surrounded by a network of capillaries and septa. The hepatic plates may be moderately thickened (two or three cells in thickness). The central scar contains fibrous connective tissue, cholangiolar proliferation with the surrounding inflammatory infiltrates, and malformed tortuous arteries with thickened walls, capillaries, and veins (Fig. 57.3). FNHs contain Kupffer cells.

Literature

1. Finley A, Hosey J, Noone T, et al. (2005) Multiple focal nodular hyperplasia syndrome: diagnosis with dynamic, gadolinium-enhanced MRI. MRM 23:511–513
2. Hussain SM, Terkivatan T, Zondervan PE, et al. (2004) Focal nodular hyperplasia: a spectrum of findings at state-of-the-art MR imaging, ultrasound, CT and pathology. Radiographics 24:3–19
3. Hussain SM, Zondervan PE, Ijzermans JN, et al. (2002) Benign versus malignant hepatic nodules: MR imaging findings with pathologic correlation. Radiographics 22:1023–1036
4. Elsayes KM, Narra VR, Yin Y, et al. (2005) Focal hepatic lesions: diagnostic value of enhancement pattern approach with contrast-enhanced 3D gradient-echo MR imaging. Radiographics 25:1299–1320

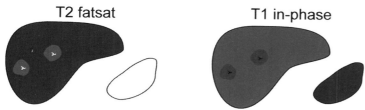 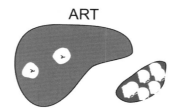 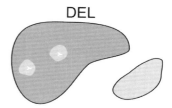

Fig. 57.1. FNH, multiple, fat containing in a fatty liver, schematic drawings. T2 fatsat: both FNHs are slightly hyperintense to the liver with brighter central scars; T1 in-phase: both FNHs are slightly hypointense to the liver;

ART: both FNHs show very intense homogeneous enhancement; DEL: both FNHs become almost isointense with enhancement of the central scars

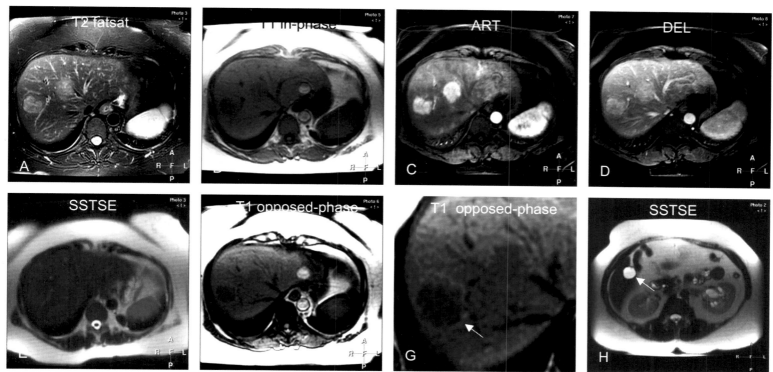

Fig. 57.2. FNH, multiple, fat containing in a fatty liver, MRI findings. A Axial fat-suppressed T2-w TSE image (T2 fatsat): both FNHs are slightly hyperintense to the liver with brighter central scars. **B** Axial in-phase image (T1 in-phase): FNHs are slightly hypointense to the liver. **C** Axial arterial phase image (ART): FNHs show very intense and homogeneous enhancement. **D** Axial delayed phase image (DEL): FNHs become almost isointense with enhancement of the central scars. **E** Axial SSTSE with an echo time (TE) of 120 ms (T2 longer than TE): both lesions are isointense to the liver. **F** Axial opposed-

phase image (T1 opposed-phase): FNHs as well as the liver decrease the signal compared to the in-phase image due to some fatty infiltration. Note the perilesional rim of high signal intensity (*arrow*) caused by compressed liver parenchyma (pseudocapsule). **G** A detailed view of the axial opposed-phase image (T1 opposed-phase) shows the pseudocapsule better (*arrow*). **H** Axial SSTSE image (SSTSE) at a lower anatomic level shows a coincidental cyst (*arrow*) that is very bright (fluid-like) compared to the liver

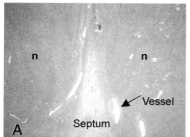 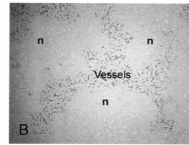 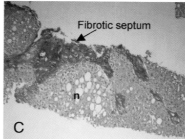 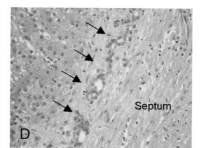

Fig. 57.3. FNH, MR pathology correlation. A Photomicrograph shows FNH nodules (*n*) separated by a septum and large vessels (*arrow*). H&E ×100. **B** Photomicrograph shows nodules (*n*) surrounded by an extensive network of vessels. CD34 stain, ×10. **C** Photomicrograph shows fibrotic septa around

nodules (*n*) with fatty infiltration. Elastica-von Giesen stain, ×4. **D** Photomicrograph shows bile duct proliferation (*arrows*) within a septum, a classic finding of FNH. H&E stain, ×200

58 Focal Nodular Hyperplasia V – Fatty FNH with Concurrent Fatty Adenoma

Focal nodular hyperplasia (FNH) is a common benign liver lesion and may concur with other benign or malignant liver lesions including hepatocellular adenoma (HCA). It is important to distinguish between FNH and HCA. HCA is considered a premalignant lesion which is associated with risk of life-threatening hemorrhage. In some patients, HCA may show an oral contraceptive (OC)-dependent change in diameter. FNH is a benign lesion which is not OC dependent. HCA does not need follow-up or treatment in the majority of cases.

MR Imaging Findings

At MR imaging, FNH and HCA share several *similarities:* (1) the lesions are nearly isointense on T1- and T2-weighted images; and (2) both entities show intense enhancement in the arterial phase and fade to near isointensity in the delayed phase. There are however a number of *differences:* (1) FNHs are more often isointense or hypointense whereas HCAs are more often hyperintense on the pre-contrast T1-weighted images; (2) FNHs show a central scar and septa in most cases whereas HCAs lack these; (3) FNHs may display evidence of fat on imaging in about 6 % of cases whereas HCAs contain fat in up to 78 % of cases; (4) FNHs show more intense enhancement with central scar and septal sparing whereas HCAs show less intense and more homogeneous enhancement; and (5) FNHs do not show any change in size or appearance after stopping the OC whereas OC-dependent HCAs become smaller after cessation of OC (Figs. 58.1 – 58.3).

Management

Because many of the differences are related to the intrinsic soft tissue contrast, MR imaging should be the modality of choice for detection, characterization, and follow-up of patients with concurrent FNH and HCA.

Literature

1. Edmondson HA, Henderson B, Benton B (1976) Liver-cell adenomas associated with use of oral contraceptives. N Engl J Med 294:470 – 472
2. Gordon SC, Reddy KR, Livingstone AS, et al. (1986) Resolution of a contraceptive-steroid-induced hepatic adenoma with subsequent evolution into hepatocellular carcinoma. Ann Intern Med 105:547 – 549
3. Terkivatan T, Van den Bos IC, Hussain SM, et al. (2006) Focal nodular hyperplasia: lesion characteristics on state-of-the-art MRI including dynamic gadolinium-enhanced and superparamagnetic iron-oxide-uptake sequences in a prospective study. JMRI 24:864 – 872
4. Hussain SM, Van den Bos IC, Dwarkasing S, et al. (2006) Hepatocellular adenoma: findings at state-of-the-art magnetic resonance imaging, ultrasound, computed tomography and pathologic analysis. Eur Radiol 16: 1873 – 1886

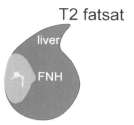 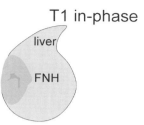 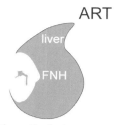 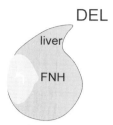

Fig. 58.1. FNH, drawings. T2 fatsat: FNH is hyperintense to the liver with a brighter central scar; **T1 in-phase**: FNH is hypointense to the liver with a darker central scar; **ART**: FNH shows a very intense homogeneous enhance-

ment of the entire lesion, except the central scar; **DEL**: FNH becomes almost isointense with enhanced central scar

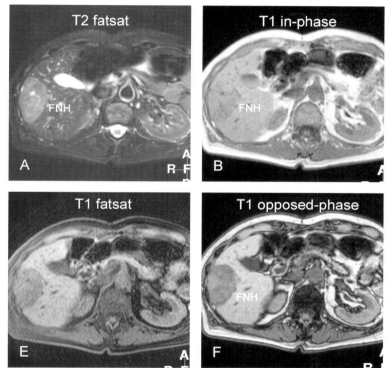 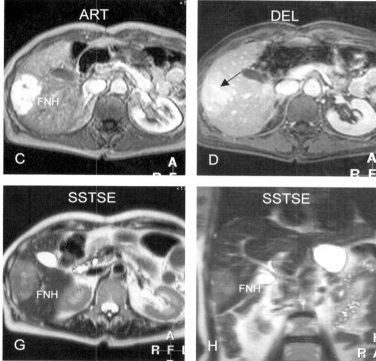

Fig. 58.2. FNH, typical MRI findings. A Axial fat-suppressed TSE image (T2 fatsat): FNH is hyperintense to the liver with a brighter central scar. **B** Axial in-phase image (T1 in-phase): FNH is slightly hypointense to the liver with a darker central scar. **C** Axial arterial phase image (ART): FNH shows very intense and homogeneous enhancement, except the central scar. **D** Axial delayed phase image (DEL): FNH becomes almost isointense with enhancement of the central scar (*arrow*). **E** Axial fat-suppressed T1-w GRE image

(T1 fatsat) FNH is markedly hypointense, most likely due to fat suppression pulse. **F** Axial opposed-phase image (T1 opposed-phase) shows decreased signal within FNH indicating moderate to strong fatty infiltration. **G** Axial SSTSE image (SSTSE): FNH is hyperintense. **H** Coronal SSTSE image (SSTSE): FNH is slightly hyperintense to the liver. (This MR imaging examination was performed in 2005 as a follow-up in a patient known with FNH and HCA)

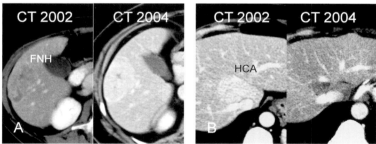 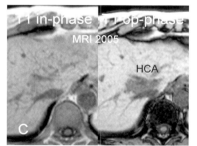 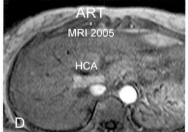

Fig. 58.3. FNH, follow-up in the same patient known with FNH and HCA, CT and MRI findings. A CTs in 2002 and 2004 show unchanged FNH. **B** CTs in 2002 and 2004 show decrease in size of HCA after stopping oral contraceptives.

C Axial in- and opposed-phase images (T1 in-phase and T1 op-phase) shows HCA with fatty infiltration. **D** Axial arterial phase image (ART): HCA shows less intense enhancement than FNH

59 Focal Nodular Hyperplasia VI – Atypical with T2 Dark Central Scar

Focal nodular hyperplasia (FNH) may show more than one atypical feature at MR imaging and cause difficulty in diagnosis. Such lesions may mimic other primary liver lesions including hepatocellular carcinoma (HCC) in a non-cirrhotic liver. In Europe and North America, a large percentage (up to 40%) of HCCs may occur in non-cirrhotic livers and form a differential diagnostic problem with atypical benign primary liver lesions including atypical FNH. HCC in non-cirrhotic liver often presents as a solitary large lesion with a central scar with variable signal intensity on T2-weighted images. Knowledge of the appearance of atypical FNH may help to avoid unnecessary anxiety, follow-ups with US and CT, and surgery for the patient.

MR Imaging Findings

At MR imaging, atypical FNH may have exceptionally high signal intensity on T2-weighted images with suggestion of lamella, a central scar with low signal intensity on T2-weighted images, a prominent pseudocapsule, and incomplete intense enhancement of the lesion (Figs. 59.1, 59.2). In such cases, the application of the specific type of contrast media may confirm the hepatocellular origin of the lesion. With an homogeneous uptake of such agents in combination with a normal alpha-fetoprotein and viral serology, the patients may be followed with MR imaging safely. If any doubt remains, US-guided biopsy should be carried out of the lesion as well as the surrounding liver to exclude malignancy and cirrhosis.

Management

HCC in non-cirrhotic liver and fibrolamellar carcinoma should be excluded in atypical FNH by means of follow-up with MR imaging and US-guided biopsy. HCC in non-cirrhotic livers may show a T2-dark central scar, but signal intensity on T1- and T2-weighted images, as well as the enhancement pattern, is quite different from atypical FNH, which may rarely resemble the MR imaging appearance of an orange (Fig. 59.3). Surgery is justified in patients with inconclusive imaging findings or biopsy.

Literature

1. Terkivatan T, Van den Bos IC, Hussain SM, et al. (2006) Focal nodular hyperplasia: lesion characteristics on state-of-the-art MRI including dynamic gadolinium-enhanced and superparamagnetic iron-oxide-uptake sequences in a prospective study. JMRI 24:864–872
2. Hussain SM, Zondervan PE, et al. (2002) Benign versus malignant hepatic nodules: MR imaging findings with pathologic correlation. Radiographics 22:1023–36
3. Hussain SM, Semelka RC, Mitchell DG (2002) MR imaging of hepatocellular carcinoma. Magn Reson Imaging Clin N Am 10:31–52

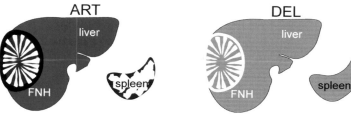

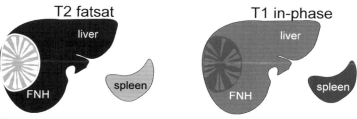

Fig. 59.1. FNH, very bright on T2 and with a dark central scar, drawings. T2 fatsat: FNH is very bright to the liver with a spoke-wheel configuration; note also the bright pseudocapsule and a dark central scar; **T1 in-phase:** FNH is pre-dominantly isointense to the liver; **ART:** FNH shows in part intense enhancement; **DEL:** FNH shows almost homogeneous enhancement, including the central scar and the pseudocapsule

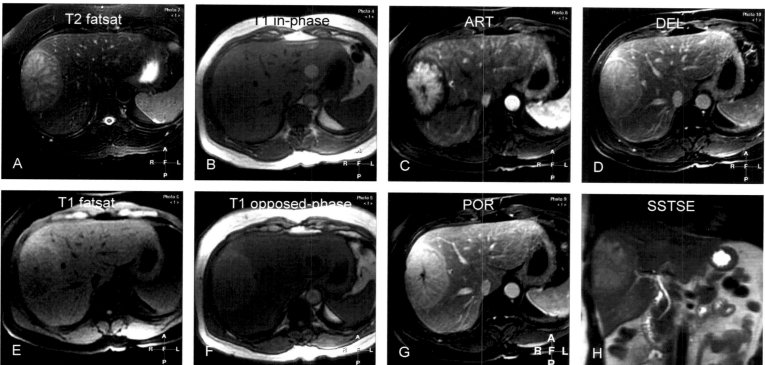

Fig. 59.2. FNH, very bright on T2 with a dark central scar, MRI findings. A Axial TSE image (T2 fatsat): FNH is very bright to the liver with a spoke-wheel configuration; note also the bright pseudocapsule and a dark central scar. **B** Axial in-phase image (T1 in-phase): FNH is predominantly isointense to the liver. **C** Axial arterial phase image (ART): FNH shows intense enhancement in the spoke-wheel part. **D** Axial delayed phase image (DEL): FNH shows almost homogeneous enhancement, including the central scar and the pseudocapsule. **E** Axial fat-suppressed GRE image (T1 fatsat): FNH is

slightly hypointense to the liver. **F** Axial opposed-phase image (T1 opposed-phase) shows diffuse fatty infiltration in the liver; therefore FNH appears relatively brighter. **G** Axial portal phase image (POR): The central scar is not fully enhanced yet and is still visible. **H** Coronal SSTSE image (SSTSE) shows the FNH within a normal liver with smooth contours and normal bile ducts. During a 2-year follow-up, FNH remained completely unchanged and showed uptake of SPIO on one of the MRI examinations

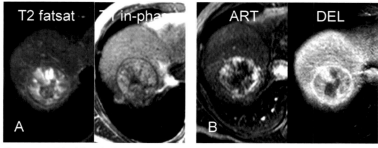

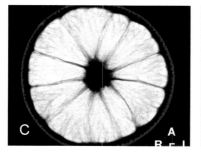

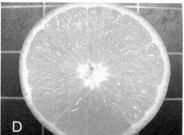

Fig. 59.3. HCC with a dark central scar (another patient), MRI findings, and MR-orange correlation. A Axial TSE image (T2 fatsat): HCC is heterogeneous and shows a dark central scar; T1 in-phase image shows HCC surrounded by dark tumor capsule. **B** Axial arterial (ART) and delayed (DEL) phase images

show heterogeneous enhancement with washout and capsular enhancement. **C** and **D** show a T2-weighted MR image and the cross section of an orange with striking similarity to the FNH shown above

60 Hepatic Angiomyolipoma – MR-CT Comparison

Angiomyolipoma (AML) is a benign, unencapsulated mesenchymal tumor that is composed of varying proportions of three elements: smooth muscle cells, thick-walled blood vessels, and mature adipose tissue. Renal AMLs are associated with tuberous sclerosis in 20% of patients, whereas hepatic AMLs are associated with tuberous sclerosis in only 6%. Hepatic AMLs may mimic other primary hypervascular, fat-containing hepatic lesions including hepatocellular adenomas (may contain fat in up to 78%) and hepatocellular carcinomas (may contain fat in up to 10%). However, hepatic AMLs often occur in conjunction with renal AMLs. Chemical shift MR imaging was recently shown to have high sensitivity and specificity (96% and 93%, respectively) for renal AMLs with minimal fat. Therefore, MR imaging should also be applied in patients who are known to have renal AMLs and present with hepatic lesions.

MR Imaging Findings

At MR imaging, multiple lesions may be present with somewhat variable but predominantly high signal intensity on T2-weighted sequences. In addition, on fat-suppressed T2-weighted images the lesions contain areas with low signal intensity likely due to muscle and fat components. Chemical shift (in- and opposed-phase) imaging however provides specific information by showing a small amount of fat in the lesions which lowers the signal intensity on the opposed-phase imaging. The lesions show intense heterogeneous enhancement in the arterial phase. The enhancement may be somewhat decreased but grossly persists in the delayed phase (Figs. 60.1, 60.2). The findings on CT are often non-specific mainly because CT is insensitive to the small amount of fat with hepatic AMLs (Fig. 60.3).

Differential Diagnosis

Fatty hepatocellular adenomas (HCAs) and carcinomas (HCCs) differ considerably in tumor morphology and enhancement from hepatic AMLs. HCAs are near isointense on T1- and T2-weighted images, and show homogeneous enhancement, fading to isointensity in the delayed phase. Small multiple fat-containing HCCs typically occur in cirrhotic livers, have a mosaic pattern on T1- and T2-weighted images, and show washout with capsular enhancement in the delayed phase. Liposarcoma and teratoma are very rare fat-containing hepatic tumors.

Literature

1. Worawattanakul S, Semelka RC, Kelekis NL, et al. (1996) Hepatic angiomyolipoma with minimal fat content: MR demonstration. MRM 14: 687–689
2. Ahmadi T, Itai Y, Takahashi M, et al. (1998) Angiomyolipoma of the liver: significance of CT and MR dynamic study. Abdom Imaging 23:520–526
3. Balci NC, Akinci A, Akun E, et al. (2002) Hepatic angiomyolipoma: demonstration by out of phase MRI. Clin Imaging 26:418–420
4. Kim JK, Kim SH, Jang YJ, et al. (2006) Renal angiomyolipoma with minimal fat: differentiation from other neoplasms at double-echo chemical shift FLASH MR imaging. Radiology 239:174–180

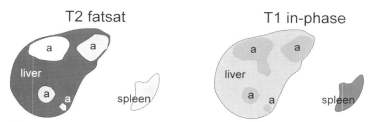
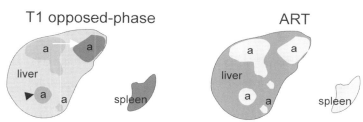

Fig. 60.1. Hepatic angiomyolipoma (*a*), drawings. T2 fatsat: multiple angiomyolipomas show predominantly hyperintense signal to the liver; **T1 in-phase:** lesions show predominantly hypointense signal to the liver; **T1 opposed-** phase: one lesion shows marked (*solid arrow*) and another mild (*arrowhead*) signal loss due to variable fatty content; **ART:** angiomyolipomas show intense heterogeneous enhancement

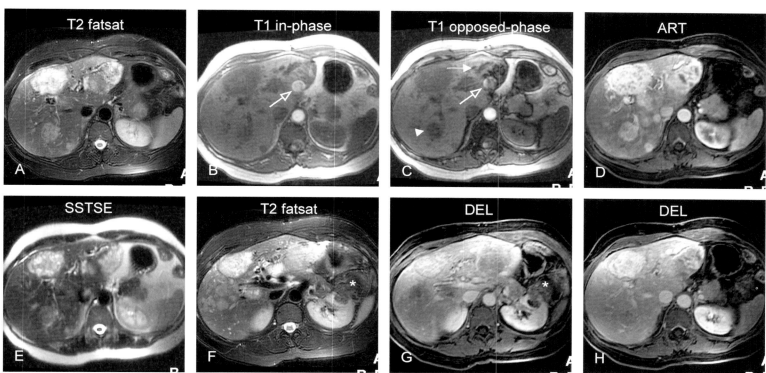

Fig. 60.2. Hepatic angiomyolipoma, MRI findings. A Axial TSE image (T2 fatsat): multiple angiomyolipomas show predominantly hyperintense signal to the liver. **B** Axial in-phase image (T1 in-phase): lesions show predominantly hypointense signal to the liver. Aortic pulsation artifact (*open arrow*). **C** Axial opposed-phase image (T1 opposed-phase): One lesion shows marked (*solid arrow*) and another mild (*arrowhead*) signal loss due to variable fatty content. Aortic pulsation artifact (*open arrow*). **D** Axial arterial phase image (ART): angiomyolipomas show intense heterogeneous enhancement. **E** Axi- al SSTSE image (SSTSE) image: multiple angiomyolipomas show predominantly hyperintense signal to the liver. **F** Axial TSE image (T2 fatsat) image at a different level: Note a large fat-containing renal angiomyolipoma (*). **G** Axial delayed phase image (DEL): hepatic and renal (*) angiomyolipomas show similar enhancement. **H** Axial delayed phase image (DEL) image at a different level: hepatic angiomyolipomas show similar enhancement in parts of the tumors

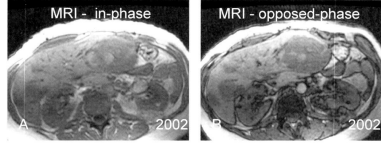
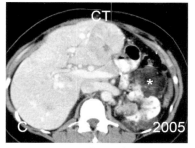
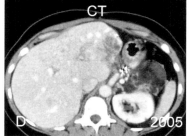

Fig. 60.3. Hepatic angiomyolipoma, MRI findings (same examination as above) with follow-up CT. A, B Axial in- and opposed-phase images show multiple angiomyolipomas with more fatty content and signal loss in renal lesions.

C, D Contrast-enhanced CTs (3 years after MRI examination) at two different levels show the essentially unchanged size and appearance of the renal (*) and hepatic lesions

61 Hepatic Lipoma – MR-CT-US Comparison

Hepatic lipomas are extremely uncommon lesions. Histologically, these lesions consist of mature adipose tissue, and usually, these tumors do not cause symptoms and present as an incidental finding at imaging. Lipomas have characteristic findings at CT and MR imaging. If lesions present with any atypical findings such as subtle heterogeneity or unusual enhancement, other entities such as liposarcomas, teratomas, hepatocellular adenomas, and hepatocellular carcinomas should be considered as differential diagnostic possibilities. Particularly, MR imaging can provide a highly specific diagnosis.

MR Imaging Findings

At MR imaging, hepatic lipomas should behave similarly to the subcutaneous fat. The lesions show very bright signal on non-fat-suppressed T2-weighted single-shot spin-echo sequences and very dark signal on fat-suppressed T2-weighted fast spin-echo. On T1-weighted in-phase images the lesions appear very bright (similar to the subcutaneous fat) and on opposed-phase images the lesions are surrounded by the characteristic phase cancellation (India-ink) artifact. Hepatic lipomas show negligible enhancement after administration of gadolinium (Figs. 61.1, 61.2). MR imaging findings are pathognomonic for hepatic lipomas. The findings on CT are also very characteristic, whereas US shows a hyperechoic non-specific appearance (Fig. 61.3).

Literature

1. Langsteger W, Lind P, Schneider GH, et al. (1990) Lipoma of the liver: Computed tomographic, ultrasonographic and cytologic findings. Scand J Gastroenterol 25:302–306
2. Sonsuz A, Ozdemis S, Akdogan M, et al. (1994) Lipoma of the liver. Gastroenterology 32:348–350
3. Hirasaki S, Koide N, Ogawa H, et al. (1999) Tuberous sclerosis associated with multiple hepatic lipomatous tumors and hemorrhagic renal angiomyolipoma. Intern Med 38:345–348
4. Prasad SR, Wang H, Rosas H, et al. (2005) Fat-containing lesions of the liver: radiologic-pathologic correlation. Radiographics 25:321–331
5. Henkelman RM, Hardy PA, Bishop JE, et al. (1992) Why fat is bright in RARE and fast spin-echo imaging. JMRI 2:533–540

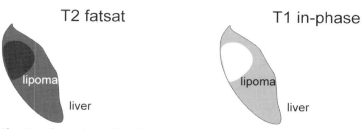
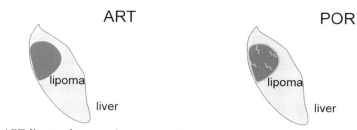

Fig. 61.1. Lipoma in the liver, drawings. T2 fatsat: lipoma is much darker than the liver due to fat suppression (lipoma behaves like the subcutaneous fat); **T1 in-phase:** lipoma is as bright as the intra-abdominal and subcutaneous fat; **ART:** lipoma does not show much enhancement and appears dark due to fat suppression; **POR:** lipoma shows faint enhancement of intratumoral septa. (Courtesy of Dr. Franz Sulzer)

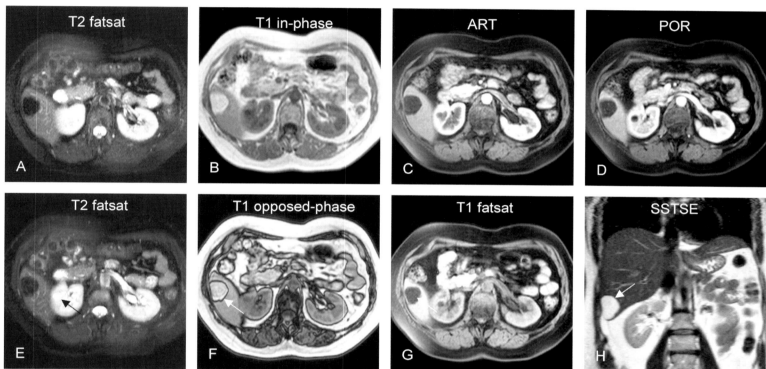

Fig. 61.2. Lipoma in the liver, MRI findings. A Axial TSE image (T2 fatsat): lipoma is much darker than the liver due to fat suppression. **B** Axial in-phase image (T1 in-phase): lipoma is very bright and comparable to the intra-abdominal and subcutaneous fat. **C** Axial arterial phase image (ART): lipoma does not show much enhancement and appears dark due to fat suppression. **D** Axial portal phase image (POR): lipoma shows faint enhancement. **E** Axial TSE image (T2 fatsat) at a different anatomic level: lipoma appears dark; a simple cyst in the right kidney is bright signal (*arrow*). **F** Axial opposed-phase image (T1 opposed-phase): lipoma is surrounded by a dark line (*arrow*) caused by the phase cancellation (artifact), which can only be present at the interfaces between fatty and non-fatty tissues. **G** Axial T1-w fat-suppressed GRE image (T1 fatsat): the signal in lipoma is suppressed due to fatty content. **H** Coronal SSTSE image (SSTSE): on this heavily T2-weighted sequence lipoma shows similarity with non-solid lesions such as cysts and hemangiomas. (Courtesy of Dr. Franz Sulzer)

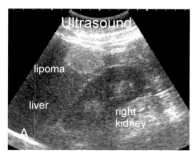
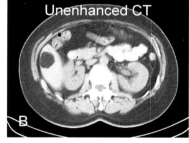
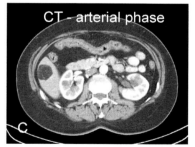
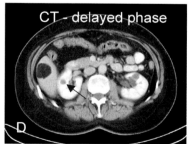

Fig. 61.3. Lipoma in the liver, US and CT findings in the same patient as above. A Ultrasound shows a hyperechoic (non-specific) lesion. **B** Unenhanced CT shows lipoma as dark as the subcutaneous fat (with comparable negative Hounsfield units). **C** CT in the arterial phase shows negligible enhancement. **D** CT in the delayed phase shows a similar appearance to in the arterial phase; renal cyst shows no enhancement (*arrow*). (Courtesy of Dr. Franz Sulzer)

62 Hepatocellular Adenoma I – Typical with Pathologic Correlation

With the introduction of oral contraceptives (OC) during the late 1960s, a sudden increase in the number of hepatocellular adenomas (HCAs) was observed. Later (in 1979), others confirmed the positive relationship between the OC use and HCA. HCAs develop at an annual rate of about 0.1 – 0.13 per 100,000 without OC use, whereas the long-term users of OC have an estimated annual incidence of HCA of 3.4 per 100,000. The incidence of HCA with OC is reported to be more than 25-fold higher than without OC use. Non-OC-related causes of HCA include glycogen storage diseases, and hormonal stimulation from other sources, for instance anabolic steroid use by body builders, gynecological tumors, and pregnancy. HCA is reported rarely in males, probably from using anabolic steroids or based on abnormal stimulus from an endogenous source.

MR Imaging Findings

At MR imaging, typical HCAs often have the following characteristics: (1) near isointense or slightly hyperintense to the surrounding liver on T1-weighted in-phase gradient-echo images (indicating the hepatocellular nature of the lesions), (2) slightly hyperintense or hypointense on fat-suppressed T2-weighted images (depending mainly on whether HCA is surrounded by fatty liver or the lesion itself contains abundant fat or fibrosis, respectively), (3) faint homogeneous enhancement (blush) in the arterial phase, and (4) fading to isointensity in the delayed phase without any washout of contrast or enhanced tumor capsule, central scar, or septa (Figs. 62.1, 62.2).

Pathology

At gross pathology, HCAs are unencapsulated well-delineated yellow or tan lesions. The consistency is soft or friable, and areas of necrosis and hemorrhage may be present. Tumors are highly vascular. Areas of scarring indicate previous episodes of infarction. At histology, HCA solely consists of liver cells that are arranged in plates that are not thicker than two to three cells, devoid of lobular pattern due to absence of portal areas. The plates are separated by slit-like sinusoids lined by epithelium. HCAs lack portal circulation. Lack of bile ductules facilitates distinction from FNH at histology (Fig. 62.3). Kupffer cells are always present in HCA.

Literature

1. Baum JK, Holtz F, Bookstein JJ, et al. (1973) Possible association between benign hepatoma and oral contraceptives. Lancet 2:926–929
2. Edmondson HA, Henderson B, Benton B (1976) Liver-cell adenomas associated with use of oral contraceptives. NEJM 294:470–472
3. Hussain SM, Van den Bos IC, Dwarkasing S, et al. (2006) Hepatocellular adenoma: findings at state-of-the-art magnetic resonance imaging, ultrasound, computed tomography and pathologic analysis. Eur Radiol 16: 1873–1886

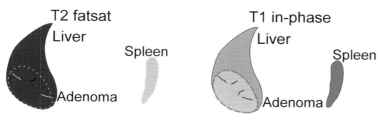 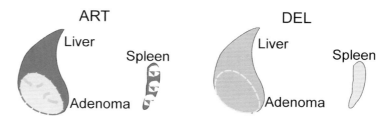

Fig. 62.1. Adenoma, drawings. T2 fatsat: adenoma is isointense with a thin bright pseudocapsule; **T1 in-phase**: adenoma is slightly hyperintense to the liver; ART: adenoma shows a moderately intense homogeneous enhance-ment of the entire lesion; **DEL**: adenoma becomes isointense to the liver with enhancement of the pseudocapsule (compressed liver tissue and vessels)

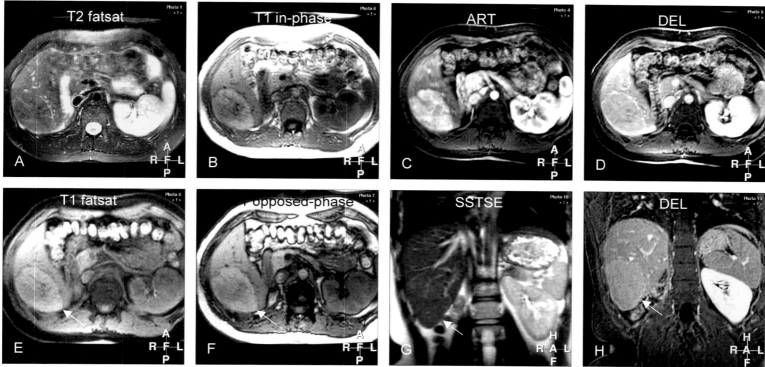

Fig. 62.2. Adenoma, typical MRI findings. A Axial fat-suppressed T2-w TSE image (T2 fatsat): Adenoma is isointense to the liver and surrounded by a bright pseudocapsule. **B** Axial in-phase T1-w GRE (T1 in-phase): Adenoma is slightly hyperintense to the liver. **C** Axial arterial phase post-Gd 3D T1-w GRE image (ART): Adenoma shows moderately intense and homogeneous enhancement. **D** Axial delayed post-Gd T1-w GRE image (DEL): Adenoma becomes isointense with some enhancement of the pseudocapsule. **E** Axial 2D fat-suppressed T1-w GRE image (T1 fatsat): Adenoma is slightly hyperintense with low signal pseudocapsule (*arrow*). **F** Axial opposed-phase 2D T1-w GRE image (T1 opposed-phase): Adenoma shows no evidence of fatty infiltration (*arrow*). **G** Coronal T2-w SSFSE image (T2 coronal): Adenoma is slightly brighter than the liver (*arrow*). **H** Coronal delayed phase post-Gd T1-w GRE image (DEL coronal): Adenoma has become isointense with the liver without any central scar (*arrow*)

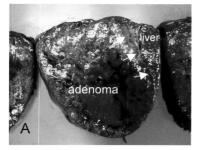 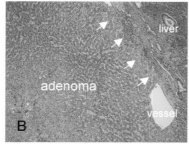 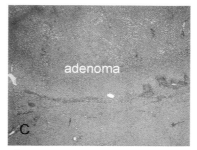 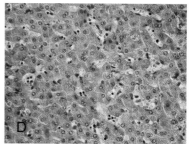

Fig. 62.3. Adenoma, direct MR-pathology correlation. A Photograph of the re-sected specimen: adenoma is very similar to the liver, with sharp demarca-tion and without any tumor capsule (*arrows*). **B** Photomicrograph shows al-most normal hepatocytes arranged in plates with large vessels. The inter-face shows with compressed liver parenchyma (*arrows*). H&E, × 200. **C** Pho-tomicrograph shows adenoma that is surrounded by the compressed liver tissue. H&E, × 100. **D** Photomicrograph shows almost normal hepatocytes arranged in plates that are up to two cell layers thick. H&E, × 400

63 Hepatocellular Adenoma II – Large Exophytic with Pathologic Correlation

Hepatocellular adenoma (HCA) contains fat in up to 78 % of cases. The size may vary between a few millimeters and several centimeters. Occasionally, the lesions may be exophytic and contain large vessels.

MR Imaging Findings

At MR imaging, fat-containing HCAs are bright on T1-weighted in-phase images and decrease their signal intensity on T1-weighted opposed-phase images due to the presence of a small amount of fat. Some areas within fatty HCAs may appear dark on fat-suppressed T2-weighted images as well as on three-dimensional gadolinium-enhanced gradient-echo images in the delayed phase because the amount of fat may be sufficient to be affected by the fat-suppression pulse. On the delayed images, this finding may mimic washout (Figs. 63.1, 63.2). At gross pathology, fat-containing HCAs have yellowish areas. At histology, the lesions resemble liver tissue and are often surrounded by a pseudocapsule which consists of compressed liver parenchyma (Fig. 63.3).

Management

The management of HCAs should be individualized based on their size and mode of presentation. The initial step should be to stop any oral contraceptive use. Patients should be informed about the increased risk of hemorrhage, the potential risk of malignant transformation, and the increased risk of rupture particularly during pregnancy. Patients with lesions smaller than 5 cm and normal alpha-fetoprotein can be safely observed and followed by MR imaging. HCAs >5 cm should be considered for surgical or other types of treatment due to the risk of malignancy. Surgery is controversial, particularly in patients with multiple lesions and lesions located at difficult anatomic locations. In patients with multiple adenomas or liver adenomatosis, surgical resection or other local treatment may be technically impossible. Interval growth and/or elevated serum alpha-fetoprotein levels in patients with a known hepatocellular adenoma suggest malignant transformation. HCAs with hemorrhage may be treated with hepatic arterial embolization to control the hemorrhage.

Literature

1. Baum JK, Holtz F, Bookstein JJ, et al. (1973) Possible association between benign hepatoma and oral contraceptives. Lancet 2:926–929
2. Terkivatan T, de Wilt JH, de Man RA, et al. (2001) Indications and long-term outcome of treatment for benign hepatic tumors: a critical appraisal. Arch Surg 136:1033–1038
3. Hussain SM, Van den Bos IC, Dwarkasing S, et al. (2006) Hepatocellular adenoma: findings at state-of-the-art magnetic resonance imaging, ultrasound, computed tomography and pathologic analysis. Eur Radiol 16:1873–1886

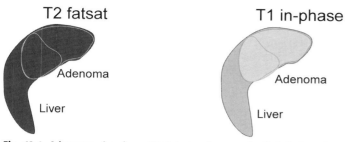

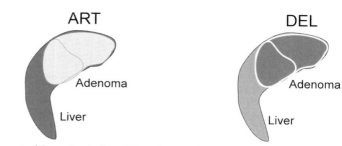

Fig. 63.1. Adenoma, drawings. T2 fatsat: adenoma is slightly hypointense to the liver; **T1 in-phase**: adenoma is almost isointense to slightly hyperintense to the liver; **ART**: adenoma shows a moderately intense homogeneous en-hancement of the entire lesion; **DEL**: adenoma becomes almost isointense to slightly hypointense

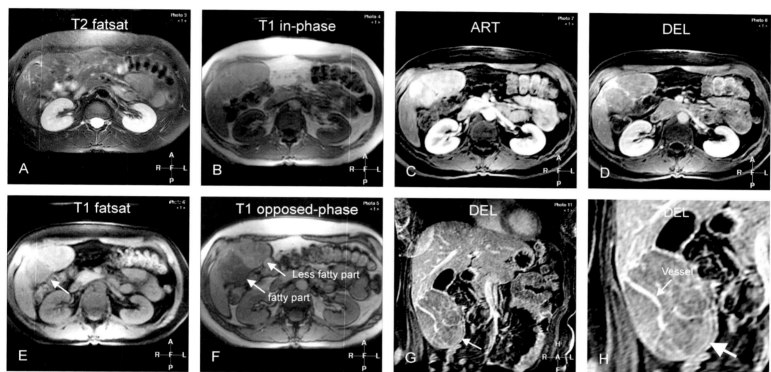

Fig. 63.2. Adenoma with fatty infiltration. A Axial fat-suppressed T2-w TSE image (T2 fatsat): adenoma is isointense to the liver. **B** Axial in-phase T1-w GRE (T1 in-phase): adenoma is slightly hyperintense to the liver. **C** Axial arterial phase post-Gd 3D T1-w GRE image (ART): adenoma shows moderately intense and homogeneous enhancement. **D** Axial delayed phase GRE image (DEL): adenoma becomes slightly hypointense to the liver, likely due to the fatty contents of the lesion. **E** Axial 2D T1-w GRE image (T1 fatsat): a part of the adenoma that is most fatty has a lower signal (*arrow*). **F** Axial op-posed-phase 2D T1-w GRE image (T1 opposed-phase): some parts of the lesion lose their signal more than other parts, indicating a variable amount of fatty infiltration (*arrows*). **G** Coronal delayed phase post-Gd 3D GRE image (DEL) with high spatial resolution clearly shows the adenoma as an exophytic lesion (*arrow*). **H** A detailed view of the previous image (DEL) shows the tumor anatomy better (*arrow*) with a large intratumoral vessel, most likely with accompanying fibrotic tissue

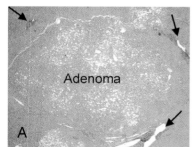

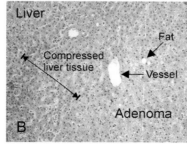

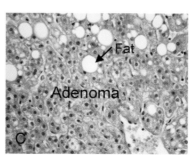

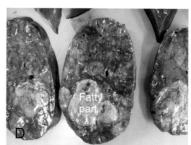

Fig. 63.3. MR-pathology correlation. A Photomicrograph shows a small fatty adenoma surrounded by large vessels (*arrows*). H&E, ×40. **B** Photomicrograph from the resected adenoma shown above: note normal appearing hepatocytes with fat, large vessels, and compressed parenchyma. H&E, ×200.

C Photomicrograph shows the findings in more detail. H&E, ×400. **D** Photo-graph of the gross specimen: large parts of the tumor contain fat and appear yellowish

64 Hepatocellular Adenoma III – Typical Fat-Containing

Fat-containing hepatocellular adenomas (HCAs) are among a variety of other fat-containing tumors of the liver with characteristic histologic features and variable imaging findings. Other common liver lesions that contain fat include focal fatty infiltration (steatosis), focal nodular hyperplasia (FNH), and hepatocellular carcinoma (HCC). Uncommon fat-containing liver lesions include angiomyolipoma, lipoma, liposarcoma, and teratoma. Identification of fat within a liver lesion can be critical in the characterization of the lesion. The imaging characteristics of a lesion such as enhancement pattern combined with the pattern of fatty content and the presence of Kupffer cells are helpful in narrowing the differential diagnosis. Computed tomography or ultrasound may indicate the presence of a within hepatic lesion, and MR imaging is the most specific imaging technique for demonstration of both microscopic and macroscopic fat based on the chemical shift imaging and fat suppressed sequences.

MR Imaging Findings

At MR imaging, minimally fat-containing HCAs are near isointense on the T1- and T2-weighted sequences, drop their signal on opposed-phase images, show homogeneous enhancement in the arterial phase, and fade to isointensity on the delayed phase images. HCAs show uptake of the superparamagnetic iron-oxide (SPIO) based contrast media and reveal the presence of a small amount of Kupffer cells. Such contrast media can be used to distinguish between primary and secondary liver lesions. Specific contrast media such as SPIO cannot replace dynamic gadolinium-enhanced imaging because the enhancement patterns play an essential role in the characterization of liver lesions at MR imaging (Figs. 64.1, 64.2). At histology, fat-containing liver lesions may show striking similarity (Fig. 64.3).

Differential Diagnosis

Focal fatty infiltration is often geographic, shows signal drop on the opposed phased imaging and does not show washout on the gadolinium-enhanced delayed phase images. FNH contains fat in approximately 6% and HCC in about 10% of cases and they have tumor morphology and enhancement patterns distinct from HCA at MR imaging.

Literature

1. Prasad SR, Wang H, Rosas H, et al. (2005) Fat-containing lesions of the liver: radiologic-pathologic correlation. Radiographics 25:321–331
2. Wang YX, Hussain SM, et al. (2001) Superparamagnetic iron oxide contrast media: physicochemical characteristics and applications in MR imaging. Eur Radiol 11:19–31
3. Hussain SM, Van den Bos IC, Dwarkasing S, et al. (2006) Hepatocellular adenoma: findings at state-of-the-art magnetic resonance imaging, ultrasound, computed tomography and pathologic analysis. Eur Radiol 16:1873–1886

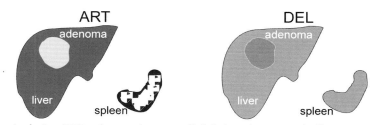

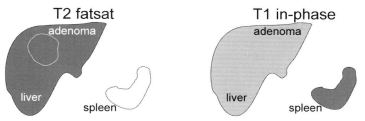

Fig. 64.1. Adenoma, fat containing, drawings. T2 fatsat: adenoma is isointense with a thin bright pseudocapsule; **T1 in-phase:** adenoma is isointense to the liver; **ART:** adenoma shows an intense homogeneous enhancement of the entire lesion; **DEL:** adenoma becomes slightly hypointense to the liver most likely due to fat suppression and not due to washout of contrast material. Note the enhancement of the pseudocapsule

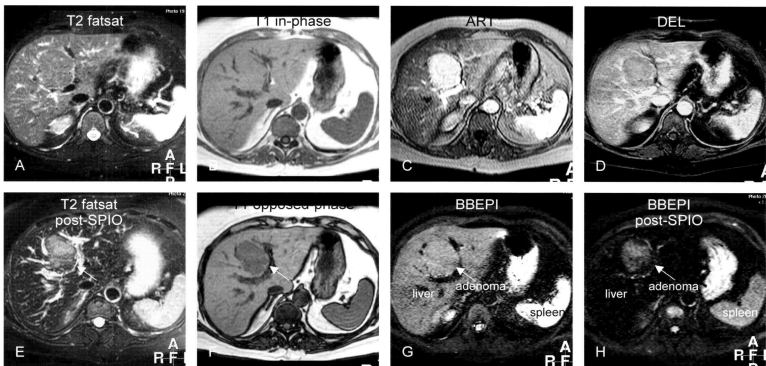

Fig. 64.2. Adenoma, typical, fat containing, MRI findings. A Axial fat-suppressed T2-w TSE image (T2 fatsat): Adenoma is isointense and only visible due to mass effect and a bright pseudocapsule. **B** Axial in-phase GRE (T1 in-phase): Adenoma is isointense to the liver. **C** Axial arterial phase GRE image (ART): Adenoma shows homogeneous enhancement. **D** Axial delayed GRE image (DEL): Adenoma becomes slightly hypointense due to fat suppression and not due to washout. Note the enhanced pseudocapsule. **E** Axial TSE image after SPIO (T2 fatsat post-SPIO): Adenoma shows drop in signal in the periphery of the lesion, indicating its hepatic origin (*arrow*). **F** Axial opposed-phase GRE image (T1 opposed-phase): Adenoma drops its signal due to homogeneous fatty infiltration (*arrow*). **G** Axial fat-suppressed T2-w black-blood echoplanar image (BBEPI): Adenoma is isointense to the liver (*arrow*). **H** Axial BBEPI after SPIO (BBEPI post-SPIO): Adenoma shows drop in signal particularly in the periphery of the lesion due to the presence of the Kupffer cells (*arrow*)

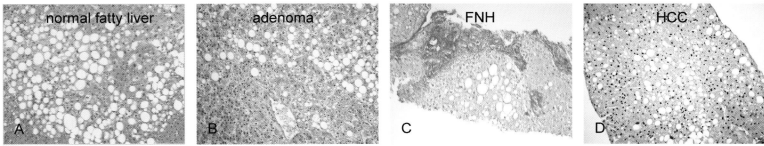

Fig. 64.3. Adenoma, and other fatty tissues and tumors, histology findings. A Photomicrograph of a focal fatty infiltration of the liver visible as a lesion at imaging. H&E, ×200. **B** Photomicrograph from a fatty adenoma (note the similarity with the previous image). H&E, ×200. **C** Photomicrograph of bi-opsy from a fatty focal nodular hyperplasia (FNH). H&E, ×100. **D** Photomicrograph of biopsy from a fatty hepatocellular carcinoma (HCC). H&E, ×200

65 Hepatocellular Adenoma IV – With Large Hemorrhage

Patients with hepatocellular adenomas (HCAs) can present with a number of symptoms, including pain (32–70%), hemorrhage (15–42%), an incidental finding at imaging (15–21%), or mass on physical or surgical examination (0–26%). Some women with HCA may present intrahepatic or intraperitoneal (life-threatening) hemorrhage around the menstrual period, which suggests a common hormonal influence on the vasculature of the endometrium and shredding of the endometrial tissue as well as vessels within the HCA and hemorrhage. With increasing use of the cross-sectional imaging modalities, including US, CT, and MR imaging, in the assessment of upper abdomen complaints, it is likely that HCA will be discovered as an incidental finding in more patients in the near future.

MR Imaging Findings

At MR imaging, hemorrhage has a characteristic appearance on T1-weighted images with predominantly high signal intensity due to the presence of methemoglobin. A thin rim of low signal intensity indicates the presence of hemosiderin. On T2-weighted images, recent hemorrhage has a high signal with low signal intensity areas centrally with lower signal intensity in the periphery mainly caused by the hemosiderin. The underlying HCA may be small and may remain latent until the resolution of most of the hematoma (Figs. 65.1, 65.2). At ultrasound, the appearance is non-specific; however, at CT the hematomas present with fluid collections with relatively high density (Fig. 65.3A, B).

Management

In the case of acute hemorrhage with an underlying HCA, usually patients are carefully observed and followed with imaging. Hepatic arterial embolization can be an alternative treatment. Digital subtraction angiography prior to embolization may reveal the underlying HCA with an arterial blush and tortuous abnormal tumor vessels (Fig. 65.3C, D). Embolization may be used to control the ongoing hemorrhage but the underlying HCA can recur after a successful treatment.

Literature

1. Rooks JB, Ory HW, Ishak KG, et al. (1979) Epidemiology of hepatocellular adenoma: the role of oral contraceptive use. JAMA 242:644–648
2. Terkivatan T, de Wilt JH, de Man RA, et al. (2001) Indications and long-term outcome of treatment for benign hepatic tumors: a critical appraisal. Arch Surg 136:1033–1038
3. Mathieu D, Bruneton JN, Drouillard J, et al. (1986) Hepatic adenomas and focal nodular hyperplasia: dynamic CT study. Radiology 160:53–58
4. Hussain SM, Van den Bos IC, Dwarkasing S, et al. (2006) Hepatocellular adenoma: findings at state-of-the-art magnetic resonance imaging, ultrasound, computed tomography and pathologic analysis. Eur Radiol 16:1873–1886

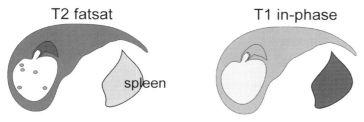
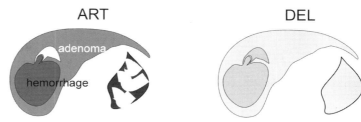

Fig. 65.1. Adenoma, drawings. T2 fatsat: adenoma is isointense with a thin bright pseudocapsule; T1 in-phase: adenoma is slightly hyperintense to the liver; ART: adenoma shows a moderately intense homogeneous enhance- ment of the entire lesion; DEL: adenoma becomes isointense to the liver with enhancement of the pseudocapsule (compressed liver tissue and vessels)

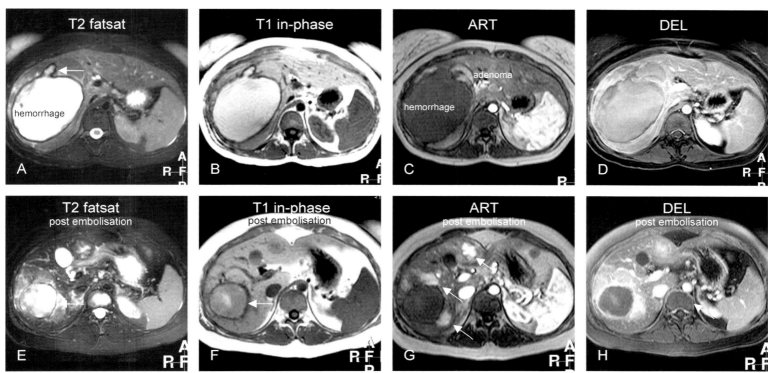

Fig. 65.2. Twenty-four-year-old female – ruptured adenoma, MRI findings before and after embolization. A Axial fat-suppressed T2-w TSE image (T2 fatsat): A large hematoma is predominantly bright with a dark rim of hemosiderin and a stalk-like structure indicating the origin of the hematoma (*arrow*). **B** Axial in-phase T1-w GRE (T1 in-phase): Hematoma is bright to the liver. **C** Axial arterial phase post-Gd T1-w GRE image (ART): Adenoma shows homogeneous enhancement around the stalk-like structure. **D** Axial delayed phase image (DEL): Adenoma becomes almost isointense to the liver. **E** Axial fat-suppressed T2-w image after embolization (T2 fatsat): Hematoma has decreased in size (*arrow*). **F** Axial in-phase image (T1 in-phase): Hematoma has lost most of its high signal (*arrow*). **G** Axial arterial phase image (ART): Multiple (residual or recurrent) adenomas become apparent with homogeneous enhancement (*arrows*). **H** Axial delayed phase image (DEL): Adenomas become almost isointense to the liver

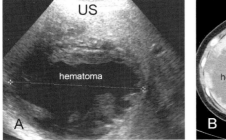
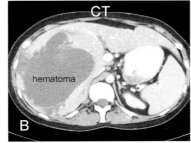
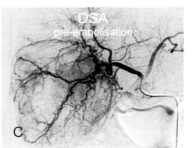
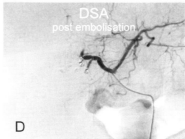

Fig. 65.3. Ruptured adenoma: US, CT, and DSA. A Ultrasound (US) shows a large hematoma. **B** Computed tomography (CT) shows the relatively dense hematoma. **C** Selective digital subtraction angiography (DSA) prior to embolization (4 months after the initial MRI) shows multiple areas with extensive arterial enhancement (blush) of adenoma with multiple abnormal tortuous tumor arteries surrounding the lesion. **D** DSA after completion of the embolization procedure shows no evidence of adenomas

66 Hepatocellular Adenoma V – Multiple in Fatty Liver (Non-OC-Dependent)

Multiple HCA's often occur in a fatty liver with altered shape and size. Multiple HCA's may also be found in non-fatty livers. Small lesions may mimic metastases with fatty liver. Multiple lesions may occur with type 1 glycogen storage disease and liver adenomatosis (usually > 10 HCA). At gross pathologic sectioning, HCA's are well demarcated yellow or tan lesions that are seldom encapsulated. The consistency is soft or friable, and areas of necrosis and hemorrhage are frequently present. All tumors are highly vascular.

MR Imaging Findings

At MR imaging, very small liver lesions within fatty or non-fatty liver can be characterized with much higher accuracy because of the high intrinsic soft tissue contrast based on the T2 characteristics and chemical shift imaging, and the ability to visualize enhancement patterns on the routine gadolinium-enhanced dynamic imaging. On follow-up after stopping oral contraceptives (OC), the lesions may remain unchanged. Large exophytic lesion may be characterized as hepatic lesions by identifying the feeding vessels (Figs. 66.1, 66.2). At US, HCA's within a fatty liver will appear hypoechoic due to the increased echogenecity of the bachground liver, and may mimic a wide variety of lesions, including liver metastases. At CT, multiple HCA's may appear hyperdense on the unenhanced as well as enhanced scans because of the low density of the fatty liver.

Pathology

Histologically, there is no difference among the adenomas arising as single lesions, multiple lesions (2-6 lesions), and liver adenomatosis (> 10 lesions) (Fig. 66.3). The difference between "multiple" and "adenomatosis" is arbitrary. Previously, some reports had suggested that liver adenomatosis occurred in a different population and the change in size of these adenomas did not depend on the OC use. Recent reports as well as our own experience contradict this. Therefore, it is likely that "hepatocellular adenomas" and "liver adenomatosis" are two manifestations of the same underlying disease.

Literature

1. International Working Party (1995) Terminology of nodular hepatocellular lesions. Hepatology 22:983–993
2. Anthony PP (2002) Tumours and tumour-like lesions of the liver and biliary tract: aetiology, epidemiology and pathology. In: MacSween RNM, Burt AD, Portmann BC, et al. (editors). Pathology of the liver. Fourth edition. Churchill Livingstone pp. 711–775
3. Flejou JF, Barge J, Menu Y, et al. (1985) Liver adenomatosis. An entity distinct from liver adenoma? Gastroenterology 89:1132–1138
4. Hussain SM, Van den Bos IC, Dwarkasing S, et al. (2006) Hepatocellular adenoma: findings at state-of-the-art magnetic resonance imaging, ultrasound, computed tomography and pathologic analysis. Eur Radiol 16: 1873–1886

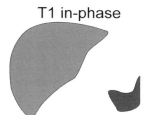
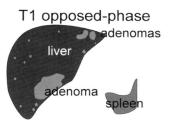
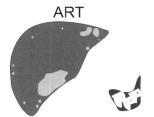
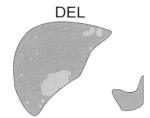

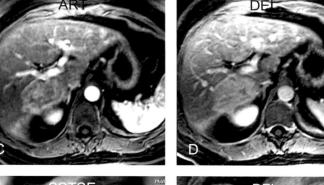
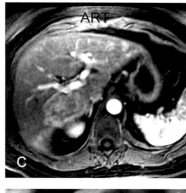
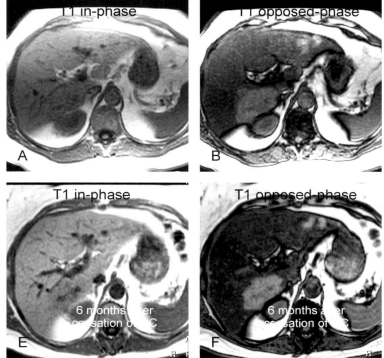
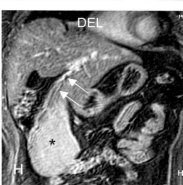

Fig. 66.1. Multiple adenomas, drawings. T1 in-phase: no lesions are visible. Adenomas are isointense to the liver; **T1 opposed-phase**: multiple larger as well as very small adenomas are present in the entire liver, which shows strong fatty infiltration; **ART**: adenomas show homogeneous enhancement; **DEL**: adenomas become almost isointense to the liver. Note that none of lesions shows tumor capsule

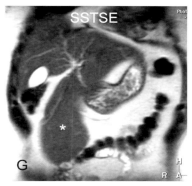
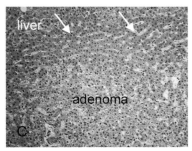
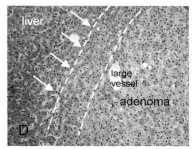

Fig. 66.2. Multiple adenomas, before and after OC: MRI findings. A Axial in-phase T1-w GRE (T1 in-phase): Adenomas are isointense to the liver. **B** Axial opposed-phase T1-w GRE (T1 opposed-phase): Multiple larger and smaller adenomas become visible due to strong signal drop in the fatty liver. **C** Axial arterial phase T1-w GRE image (ART): Adenomas show homogeneous enhancement. **D** Axial delayed phase GRE image (DEL): Adenomas become isointense to the liver. **E** Axial in-phase T1-w GRE (T1 in-phase): 6 months follow-up after stopping OC. No change is visible. **F** Axial opposed-phase T1-w GRE (T1 opposed-phase): 6 months follow-up after stopping OC. Adenomas remain unchanged in size, number, and signal intensity. **G** Coronal T2-w SSTSE (SSTSE): A large exophytic adenoma is visible originating from segment IVB of the liver (*). **H** Coronal delayed phase (DEL): Adenoma (*) clearly receives its vasculature from the liver (*arrows*)

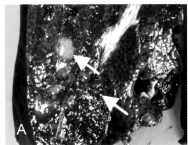
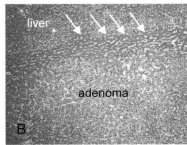

Fig. 66.3. Pathology and histology of multiple adenomas (from a different patient). A Photograph of a resected specimen shows multiple adenomas (*arrows*) within normal liver. **B** Photomicrograph shows the transition with compressed liver (between the lines indicated by *arrows*), surrounding the adenoma. H&E, ×100. **C** Photomicrograph shows an adenoma with mononuclear cells, surrounded by compressed liver (*arrows*). H&E, ×200. **D** Photomicrograph: The pseudocapsule is formed by compressed liver (*lines and arrows*). H&E, ×200

67 Hepatocellular Adenoma VI – Multiple in Fatty Liver (OC-Dependent)

The exact pathogenesis of HCA is not known. Based on a detailed pathologic analysis of various types of lesions that occur in patients with liver adenomatosis, a number of different types of lesions were observed in the same liver. Based on these observations, the following sequence of events was hypothesized: focus → group of foci → nodule → microadenoma → adenoma.

Malignant transformation of HCA into HCC has been described in the literature by several groups. Most authors have reported transformation of an existing HCA into HCC. At this point in time, it is not quite clear if all HCAs eventually can transform into HCCs. Also the exact characteristics of HCAs that eventually may undergo malignant transformation are not well known. Currently, most authors consider increase in size of the lesion at imaging, increased serum alpha-fetoprotein, and suspicious findings at fine-needle aspiration biopsy as signs of malignant transformation of HCA. According to some authors, some HCAs can undergo changes similar to liver cell dysplasia (LCD). In principle, HCA is not pre-malignant and may undergo reversible change after withdrawal of oral contraceptive (OC), whereas LCD is an irreversible, pre-malignant change and will eventually progress to HCC (HCA-LCD-HCC sequence). After stopping OC, HCAs may show a decrease in size.

MR Imaging Findings

At MR imaging, multiple HCA within a single liver may vary in signal intensity on T2-weighted images. The liver as well as the lesions may contain a variable amount of fat on opposed-phase images. Arterial phase is perhaps the most sensitive sequence to detect lesions. On the delayed phase images, the lesions should not show any washout or enhanced tumor capsule (Figs. 67.1, 67.2). MR imaging can display many faces of hepatocellular adenomas. (1) A non-fatty single lesion in a non-fatty liver: the lesion appears very similar to the surrounding liver. (2) Multiple HCAs within a fatty liver. (3) Fatty HCA and small HCAs associated with intra- and extrahepatic hematomas. (4) Hepatocellular carcinomas (HCC) may arise from HCAs or at the same anatomic location after regression of HCA. Note the confluent nodules of HCC contained within a thick fibrous tumor capsule (Fig. 67.3).

Literature

1. Gyorffy EJ, Bredfeldt JE, Black WC (1989) Transformation of hepatic cell adenoma to hepatocellular carcinoma due to oral contraceptive use. Ann Intern Med 110:489–490
2. Tao LC (1991) Oral contraceptive-associated liver cell adenoma and hepatocellular carcinoma: cytomorphology and mechanism of malignant transformation. Cancer 68:341–347
3. Ferrell LD (1993) Hepatocellular carcinoma arising in a focus of multilobular adenoma: a case report. Am J Surg Pathol 17:525–529
4. Foster JH, Berman MM (1994) The malignant transformation of liver cell adenomas. Arch Surg 129:712–717
5. Lepreux S, Laurent C, Blanc JF, et al. (2003) The identification of small nodules in liver adenomatosis. J Hepatol 39:77–85

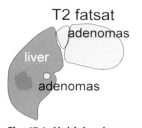
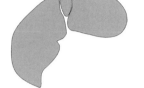
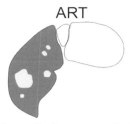
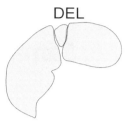

Fig. 67.1. Multiple adenomas, drawings. T2 fatsat: some adenomas are hyperintense, others isointense and at least one is slightly hypointense to the liver;

T1 in-phase: all adenomas are isointense; ART: multiple adenomas show homogeneous enhancement; DEL: all adenomas become isointense to the liver

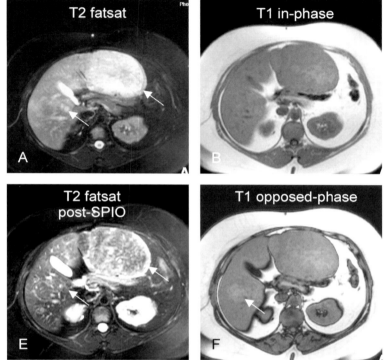
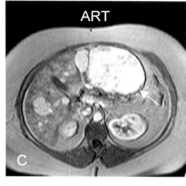
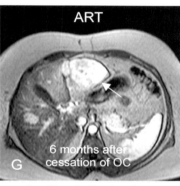
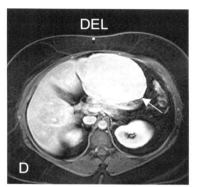
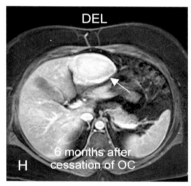

Fig. 67.2. Forty-three-year-old female – multiple adenomas, before and after OC: MRI findings. A Axial fat-suppressed TSE image (T2 fatsat): Multiple adenomas (*arrows*) are slightly hyperintense to the liver. **B** Axial in-phase T1-w GRE (T1 in-phase): Adenomas are isointense to the liver. **C** Axial arterial phase post-Gd T1-w GRE image (ART): Adenomas show homogeneous intense enhancement. **D** Axial delayed post-Gd T1-w GRE image (DEL): Adenomas become isointense without any central scar or capsular enhancement. **E** Axial fatsat T2-w TSE after SPIO (SPIOT2 fatsat): Adenomas show

uptake of iron indicating the presence of Kupffer cells and primary origin of the lesions (*arrow*). **F** Axial opposed-phase T1-w image (T1 opposed-phase): The liver shows some fatty infiltration rendering some of the lesions hyperintense (*arrow*). **G** Axial arterial phase post-Gd T1-w image 6 months after stopping OC (ART): Adenomas show significant decrease in size (*arrow*). **H** Axial delayed post-Gd T1-w GRE image (DEL): Adenomas remain homogeneous in delayed phase (*arrow*)

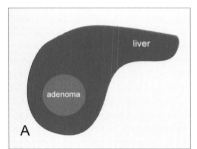
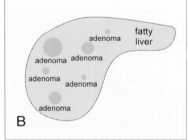
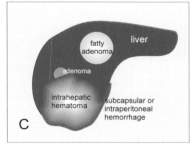
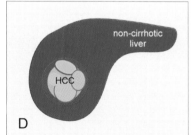

Fig. 67.3. The many faces of hepatocellular adenoma (HCA). A Single HCA that is very similar to the surrounding liver parenchyma, and hence difficult to recognize on imaging. **B** Multiple HCA (adenomatosis) in a fatty liver. **C** Fat-

ty HCA and HCA associated with intra- and extrahepatic hemorrhage. **D** Adenoma-like HCC may arise as a complication of HCA or long-term oral contraceptive use

68 HCC in Non-Cirrhotic Liver I – Small with MR-Pathologic Correlation

Hepatocellular carcinomas (HCCs) usually occur in patients with cirrhosis with an underlying viral hepatitis or alcohol abuse. HCC in cirrhosis typically shows a stepwise carcinogenesis (regenerative nodule-dysplastic nodule-HCC). In Europe and North America, HCC in non-cirrhotic livers may be present in up to 40 % of patients with HCC. HCC in non-cirrhotic livers is believed to occur according to de-novo carcinogenesis: a microscopic focus of HCC gradually develops into full-grown HCC. HCCs in non-cirrhotic livers are likely to be a solitary and relatively large dominant encapsulated mass with a central scar. However, mid-sized lesions do occur at imaging. It is important to recognize HCC in non-cirrhotic liver because these lesions are amenable to surgery even with a large size with good clinical outcome.

MR Imaging Findings

At MR imaging, HCCs in non-cirrhotic livers have often moderately high signal intensity on T2-weighted images and low signal intensity on T1-weighted images, and in this respect may resemble metastases. The lesions show heterogeneous enhancement in the arterial phase, and washout with capsular enhancement in the delayed phase (Figs. 68.1, 68.2).

Pathology

At gross pathology, midsized HCC in non-cirrhotic liver appears as a yellowish dominant nodule in a normal liver with smooth edges and normal color. At histology, the nodule may have great similarities to their cirrhotic counterparts and may contain subnodules with variable amounts of fat and a fibrous tumor capsule (Fig. 68.3).

Literature

1. Okuda K, Nakashima T, Sakamoto K, et al. (1982) Hepatocellular carcinoma arising in noncirrhotic and highly cirrhotic livers: a comparative study of histopathology and frequency of hepatitis B markers. Cancer 49:450–455
2. Nakayama M, Kamura T, Kimura M, et al. (1998) Quantitative MRI of hepatocellular carcinoma in cirrhotic and noncirrhotic livers. Clin Imaging 22:280–283
3. Winston CB, Schwartz LH, Fong Y, et al. (1999) Hepatocellular carcinoma: MR imaging findings in cirrhotic and noncirrhotic livers. Radiology 210:75–79
4. Hussain SM, Semelka RC, Mitchell DG (2002) MR imaging of hepatocellular carcinoma. Magn Reson Imaging Clin N Am 10:31–52

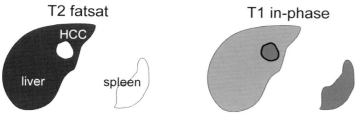
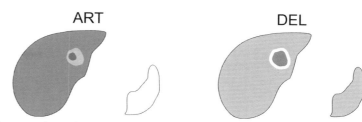

Fig. 68.1. HCC, non-cirrhotic liver, medium-sized, drawings. T2 fatsat: HCC is hyperintense compared to the liver; **T1 in-phase**: HCC is hypointense with a dark tumor capsule; **ART**: HCC is more enhanced in the peripheral than in the central part (mosaic pattern); **DEL**: HCC shows washout with enhancement of the tumor capsule

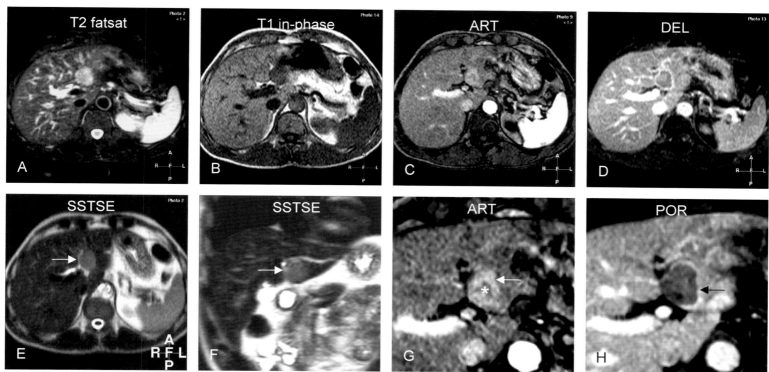

Fig. 68.2. HCC, non-cirrhotic, medium-sized, MRI findings. A Axial fat-suppressed T2-w TSE image (T2 fatsat): HCC is hyperintense compared to the liver. **B** Axial in-phase T1-w GRE (T1 in-phase): HCC is slightly hypointense compared to the liver with a darker tumor capsule. **C** Axial arterial phase post-Gd 2D T1-w GRE image (ART): HCC is more enhanced in the peripheral than in the central part. **D** Axial delayed phase 3D T1-w GRE image (DEL): HCC shows washout with enhancement of the tumor capsule. **E** Axial T2-w SSTSE image (SSTSE): HCC is slightly hyperintense compared to the liver (*arrow*). **F** Coronal SSTSE image (SSTSE): HCC becomes more hypointense due to its solid nature (*arrow*). **G** Axial arterial phase GRE image (ART): HCC is more enhanced in the peripheral (*arrow*) than in the central part (*). **H** Axial delayed phase GRE image (POR): HCC shows washout with enhancement of the tumor capsule (*arrow*)

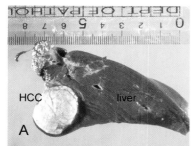
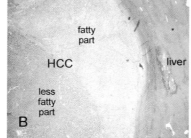
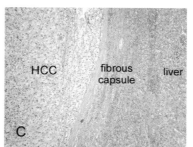
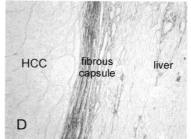

Fig. 68.3. HCC, non-cirrhotic liver, medium-sized, direct MR-pathology correlation. A Photograph of the resected specimen with the normal liver (non-cirrhotic liver) and an HCC. **B** Photomicrograph of the HCC shows two parts of the HCC with a thick capsule. H&E, ×40. **C** Photomicrograph shows HCC surrounded by a thick capsule. H&E, ×100. **D** Photomicrograph more clearly shows the stained fibrous tissue composing the thick tumor capsule. Sirius red stain, ×100

69 HCC in Non-Cirrhotic Liver II – Large with MR-Pathologic Correlation

Hepatocellular carcinomas (HCCs) in non-cirrhotic patients are more likely to be solitary than in patients with cirrhosis (72% vs. 27%). The lesions are significantly larger than in cirrhotic livers and are well-circumscribed masses in 57% of cases (median size: 8.8 cm). Central scar is more frequent in HCC in non-cirrhotic than in cirrhotic liver (50% vs. 6%). Smaller satellite nodules are present in only 6% of cases. Venous invasion is substantially more common in patients with cirrhosis (41%) than in patients without underlying liver disease (15%) and thus potentially promotes transhepatic hematogenous tumor spread. HCC originating in a non-cirrhotic liver is more likely to involve lymph nodes.

MR Imaging Findings

At MR imaging, HCC in non-cirrhotic liver will typically present as a large hyperintense lesion on T2-weighted images. Unencapsulated lesions are likely to show satellite nodules. On opposed-phase T1-weighted images, the lesions may be surrounded by a rim of compressed, non-fatty, liver parenchyma within a fatty liver. Due to neoangiogenic activity, the lesions contain large tumor vessels which can be seen on gadolinium-enhanced images in the arterial phase, particularly after postprocessing (Figs. 69.1, 69.2). MR imaging can provide an exact road-map for surgical resection. MR-pathologic correlation may provide evidence for the vasoinvasive growth which is most likely the basis for the satellite nodules (Fig. 69.3).

Management

For HCC in cirrhotic livers, the size of a lesion is an important variable for both treatment planning and patient outcome. Lesions larger than 5 cm in diameter have been shown to be associated with a poorer prognosis after hepatic resection. For HCC in non-cirrhotic livers this may not be true. In one study, 72% of patients with HCC in non-cirrhotic livers (median size > 8 cm) underwent partial resection. These patients may develop late recurrence, but aggressive surgery is nonetheless justified. Surgical procedures may consist of major hepatectomy (three segments or more). Operative mortality and morbidity were 2.9% and 19.0%, respectively. The 1-, 3-, 5-, and 10-year survivals and the survivals without recurrence were 74%, 52%, 40%, and 26% and 69%, 43%, 33%, and 19%, respectively.

Literature

1. Okuda K, Nakashima T, Sakamoto K, et al. (1982) Hepatocellular carcinoma arising in noncirrhotic and highly cirrhotic livers: a comparative study of histopathology and frequency of hepatitis B markers. Cancer 49:450–455
2. Winston CB, Schwartz LH, Fong Y, et al. (1999) Hepatocellular carcinoma: MR imaging findings in cirrhotic and noncirrhotic livers. Radiology 210:75–79
3. Bismuth H, Chiche L, Castaing D (1995) Surgical treatment of hepatocellular carcinoma in non-cirrhotic liver: experience in 68 liver resections. World J Surg 19:35–41
4. Smalley S, Moertel C, Hilton J, et al. (1988) Hepatoma in the noncirrhotic liver. Cancer 62:1414–1424

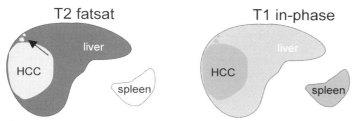
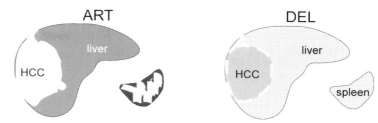

Fig. 69.1. HCC, non-cirrhotic, drawings. T2 fatsat: HCC is hyperintense to the liver; note the satellite nodule in the periphery of the tumor (*arrow*); **T1 in-phase:** HCC is hypointense to the liver; **ART:** HCC shows intense heteroge-

neous enhancement; **DEL:** HCC shows washout with enhancement of the discontinuous tumor capsule

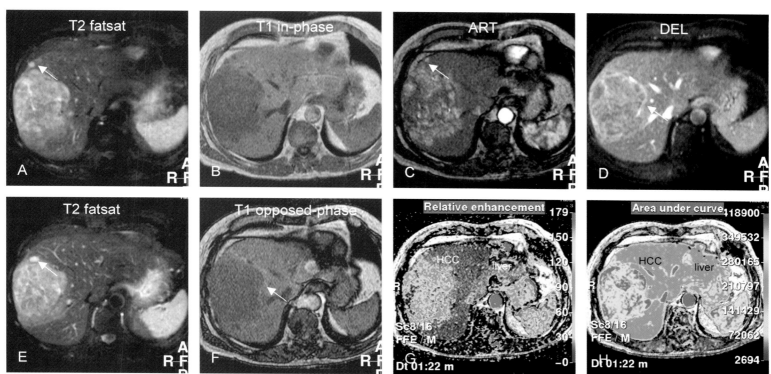

Fig. 69.2. HCC, non-cirrhotic, large, typical MRI findings. A Axial TSE image (T2 fatsat): HCC is hyperintense to the liver with similar satellite nodules (*arrow*). **B** Axial in-phase image (T1 in-phase): HCC is hypointense to the liver. **C** Axial arterial phase image (ART): HCC as well as the satellite nodules (*arrow*) show intense heterogeneous enhancement. **D** Axial delayed phase image (DEL): HCC shows washout with enhancement of the tumor capsule that partially surrounds the HCC (*arrow*). **E** Axial TSE image (T2 fatsat) at a

different anatomic level: note a satellite nodule at the level of the tumor capsule (*arrow*). **F** Axial opposed-phase image (T1 opposed-phase): Subtle fatty liver has decreased its signal with persistent high signal in the perilesional compressed liver parenchyma (*arrow*). **G** Pixelwise color-coded display of the relative enhancement shows the intratumoral arterial vessels. **H** Pixelwise color-coded display of the area-under-the-curve shows the total amount of contrast of the liver and the HCC, which is much larger

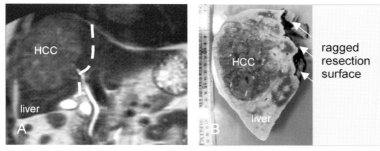
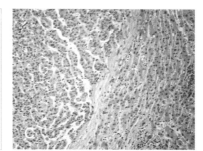
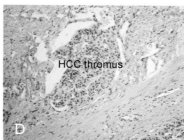

Fig. 69.3. HCC, non-cirrhotic, direct MR-pathology correlation. A Coronal SSTSE image shows the liver, HCC, and the resection surface (*white dashed line*). **B** Photograph of the right-sided hemihepatectomy specimen shows a large HCC that is – in part – surrounded by a tumor capsule. **C** Photomicrograph

shows two adjacent HCC nodules that are separated by a septum. H&E, ×100. **D** Photomicrograph shows an HCC thrombus within a large peritumoral vessel, which explains – in part – the presence of satellite nodules. H&E, ×100

70 HCC in Non-Cirrhotic Liver III – Large Lesion with Inconclusive CT

The fundamental limitation of CT is its lack of intrinsic soft tissue contrast and its moderate sensitivity to the presence of intravenous contrast. For detection and characterization, CT mainly relies on high in-plane spatial resolution and vascularity of liver lesions. Small liver lesions (<2 cm), which are now more often detected on current multidetector CT (MDCT) with thinner collimations, generally cannot be characterized with confidence at CT. Because of the high prevalence of benign liver lesions, the majority of these will be cysts, hemangiomas, biliary hamartomas, focal nodular hyperplasia or hepatocellular adenomas. However, there is no guarantee of this, and therefore it is incumbent on the imaging study to properly characterize these lesions. At CT, distinction between a small and a large benign liver lesion and a metastasis or HCC can be difficult. The major strength of multidetector CT is its ability to show the hepatic vascular (mainly arterial) anatomy. This, however, does not facilitate better characterization of focal or diffuse liver lesions as illustrated in the example below.

MR Imaging Findings

At MR imaging, various components of the focal liver lesions can be identified to make the correct diagnosis. MR imaging can identify the presence of (1) fat within the lesions on in- and opposed-phase imaging; (2) intratumoral nodules and tumor vessels on the gadolinium-enhanced imaging in the arterial phase; and (3) tumor capsule on the T1-weighted images as well as on the delayed phase images. In addition, (4) the liver shows no sign of cirrhosis, which includes irregular contours, atrophy of certain segments and hypertrophy of others, and intrahepatic nodules. Based on these findings, an HCC in a non-cirrhotic liver can be diagnosed confidently (Figs. 70.1, 70.2). The findings of multiphasic MDCT will be inconclusive (Fig. 70.3A–C). After resection, pathology confirms the MR imaging findings (Fig. 70.3D).

Literature

1. Winston CB, Schwartz LH, Fong Y, et al. (1999) Hepatocellular carcinoma: MR imaging findings in cirrhotic and noncirrhotic livers. Radiology 210:75–79
2. Hussain SM, Semelka RC, Mitchell DG (2002) MR imaging of hepatocellular carcinoma. Magn Reson Imaging Clin N Am 10:31–52
3. Hussain SM, Semelka RC (2005) Hepatic imaging: comparison of modalities. Radiol Clin N Am 43:929–947

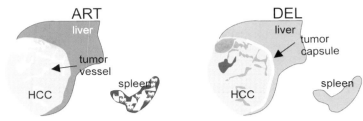

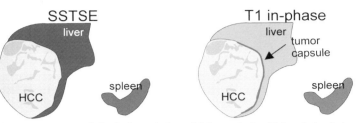

Fig. 70.1. HCC, non-cirrhotic, large lesion with inconclusive CT (see below), drawings. SSTSE: HCC is hyperintense to the liver; **T1 in-phase:** HCC is predominantly hypointense to the liver with a darker partial capsule; **ART:** HCC shows intense heterogeneous enhancement; **DEL:** HCC shows washout with enhancement of a partial tumor capsule

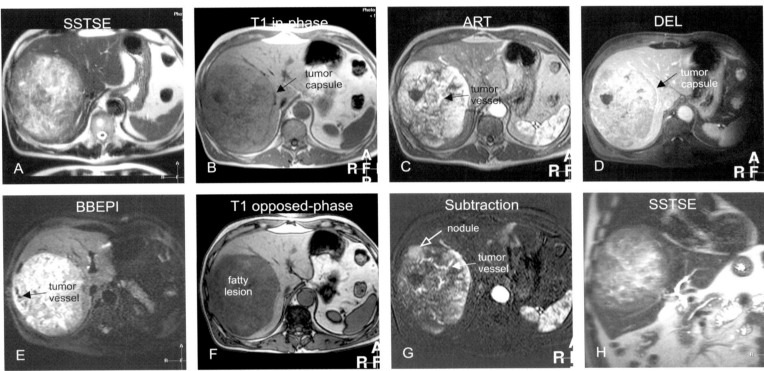

Fig. 70.2. HCC, non-cirrhotic, large fatty lesion with an inconclusive CT (see below), MRI findings. A Axial SSTSE image (SSTSE): HCC is hyperintense to the liver. **B** Axial in-phase image (T1 in-phase): HCC is predominantly hypointense to the liver with a darker tumor capsule. **C** Axial arterial phase image (ART): HCC shows intense heterogeneous enhancement with intratumoral vessels. **D** Axial delayed phase image (DEL): HCC shows washout with enhancement of a partial tumor capsule (*arrow*). **E** Axial BBEPI image (BBEPI): intratumoral vessels appear dark due to the application of diffusion gradients that dephase the signal from flowing blood. **F** Axial opposed-phase image (T1 opposed-phase): HCC appears darker compared to the in-phase image due to fatty infiltration. **G** Subtraction image based on the arterial phase shows enhanced intratumoral nodules and vessels. **H** Coronal SSTSE image (SSTSE): HCC is visible in a normal (non-cirrhotic) liver with normal signal and sharp edges

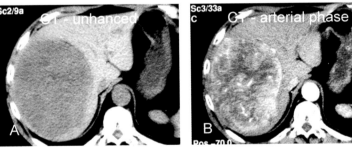

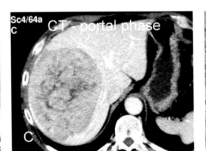

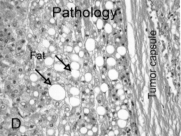

Fig. 70.3. HCC, non-cirrhotic, inconclusive CT findings, and pathology after resection. A Unenhanced CT shows a hypodense large tumor. **B** CT in the arterial phase shows a hypervascular lesion. **C** CT in the portal phase shows more homogeneous enhancement of the lesion. **D** Photomicrograph from the resected specimen shows a hepatocellular tumor with fatty infiltration that is surrounded by a fibrous tumor capsule. Pathology confirmed the MRI findings. H&E, ×200

71 HCC in Non-Cirrhotic Liver IV – Cholangiocellular or Combined Type

Combined hepatocellular-cholangiocarcinoma (cHCC-CC) is a rare form of primary liver carcinoma comprising cells with histopathologic features of both hepatocellular carcinoma (HCC) and cholangiocarcinoma (CC). cHCC-CC patients show a greater similarity to HCC patients than to CC patients with regard to male/female ratio, status of hepatitis viral infection, serum alpha-fetoprotein level, and non-tumor liver histology. The average size of tumors is about 9 cm. At presentation, the disease stage of cHCC-CC patients is more advanced than that of either HCC or CC patients. Satellite nodules and lymph node metastases are less common than in HCC in non-cirrhotic livers. The surgical approach is recommended for selected patients with cHCC-CC. The prognosis is poorer than that of HCC.

MR Imaging Findings
At MR imaging, the cholangiocellular type of HCC appears predominantly bright on T2-weighted images, most likely due to the presence fluid-filled glands. On T1-weighted images, the lesions are hypointense. The tumors show intense heterogeneous enhancement on the gadolinium-enhanced images in the arterial phase and washout in the delayed phase. A tumor capsule may faintly enhance. Apart from the high signal intensity on T2-weighted images, liver capsular retraction may be seen (Figs. 71.1, 71.2).

Pathology
Tumors often show histopathologic features intermediate between those of HCC and CC throughout or demonstrate a gradual transition from moderate to well differentiated areas of HCC toward glandular CC areas (Fig. 71.3A, B).

Management
The majority of tumors can be resected successfully. However, patients with HCC-CC are said to have a worse survival outcome after hepatic resection when compared with patients with HCC. Postoperative adjuvant therapy and multimodality treatment for recurrent disease are required to prolong the survival of these patients. Any extrahepatic or recurrent lesions will show similar increased enhancement on gadolinium-enhanced MR imaging in the arterial phase (Fig. 71.3C, D).

Literature
1. Yano Y, Yamamoto J, Kosuge T, et al. (2003) Combined hepatocellular and cholangiocarcinoma: a clinicopathologic study of 26 resected cases. Jpn J Clin Oncol 33:283–287
2. Maeda T, Adachi E, Kajiyama K, et al. (1995) Combined hepatocellular and cholangiocarcinoma: proposed criteria according to cytokeratin expression and analysis of clinicopathologic features. Hum Pathol 26:956–964
3. Jarnagin WR, Weber S, Tickoo S, et al. (2002) Combined hepatocellular and cholangiocarcinoma: demographic, clinical, and prognostic factors. Cancer 94:2040–2046
4. Liu CL, Fan ST, Lo CM, et al. (2003) Hepatic resection for combined hepatocellular and cholangiocarcinoma. Arch Surg 138:86–90

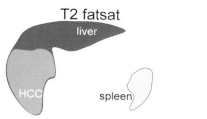 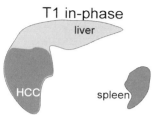 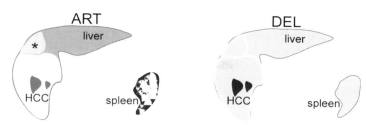

Fig. 71.1. HCC, non-cirrhotic liver, cholangiocellular type, drawings. T2 fatsat: HCC is slightly brighter and heterogeneous to the liver; **T1 in-phase:** HCC is hypointense to the liver; ART: HCC shows intense heterogeneous enhance-ment with a wedge-shaped perilesional enhancement (*); DEL: HCC shows washout and becomes almost isointense to the liver

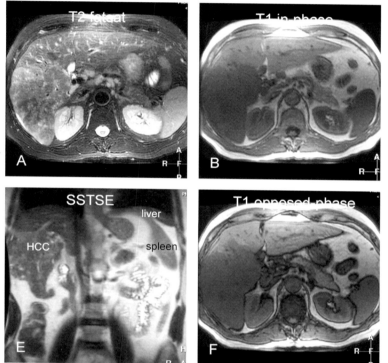 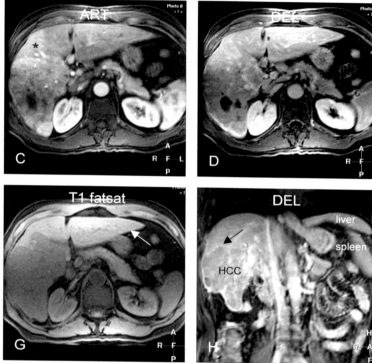

Fig. 71.2. HCC, non-cirrhotic liver, cholangiocellular type, MRI findings. A Axial TSE image (T2 fatsat): HCC is heterogeneous and predominantly hyperin-tense to the liver. **B** Axial in-phase image (T1 in-phase): HCC is hypointense to the liver. **C** Axial arterial phase image (ART): HCC shows intense hetero-geneous enhancement with a wedge-shaped perilesional enhancement (*). **D** Axial delayed phase image (DEL): HCC shows washout and becomes al-most isointense to the liver. **E** Axial SSTSE image (SSTSE): HCC is slightly hyperintense to the liver. **F** Axial opposed-phase image (T1 opposed-phase): No fatty infiltration is present. **G** Axial fat-suppressed T1 GRE image (T1 fat-sat): The liver has a normal signal and smooth edges (*arrow*), consistent with a non-cirrhotic liver. **H** Coronal delayed phase image (DEL): HCC shows washout with faintly enhanced tumor capsule (*arrow*)

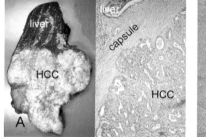 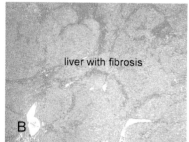 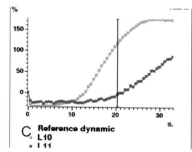 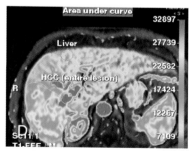

Fig. 71.3. HCC, direct MR-pathology correlation and time-intensity curves. A Pho-tograph of the resected tumor specimen shows HCC in a non-cirrhotic liver. Photomicrograph: HCC shows multiple glands (cholangiocellular type). H&E, ×100. **B** Photomicrograph: Note the liver with septa and inflamma-tion, consistent with fibrosis. H&E, ×40. **C** Time-intensity curves (single slice scanning during the first 33 s after gadolinium) of the liver (*blue*) and HCC (*green*). **D** Color-coded display of the area-under-the-curve shows the total amount of contrast of the liver and the HCC

72 HCC in Non-Cirrhotic Liver V – Central Scar and Capsule Rupture

Hepatocellular carcinoma (HCC) in non-cirrhotic livers is a large lesion which frequently shows a large malformed central scar, a tumor capsule, and satellite nodules. Particularly, the presence of a large central scar on imaging may mimic other liver lesions including giant hemangioma and focal nodular hyperplasia. These entities can be distinguished based on MR imaging.

MR Imaging Findings

At MR imaging, the liver appears normal with smooth edges and normal signal intensity. The central scar may be relatively large with coarse septa. The appearance may be very bright (fluid-like) on T2-weighted images. On T2-weighted images tumor capsule is not visible because of its low signal intensity. On T1-weighted images, the central scar appears darker than the hypointense lesion compared to the surrounding liver. Tumor capsule appears as a rim of low signal intensity surrounding the tumor. The tumor shows intense heterogeneous enhancement in the arterial phase with enhancement of one or more satellite nodules in the periphery of the lesion. In the delayed phase, the tumor shows washout with enhancement of the tumor capsule, which shows discontinuity at the level of the satellite nodules consistent with tumor rupture. At another anatomic level, the tumor capsule may appear intact (Figs. 72.1, 72.2). The size of the lesions as well as the size of the central scars may vary but the basic MR imaging appearance remains consistent (Fig. 72.3).

Differential Diagnosis

Giant hemangiomas are much brighter with an even brighter central scar on T2-weighted images, and show characteristic peripheral nodular enhancement in the arterial phase and persistent enhancement in the delayed phase. Focal nodular hyperplasias are near isointense on T1- and T2-weighted images with a well-formed smaller central scar, and show intense homogeneous enhancement in the arterial phase, fading to isointensity in the delayed phase.

Literature

1. Winston CB, Schwartz LH, Fong Y, et al. (1999) Hepatocellular carcinoma: MR imaging findings in cirrhotic and noncirrhotic livers. Radiology 210:75–79
2. Hussain SM, Semelka RC, Mitchell DG (2002) MR imaging of hepatocellular carcinoma. Magn Reson Imaging Clin N Am 10:31–52
3. Hussain SM, Zondervan PE, et al. (2002) Benign versus malignant hepatic nodules: MR imaging findings with pathologic correlation. Radiographics 22:1023–36
4. Hussain SM, Terkivatan T, Zondervan PE, et al. (2004) Focal nodular hyperplasia: a spectrum of findings at state-of-the-art MR imaging, ultrasound, CT and pathology. Radiographics 24:3–19
5. Hussain SM, Semelka RC (2005) Liver masses. Magn Reson Imaging Clin N Am 13:255–275

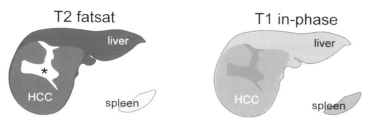

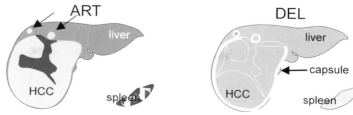

Fig. 72.1. HCC, non-cirrhotic, central scar, capsule rupture, and satellite nodules, drawings. T2 fatsat: HCC is slightly hyperintense to the liver with a brighter central scar (*); **T1 in-phase:** HCC is slightly hypointense to the liver;

ART: HCC shows intense heterogeneous enhancement; note also the satellite nodules (*arrows*); DEL: HCC shows washout and enhanced tumor capsule that is discontinuous at the site of the satellite nodules

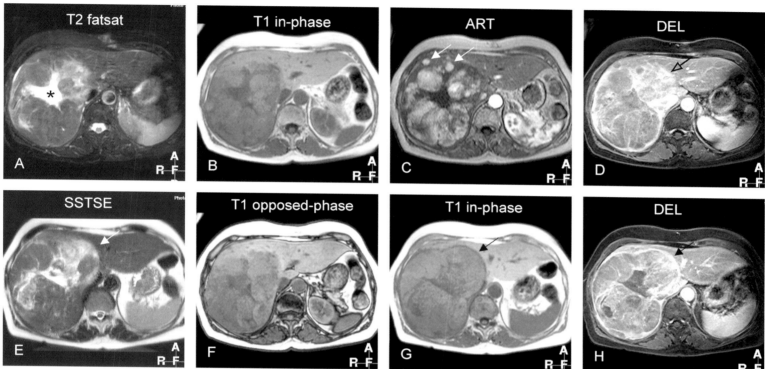

Fig. 72.2. HCC, non-cirrhotic, central scar, capsule rupture, and satellite nodules, MRI findings. A Axial TSE image (T2 fatsat): HCC is slightly hyperintense to the liver with a large, brighter central scar (*) with thick septa. **B** Axial in-phase image (T1 in-phase): HCC is slightly hypointense to the liver. **C** Axial arterial phase image (ART): HCC shows intense heterogeneous enhancement. Note also the satellite nodules (*arrows*). **D** Axial delayed phase image (DEL): HCC shows washout and enhanced tumor capsule that is discontinu-

ous at the site of the satellite nodules (*open arrow*). **E** Axial SSTSE image (SSTSE) at a different anatomic level: low signal intensity capsule completely surrounds the HCC (*arrow*). **F** Axial opposed-phase image (T1 opposed-phase): no fatty infiltration is present. **G** Axial in-phase image (T1 in-phase) at a different anatomic level: low signal intensity capsule completely surrounds the HCC (*arrow*). **H** Axial delayed phase image (DEL): HCC shows washout with enhanced septa and an intact tumor capsule (*arrow*)

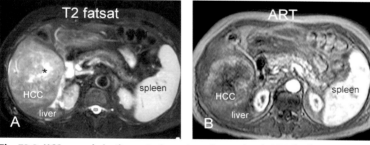

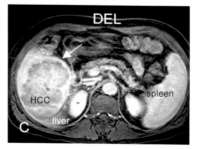

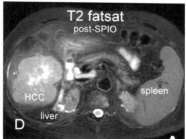

Fig. 72.3. HCC, non-cirrhotic, central scar (another patient), MRI findings. A Axial TSE image (T2 fatsat): HCC is isointense to the liver with a brighter central scar (*). **B** Axial arterial phase image (ART): HCC shows heterogeneous enhancement. **C** Axial delayed phase image (DEL): HCC shows washout and an

enhanced tumor capsule that surrounds – in part – the HCC (*arrow*). **D** Axial TSE image (T2 fatsat) after uptake of SPIO: HCC appears much brighter with better delineation due to the signal loss of the liver. Note also the signal loss in the spleen

73 HCC in Non-Cirrhotic Liver VI – Capsule with Pathologic Correlation

Tumor capsule, a characteristic sign of HCC in cirrhosis as well as in non-cirrhotic livers, is present in 60–82% of cases. Up to 75% of the lesions with a capsule will be larger than 2 cm. The tumor capsule becomes thicker with increasing tumor size. Histologically, tumor capsules are composed of two layers, an inner fibrous layer and an outer layer containing compressed vessels and bile ducts. Tumor capsule is a highly specific sign of HCC. Encapsulated lesions are associated with a better prognosis than are unencapsulated lesions after surgical resection. The recognition of the tumor capsule on imaging, particularly in non-cirrhotic liver, can facilitate the diagnosis of HCC.

MR Imaging Findings

At MR imaging, the tumor capsule is hypointense both on T1- and T2-weighted images in most cases, although capsules with a thickness of more than 4 mm can have an outer hyperintense layer on T2-weighted images. The outer layer may be composed of compressed liver parenchyma, vessels, and inflammatory cell infiltrates. The best images for recognizing tumor capsules include (1) unenhanced T1-weighted images and (2) gadolinium-enhanced T1-weighted images in the delayed phase (Figs. 73.1, 73.2).

Pathology

At gross pathology, the tumor capsule is often visible surrounding the HCC, which often consists of smaller nodules. These nodules may be interspersed by areas with old hemorrhage. The surrounding liver may show evidence of periportal fibrosis (Fig. 73.3).

Literature

1. Winston CB, Schwartz LH, Fong Y, et al. (1999) Hepatocellular carcinoma: MR imaging findings in cirrhotic and noncirrhotic livers. Radiology 210:75–79
2. Hussain SM, Semelka RC, Mitchell DG (2002) MR imaging of hepatocellular carcinoma. Magn Reson Imaging Clin N Am 10:31–52
3. Hussain SM, Zondervan PE, et al. (2002) Benign versus malignant hepatic nodules: MR imaging findings with pathologic correlation. Radiographics 22:1023–36
4. Choi BI, Takayasu K, Han MC (1993) Small hepatocellular carcinoma and associated lesions of the liver: pathology, pathogenesis, imaging findings. AJR 160:1177–1187

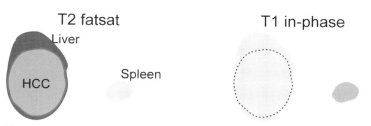
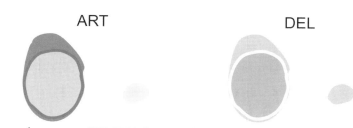

Fig. 73.1. HCC, drawings. T2 fatsat: HCC is slightly hyperintense compared to the liver with a hypointense tumor capsule; **T1 in-phase:** HCC is almost iso-intense with hypointense tumor capsule; **ART:** HCC shows faint heteroge- neous enhancement; **DEL:** HCC shows washout with enhancement of the tu- mor capsule

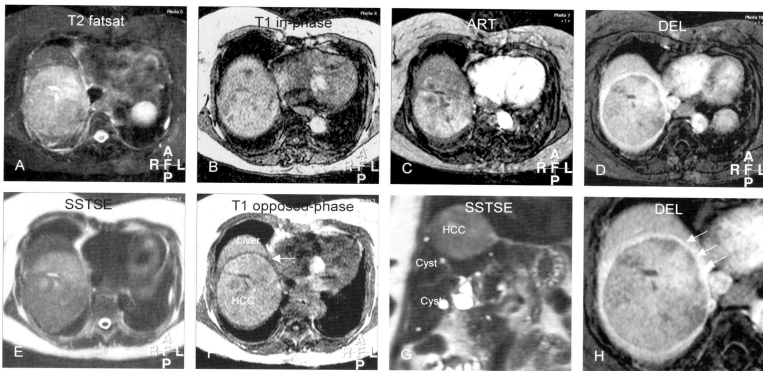

Fig. 73.2. HCC, non-cirrhotic, large, fat-containing, typical MRI findings. A Axial fat-suppressed T2-w TSE image (T2 fatsat): HCC is hyperintense to the liver with hypointense tumor capsule. **B** Axial in-phase image (T1 in-phase): HCC is slightly hypointense to the liver with a dark tumor capsule. **C** Axial arterial phase image (ART): HCC shows heterogeneous enhancement. **D** Ax- ial delayed phase image (DEL): HCC shows washout with enhancement of the tumor capsule. **E** Axial SSTSE image (SSTSE): HCC is slightly hyperin- tense to the liver. **F** Axial opposed-phase image (T1 opposed-phase): HCC as well as the liver shows a decreased signal compared to the in-phase image due to fatty infiltration. Hence the better visibility of the tumor capsule (*ar- row*). **G** Coronal SSTSE image (SSTSE): HCC is brighter than the liver in sub- phrenic location. Note the multiple, much brighter, liver cysts. **H** A detailed view of the axial delayed phase image (DEL coronal): HCC is surrounded by a thick fibrous enhanced tumor capsule (*arrows*)

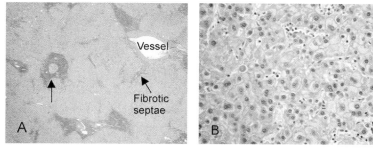
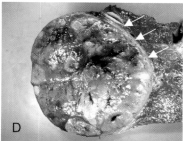

Fig. 73.3. HCC, non-cirrhotic, direct MR-pathology correlation. A Photomicro- graph of the liver shows periportal inflammation (*arrow*) indicating hepati- tis without cirrhosis. H&E, ×40. **B** Photomicrograph of the HCC shows thickened cell plates with atypical nuclei. H&E, ×400. **C** Photomicrograph shows two adjacent HCC nodules that are surrounded by a thick fibrous tu- mor capsule. H&E, ×40. **D** Photograph of the resected specimen shows a large HCC with several smaller nodules that are surrounded by a tumor cap- sule (*arrows*)

74 HCC in Non-Cirrhotic Liver VII – Very Large with Pathologic Correlation

Hepatocellular carcinomas (HCCs) in non-cirrhotic livers may present with a very large mass of up to 25 cm in diameter. Such lesions are discovered late when they become symptomatic. The massive tumors are likely to compress the normal (non-cirrhotic) liver including the vasculature and the biliary tree. Despite the massive size and the space-occupying effects, biliary obstruction is often not present. Encapsulated massive HCCs in non-cirrhotic livers are likely to displace the hepatic vessels and do not invade them. Therefore, despite their impressive appearance surgical resection should be attempted.

MR Imaging Findings

At MR imaging, the lesions may be difficult to evaluate because of their size. The multiplanar capability of MR imaging with multiple T1- and T2-weighted sequences is essential for the workup of such lesions. The lesions are predominantly heterogeneous on T1- and T2-weighted images. After injection of gadolinium, the lesions may show little, heterogeneous enhancement in the arterial phase, whereas in the delayed phase a thick tumor capsule may be seen. The presence of the tumor capsule is a very characteristic sign of HCC (Figs. 74.1, 74.2). Despite the thick fibrous tumor capsule, vasoinvasive growth may occur with the possibility of hematogenous spread through the liver (Fig. 74.3).

Literature

1. Winston CB, Schwartz LH, Fong Y, et al. (1999) Hepatocellular carcinoma: MR imaging findings in cirrhotic and noncirrhotic livers. Radiology 210:75–79
2. Hussain SM, Semelka RC, Mitchell DG (2002) MR imaging of hepatocellular carcinoma. Magn Reson Imaging Clin N Am 10:31–52
3. Hussain SM, Zondervan PE, et al. (2002) Benign versus malignant hepatic nodules: MR imaging findings with pathologic correlation. Radiographics 22:1023–36
4. de Rave S, Hussain SM (2002) A liver tumour as an incidental finding: differential diagnosis and treatment. Scand J Gastroenterol Suppl 236:81–86

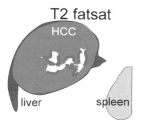
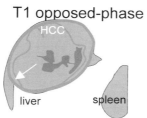
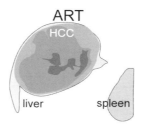
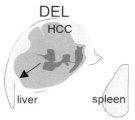

Fig. 74.1. HCC, non-cirrhotic liver with a large mass, drawings. **T2 fatsat:** HCC is slightly hyperintense to the liver with brighter central structures; **T1 opposed-phase:** HCC is almost isointense to the liver with a darker tumor capsule (*arrow*); **ART:** HCC shows faint heterogeneous enhancement; **DEL:** HCC shows washout with persistent enhancement of the peripheral parts and tumor capsule (*arrow*)

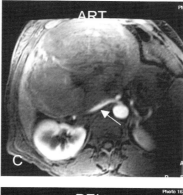
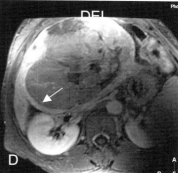
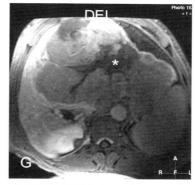
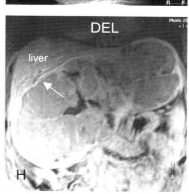

Fig. 74.2. HCC, non-cirrhotic liver with a large mass, MRI findings. **A** Axial TSE image (T2 fatsat): HCC is hyperintense to the liver with bright areas in the center. **B** Axial in-phase image (T1 opposed-phase): HCC is almost isointense to the liver with a dark tumor capsule (*arrow*). **C** Axial arterial phase image (ART): HCC shows faint heterogeneous enhancement. Note the hypertrophic common hepatic artery (*arrow*). **D** Axial delayed phase image (DEL): HCC shows washout with persistent enhancement of the peripheral parts of the tumor and the tumor capsule (*arrow*). **E** Axial SSTSE image (SSTSE): HCC is hyperintense with multiple brighter intratumoral structures. **F** Axial arterial phase image (ART) at another anatomic level shows peritumoral hypertrophic hepatic arterial branches (*arrow*). **G** Axial delayed phase image (DEL): HCC shows washout with a central scar-like less enhanced area (*). **H** Coronal delayed phase image (DEL): HCC is visible as an impressive massive lesion surrounded by a capsule (*arrow*). Note that the liver is normal with smooth edges

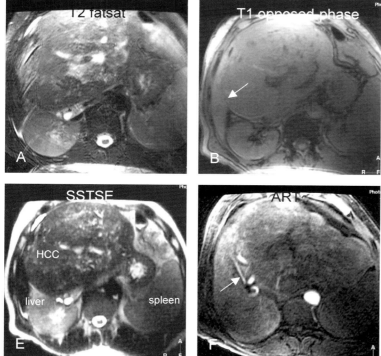
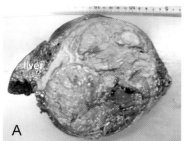
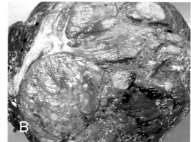
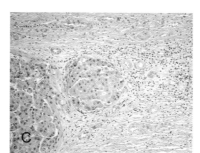
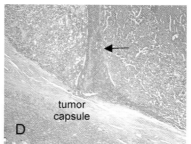

Fig. 74.3. HCC, non-cirrhotic liver with a large mass, direct MR-pathology correlation. **A** Photograph of the resected specimen shows a large massive HCC with several smaller nodules and a thick tumor capsule. **B** A detailed view of the resected specimen shows the nodules and the capsule in more detail. **C** Photomicrograph shows two nodules composed of abnormal hepatocytes. H&E, × 100. **D** Photomicrograph from the periphery of the HCC shows the tumor capsule and a large septum (*arrow*). H&E, × 40

75 HCC in Non-Cirrhotic Liver VIII – Vascular Invasion and Satellite Nodules

Vascular invasion occurs frequently in HCC and can affect both the portal and the hepatic veins. In a recent large study of HCC, 15.5% of cases showed macroscopic and 59.0% microscopic venous invasion proved on histopathology. In this study, the lesions with vascular invasion were associated with a larger tumor size, a higher α-fetoprotein level, and less frequent encapsulation. In a meta-analysis of 7 reports with 1497 patients, portal vein invasion was found in 24% of the cases with HCC. In one study, 10 of 38 patients had an extracapsular invasion. Of these, 9 were detected with MR and only 5 with CT. The presence of extracapsular invasion is one of the factors affecting recurrence after surgery.

MR Imaging Findings
At MR imaging vascular invasion can be seen as a lack of signal void on multislice T1-weighted gradient echo and flow-compensated T2-weighted fast spin-echo images. On gadolinium-enhanced MR images, the tumor thrombus typically shows enhancement on images acquired during the arterial phase and a filling defect on images acquired during later phases (Figs. 75.1, 75.2). Flow-sensitive sequences as well as black-blood echoplanar imaging may also be used to detect any vascular invasion.

Pathology
Extracapsular extension of tumor, with partial projections or formation of satellite nodules in the immediate vicinity, is present in 43–77% of HCCs (Fig. 75.3).

Literature
1. Hussain SM, Semelka RC, Mitchell DG (2002) MR imaging of hepatocellular carcinoma. Magn Reson Imaging Clin N Am 10:31–52
2. Tsai T-J, Chau G-Y, Lui W-Y, et al. (2000) Clinical significance of microscopic tumor venous invasion in patients with resectable hepatocellular carcinoma. Surgery 127:603–608
3. Lee YT, Geer DA (1987) Primary liver cancer: pattern of metastasis. J Surg Oncol 36:26–31
4. Imaeda T, Kanematsu M, Mochizuki R, et al. (1994) Extracapsular invasion of small hepatocellular carcinoma: MR and CT findings. JCAT 18:755–760

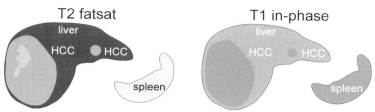
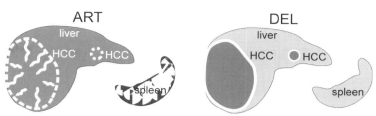

Fig. 75.1. HCC, non-cirrhotic liver, large with vascular invasion and a satellite nodule, drawings. T2 fatsat: both HCCs appear brighter than the liver: the larger contains a central scar-like area and the smaller is most likely a satellite nod-ule; **T1 in-phase:** the lesions are hypointense to the liver; **ART:** HCCs show intense peripheral heterogeneous enhancement; **DEL:** HCCs show washout with capsular enhancement

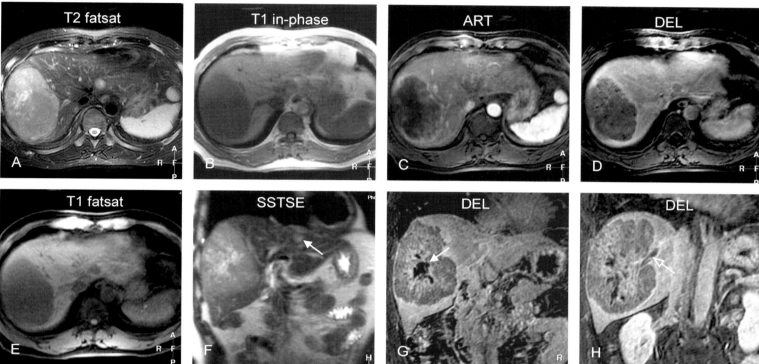

Fig. 75.2. HCC, non-cirrhotic liver, large HCC with vascular invasion and a satellite nodule, MRI findings. A Axial TSE image (T2 fatsat): Both HCCs appear brighter than the liver with sharp margins: the larger contains a central scar-like area and the smaller is most likely a satellite nodule. **B** Axial in-phase image (T1 in-phase): HCCs are hypointense to the liver. **C** Axial arterial phase image (ART): HCCs show intense peripheral heterogeneous enhancement. **D** Axial delayed phase image (DEL): HCCs show washout with capsular en-hancement. **E** Axial fat-suppressed T1 GRE image (T1 fatsat): HCCs are well-demarcated due to fat suppression and good T1-weighting. **F** Coronal SSTSE image (SSTSE): The smaller lesion is in a subphrenic/subcapsular location in the left liver (*arrow*). **G** Coronal delayed phase image (DEL) shows a less-enhanced irregular central scar (*arrow*). **H** Coronal delayed phase image (DEL) at a different anatomic level: One of the liver veins shows an extension of the tumor with abnormal enhancement (*open arrow*)

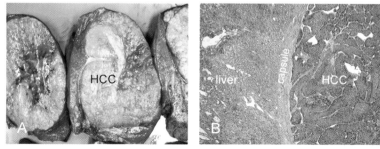
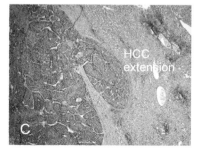
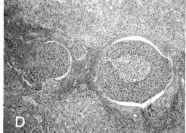

Fig. 75.3. HCC, direct MR-pathology correlation. A Photograph of the resected tumor specimen shows HCC in a non-cirrhotic liver. **B** Photomicrograph: HCC is surrounded by a fibrous tumor capsule. H&E, ×40. **C** Photomicro-graph: HCC extends with a tong-like fashion through the capsule (capsule rupture). H&E, ×40. **D** Photomicrograph shows two vessels filled with tu-mor thrombus, which most likely play a role in the formation of satellite nodules. H&E, ×40

76 HCC in Non-Cirrhotic Liver IX – Adenoma-Like HCC with Pathologic Correlation

Some hepatocellular carcinomas in non-cirrhotic livers of young and middle-aged women may have features of both hepatocellular adenomas (HCAs) and carcinomas (HCCs). These lesions may have transformed from a preexisting HCA. Malignant transformation of HCA into HCC has been described in the literature by several groups. Most authors have reported transformation of an existing HCA into HCC. Gordon et al., however, reported a case of HCC after complete regression of HCA at the same anatomic location. At this point in time, it is not quite clear if all HCAs eventually can transform into HCCs. Also the exact characteristics of HCAs that eventually may undergo malignant transformation are not well known. Tao has recently suggested that HCA is not pre-malignant and may undergo reversible change after withdrawal of OC, whereas LCD is an irreversible, pre-malignant change and will eventually progress to HCC (HCA-LCD-HCC sequence).

MR Imaging Findings

At MR imaging, the lesions occur within a non-cirrhotic liver and appear hyperintense on T2-weighted images and isointense or slightly hyperintense on T1-weighted images. A low signal intensity tumor capsule may surround the lesions. After injection of gadolinium, the lesions show enhancement of intratumoral nodules in the arterial phase, and washout with enhanced tumor capsule in the delayed phase (Figs. 76.1, 76.2).

Pathology

Recently, such a tumor was observed in our institution. Based on the MR imaging findings, an HCC in non-cirrhotic liver was diagnosed and the tumor was resected. The resected specimen was sent to three different pathologists in Europe. Two of them diagnosed the lesion as HCC and the third as HCA (Fig. 75.3). This case illustrates that the diagnoses of primary liver lesions may be challenging not only based on imaging.

Literature

1. Gordon SC, Reddy KR, Livingstone AS, et al. (1986) Resolution of a contraceptive-steroid-induced hepatic adenoma with subsequent evolution into hepatocellular carcinoma. Ann Intern Med 105:547–549
2. Gyorffy EJ, Bredfeldt JE, Black WC (1989) Transformation of hepatic cell adenoma to hepatocellular carcinoma due to oral contraceptive use. Ann Intern Med 110:489–490
3. Tao LC (1991) Oral contraceptive-associated liver cell adenoma and hepatocellular carcinoma: cytomorphology and mechanism of malignant transformation. Cancer 68:341–347
4. Ferrell LD (1993) Hepatocellular carcinoma arising in a focus of multilobular adenoma: a case report. Am J Surg Pathol 17:525–529
5. Foster JH, Berman MM (1994) The malignant transformation of liver cell adenomas. Arch Surg 129:712–717

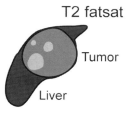
T2 fatsat

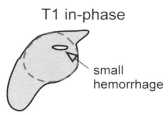
T1 in-phase

ART

DEL

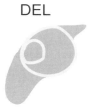

Fig. 76.1. HCC, adenoma-like and mosaic pattern, drawings. T2 fatsat: HCC is largely hyperintense to the liver; **T1 in-phase:** HCC is isointense to the liver with a darker tumor capsule; **ART:** HCC shows intralesional nodules with variable enhancement (*solid arrows*); note an additional smaller subcapsular nodule (*open arrow*); **DEL:** HCC becomes almost isointense with enhancement of tumor capsule as well as intratumoral septa

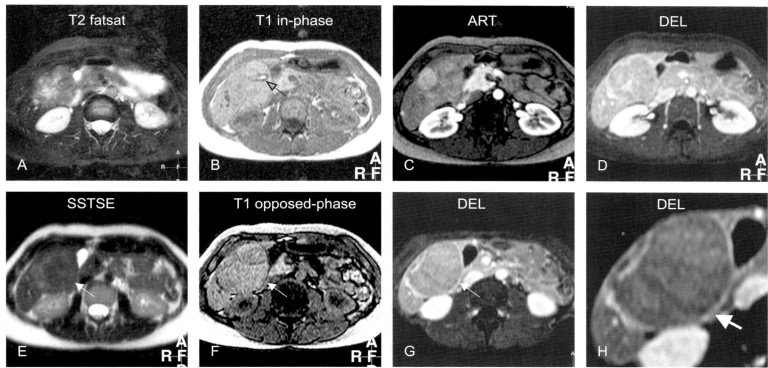

Fig. 76.2. HCC, non-cirrhotic liver, adenoma-like tumor with capsule and mosaic pattern. A Axial fatsat TSE image (T2 fatsat): Tumor is largely hyperintense to the liver. **B** Axial in-phase image (T1 in-phase): Tumor is isointense to the liver with a darker tumor capsule and a small hemorrhage (*arrow*). **C** Axial arterial phase image (ART): Tumor shows intratumoral nodules with variable enhancement (mosaic pattern). Note also an additional small subcapsular nodule (*arrow*). **D** Axial delayed phase image (DEL): Tumor shows enhancement of a tumor capsule. **E** Axial T2-w SSTSE image with long TE (SSTSE): Tumor is darker as compared to T2 fat-suppressed image (*arrow*). **F** Axial opposed-phase image (T1 opposed-phase): The tumor capsule is slightly better visible than on T1 in-phase image (*arrow*), probably due to better T1-weighting with shorter TE. **G** Axial delayed phase image (DEL) at a slightly different anatomic level shows the tumor capsule (*arrow*). **H** A detailed view of the previous image shows the tumor anatomy better with an enhancing tumor capsule (*arrow*)

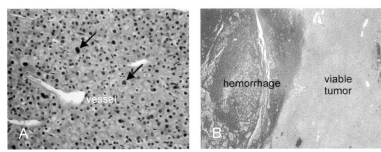
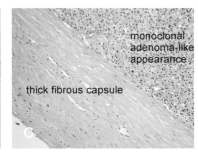
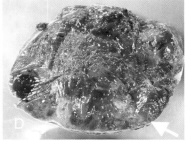

Fig. 76.3. MR-pathology correlation. A Photomicrograph shows abnormal hepatocytes with variable sized nuclei and some proliferative activity (*arrows*). Note the increased cellularity and vascularity. H&E, × 200. **B** Photomicrograph shows the solid tumor and hemorrhage. H&E, × 40. **C** Photomicrograph shows a thick fibrous capsule that correlates with the MRI findings (specific sign of HCC). The monoclonal nature though is more suggestive of adenoma. H&E, × 100. **D** Photograph of the resected specimen shows a large encapsulated tumor with multiple nodules, which is more consistent with HCC

77 Intrahepatic Cholangiocarcinoma – With Pathologic Correlation

Cholangiocarcinoma is a relatively uncommon tumor, comprising only 15% of liver cancers in the USA. Cholangiocarcinoma has been classified into three different types based on regional distribution: peripheral tumors that arise from intrahepatic ducts, Klatskin tumors that arise at the confluence of the right and left hepatic ducts, and extrahepatic tumors that arise from ducts distal to the confluence. Generally, intrahepatic tumors are mass-like. This variation in morphology has been previously shown on CT and MR images.

Between 1973 and 1997, the incidence of intrahepatic cholangiocarcinoma in the USA increased by 9.1% annually. Hepatitis B and C, cirrhosis and alcohol have been described as risk factors. Intrahepatic cholangiocarcinomas have been reported to occur more frequently in the right lobe and to arise predominately in non-cirrhotic livers. CT and MRI scans are commonly used non-invasive approaches for the detection and staging of cholangiocarcinoma.

MR Imaging Findings

At MR imaging, intrahepatic cholangiocarcinomas appear as well-circumscribed masses with moderately high signal intensity on T2-weighted images. Due to the abundant desmoplasia, the tumors appear darker centrally. In addition, desmoplasia may also cause capsular retraction. These findings give rise to the typical tumor morphology of cholangiocarcinomas at MR imaging. On gadolinium-enhanced arterial phase images, the lesions show intense enhancement of mainly the peripheral thick rim of tissue and are less intense centrally. In the delayed phase, the lesions show washout and may become somewhat heterogeneous, without any capsular enhancement. Any intrahepatic metastases show a similar appearance to the primary tumor (Figs. 77.1, 77.2). At histology, the tumor is composed of gland-like tissue interspersed within a matrix of fibrosis. Despite the presence of intrahepatic metastases, successful hepatic resection may be attempted (Fig. 77.3).

Differential Diagnosis

Hepatocellular carcinoma (HCC) in non-cirrhotic liver may show some overlapping imaging features with intrahepatic cholangiocarcinoma. HCC, however, often shows a mosaic pattern, more intense and heterogeneous enhancement with washout, and capsular enhancement.

Literature

1. Parkin DM, Ohshima H, Srivatanakul P, et al. (1993) Cholangiocarcinoma: epidemiology, mechanisms of carcinogenesis and prevention. Cancer Epidemiol Biomarkers Prev 2:537–544
2. Worawattanakul S, Semelka RC, Noone TC, et al. (1998) Cholangiocarcinoma: spectrum of appearances on MR images using current techniques. Magn Reson Imaging 16:993–1003
3. Soyer P, Bluemke DA, Reichle R, et al. (1995) Imaging of intrahepatic cholangiocarcinoma: 1. Peripheral cholangiocarcinoma. AJR 165:1427–1431
4. Patel T (2001) Increasing incidence and mortality of primary intrahepatic cholangiocarcinoma in the United States. Hepatology 33:1353–1357

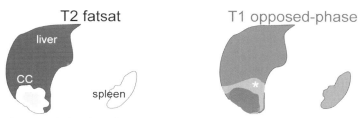

Fig. 77.1. Cholangiocarcinoma (CC), intrahepatic or central, drawings. T2 fatsat: CC is lobulated and hyperintense to the liver with a darker center due to desmoplasia; **T1 opposed-phase:** CC is surrounded by a wedge-shaped area of non-steatosis (*) in otherwise fatty liver; **ART:** CC shows intense, almost homogeneous enhancement; **DEL:** CC becomes almost isointense to the surrounding liver

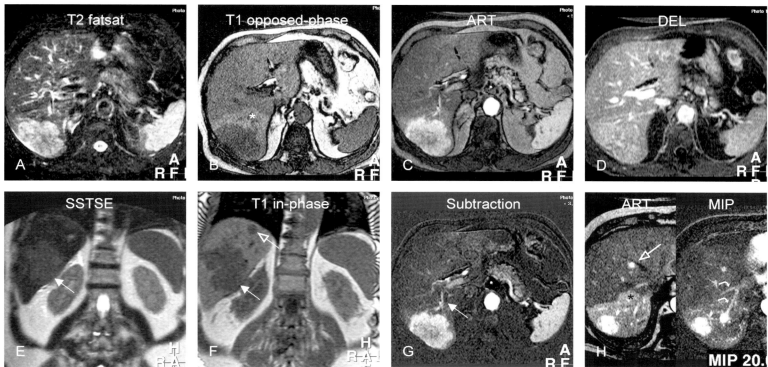

Fig. 77.2. Cholangiocarcinoma (CC), intrahepatic or central, MR findings. A Axial fat-suppressed TSE image (T2 fatsat): CC is lobulated and hyperintense to the liver with a darker center due to desmoplasia. **B** Axial T1-opposed-phase GRE image (T1 opposed-phase): CC is surrounded by a wedge-shaped area of non-steatosis in an otherwise fatty liver. **C** Axial arterial phase image (ART): CC shows intense, almost homogeneous enhancement. **D** Axial delayed phase image (DEL): CC becomes almost isointense to the liver. **E** Coronal SSTSE image (SSTSE): CC is slightly hyperintense (*arrow*). **F** Coronal T1- in-phase GRE image (T1-in-phase): CC (*solid arrow*) is accompanied by an additional lesion, most likely a metastasis (*open arrow*). **G** Subtraction of the arterial phase shows the enhanced CC as well as the feeding artery (*arrow*). **H** Axial arterial phase (ART) at a different anatomic level and a MIP: a metastasis is located close to the hepatic vein (*open arrow*). The early enhancing liver veins (*curved arrows*) and the wedge-shaped perilesional enhancement (*) indicate shunting caused by the tumor

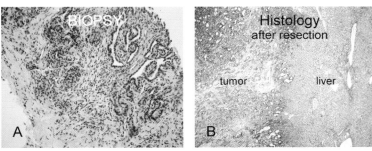
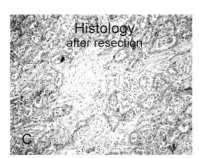
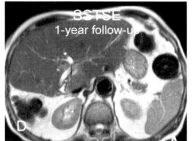

Fig. 77.3. Cholangiocarcinoma (CC), MR-pathology correlation and follow-up. A Photomicrograph of biopsy (prior to MRI) shows glands within stroma, consistent with a CC. H&E, ×200. **B** Photomicrograph of the tumor specimen shows a sharp demarcation between the tumor and the surrounding liver, without any tumor capsule. H&E, ×100. **C** Photomicrograph shows large glands that explain the high T2 signal. H&E, ×200. **D** Axial SSTSE image (follow-up after curative right-sided hepatectomy) shows regenerated liver without any residual or recurrent disease

78 Telangiectatic Hepatocellular Lesion

Telangiectatic hepatocellular lesion (also known as telangiectatic adenoma and formerly known as „telangiectatic" focal nodular hyperplasia, FNH) is now considered a variant of adenoma because a recent study showed that the molecular profile of „telangiectatic FNH" at DNA, gene, and protein expression level is much closer to that of hepatocellular adenomas than typical FNH. Histologically, telangiectatic HCAs are monoclonal, with regular-sized liver plates, a mild degree of inflammation, small isolated, thin dystrophic arteries, and signs of congestion including sinusoidal dilatation. Paradis and colleagues also indicated that FNHs are typically regenerative and polyclonal, whereas HCAs are lesions with a neoplastic and monoclonal nature. However, they did not clarify the significance of a very confusing finding in their study, namely the presence of mild to moderate ductular proliferation in most „telangiectatic FNHs" as well as typical FNHs. In addition, ductular proliferation was absent in five of six classical HCAs. On pathology, the presence of ductular proliferation is one of the hallmarks of FNH and practically excludes HCA. Until more data become available, „telangiectatic FNH" should be considered as „telangiectatic adenoma or lesion," mainly because their biological behavior is similar to the classical HCA.

MR Imaging Findings

At MR imaging, multiple lesions may be present with a variable but predominantly heterogeneous appearance on T2-weighted images. Some lesions may show evidence of fat on chemical shift imaging. The enhancement is often (persistent) heterogeneous. The presence of Kupffer cells, which is the proof for the primary hepatic nature of these lesions, shows uptake with decreased signal on the T2*-weighted images (Figs. 78.1–78.3). The heterogeneity as well as the tumor morphology differ considerably from both classical FNH and HCA. Therefore, we have grouped this lesion separately.

Differential Diagnosis

On follow-up, the lesions do not show any detectable signs of growth, hence suggesting their benign nature. Otherwise, the appearance may easily resemble primary malignant liver lesion, including multifocal hepatocellular carcinoma.

Literature

1. Paradis V, Benzekri A, Dargere D, et al. (2004) Telangiectatic focal nodular hyperplasia: a variant of hepatocellular adenoma. Gastroenterology 126:1323–1329
2. Hussain SM, Terkivatan T, Zondervan PE, et al. (2004) Focal nodular hyperplasia: a spectrum of findings at state-of-the-art MR imaging, ultrasound, CT and pathology. Radiographics 24:3–19
3. Terkivatan T, Van den Bos IC, Hussain SM, et al. (2006) Focal nodular hyperplasia: lesion characteristics at state-of-the-art MR imaging including dynamic gadolinium-enhanced and superparamagnetic iron-oxide-uptake sequences in a prospective study. JMRI (in press)
4. Hussain SM, Van den Bos IC, Dwarkasing S, et al. (2006) Hepatocellular adenoma: findings at state-of-the-art magnetic resonance imaging, ultrasound, computed tomography and pathologic analysis. Eur Radiol 16: 1873–1886

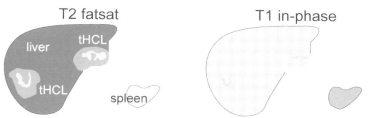
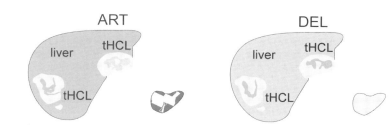

Fig. 78.1. Telangiectatic hepatocellular lesion (tHCL), drawings. T2 fatsat: tHCL is moderately hyperintense to the liver with a brighter center; **T1 in-phase:** tHCL is almost isointense to the liver; **ART:** tHCL shows heterogeneous enhancement, more in the periphery; **DEL:** both tHCLs show persistent enhancement without any capsule or washout of contrast

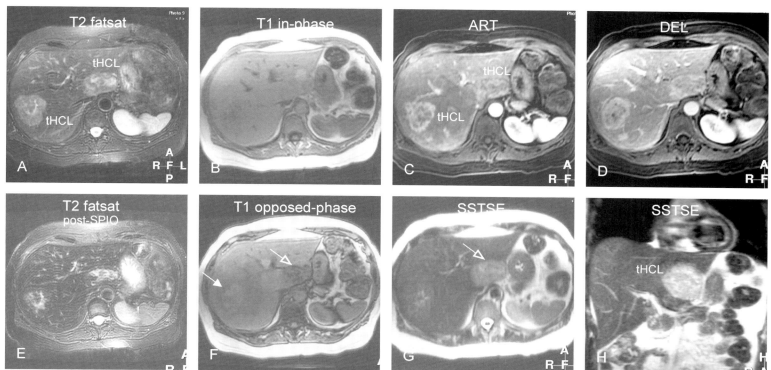

Fig. 78.2. Telangiectatic hepatocellular lesion (tHCL), MRI findings. A Axial fat-suppressed TSE image (T2 fatsat): tHCLs are moderately hyperintense to the liver with brighter centers. **B** Axial in-phase image (T1 in-phase): tHCLs are isointense to the liver. **C** Axial arterial phase image (ART): tHCLs show heterogeneous enhancement, mainly in the peripheral parts. **D** Axial delayed phase image (DEL): tHCLs show persistent enhancement without any capsule or washout. **E** Axial TSE image (T2 fatsat) after uptake of SPIO: tHCLs show similar uptake to the liver (except in the central parts) and become isointense to the liver. **F** Axial opposed-phase image (T1 opposed-phase) shows more fatty infiltration in the left (*open arrow*) than the right lesion (*solid arrow*). **G** Axial SSTSE image (SSTSE): More fatty tHCL appears brighter (*open arrow*). **H** Coronal SSTSE image (SSTSE): Bright appearance of one of the tHCLs may be due to higher fluid as well as fatty content

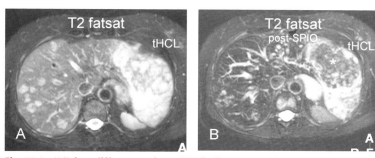
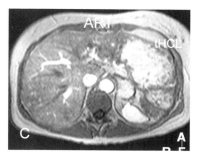
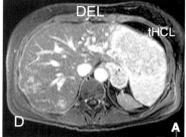

Fig. 78.3. tHCL in a different patient, MRI findings. A Axial TSE image (T2 fatsat): One large and several smaller tHCLs appear heterogeneous and bright. **B** Axial post-SPIO TSE image (T2 fatsat): Most tHCLs, including a nodule (*) within the largest lesion, show decreased signal and indicate hepatocellular origin. **C** Axial arterial phase image (ART): tHCLs show heterogeneous intense enhancement. **D** Axial delayed phase image (DEL): tHCLs show persistent enhancement without any capsule or washout

Part III

Diffuse (Depositional) Liver Diseases

III

79 Focal Fatty Infiltration Mimicking Metastases

Hepatic steatosis is one of the most common morphological abnormalities identified on liver biopsy. Detection and quantification of fat within the liver is important in patients with suspected non-alcoholic steatohepatitis, liver donors or liver transplants. Multifocal hepatic steatosis or multifocal nodular fatty infiltration of the liver is an incidental finding at imaging and can cause misleading findings in the differential diagnosis when using ultrasound (US) and computed tomography (CT). Particularly, at US the lesions appear as hyperechoic nodules which cannot be distinguished from metastatic lesions. MR imaging allows accurate differentiation. Chemical shift MR imaging is a simple and effective method to characterize multifocal nodular fatty infiltration.

MR Imaging Findings

At MR imaging, multifocal nodular fatty infiltration is visible only on the opposed-phase images as focal hepatic areas with signal loss compared to the in-phase images. On T2-weighted images, the liver should appear completely normal without any sign of hyperintense focal lesions. The liver shows normal enhancement in the delayed images (Figs. 79.1, 79.2). Currently, in- and opposed-phase sequences can be acquired in a single breath-hold with two echo time (TE) values (at 1.5T, shortest opposed-phase TE is 2.3 ms and shortest in-phase 4.6 ms). The resultant set of images is identical and displays signal loss only in the pixels with fatty infiltration.

Some patients may have strong fatty infiltration in certain areas. Such areas can show increased signal on in-phase images and show strong signal loss on opposed-phase images (Fig. 79.3).

Literature

1. Mitchell DG (1992) Focal manifestations of diffuse liver disease at MR imaging. Radiology 185:1–11
2. Martin J, Puig J, Falco J, et al. (1998) Hyperechoic liver nodules: characterization with proton fat-water chemical shift MR imaging. Radiology 207:325–330
3. Kronkce TJ, Taupitz M, Kivelitz D, et al. (2000) Multifocal nodular fatty infiltration of the liver mimicking metastatic disease on CT: imaging findings and diagnosis using MR imaging. Eur Radiol 10:1095–1100
4. Kemper J, Poll LW, Jonkmanns C, et al. (2002) CT and MRI findings of multifocal hepatic steatosis mimicking malignancy. Abdom Imaging 27:708–710
5. Pilleul F, Chave G, Dumortier J, et al. (2005) Fatty infiltration of the liver: detection and grading using dual T1 gradient echo sequences on clinical MR system. Gastroenterol Clin Biol 29:1143–1147

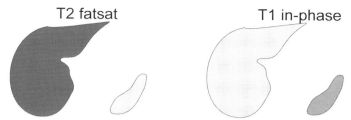

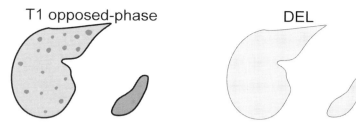

Fig. 79.1. Focal fatty infiltration mimicking metastases, drawings. T2 fatsat: the signal intensity of the liver is homogeneous and normal; **T1 in-phase:** the liver has a normal appearance; **T1 opposed-phase:** decreased focal signal in the entire liver indicates focal fatty infiltration; **DEL:** the liver shows normal homogeneous enhancement without any liver lesions

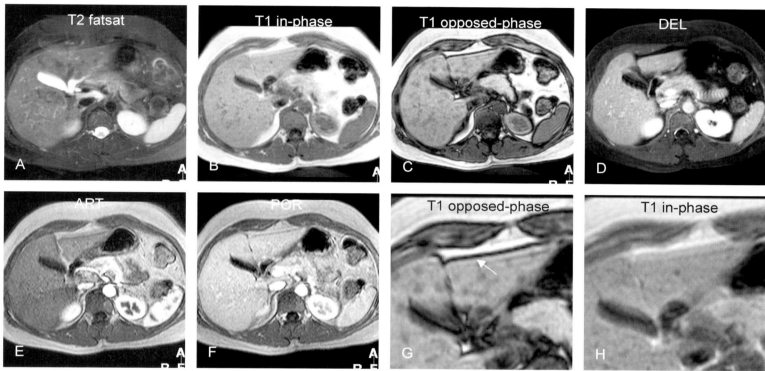

Fig. 79.2. Focal fatty infiltration mimicking metastases, MRI findings. A Axial fat-suppressed turbo spin echo (TSE) image (T2 fatsat) shows no bright lesions. **B** Axial in-phase image (T1 in-phase) shows homogeneous liver without any liver lesions. **C** Axial opposed-phase image (T1 opposed-phase) shows decreased focal signal in the entire liver caused by focal fatty infiltration, mimicking liver lesions. **D** Axial delayed phase image (DEL) shows homogeneous enhancement of the liver without any lesions. **E** Axial arterial phase image (ART) shows no enhancing lesions. **F** Axial portal phase image (POR) shows homogeneous enhancement of the liver without any sign of liver lesions. **G** A detailed view of the opposed-phase image (T1 opposed-phase) shows clearly the focal fatty infiltration with the phase cancellation artifact at the interface between the liver and the surrounding fat (*arrow*). **H** A detailed view of the in-phase image (T1 in-phase) shows homogeneous liver without any liver lesions

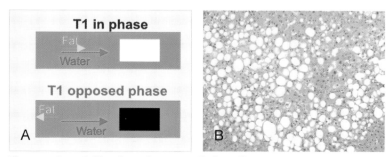

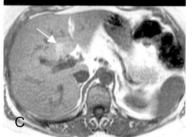

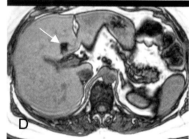

Fig. 79.3. Fatty infiltration, phase cancellation effect based on chemical shift. A Drawing explaining phase cancellation: at 1.5T, water and fat are in-phase at a minimum TE of 4.6 ms and opposed-phase at a minimum TE of 2.3 ms. **B** Photomicrograph from a liver with fatty infiltration. H&E, ×200. **C** Axial in-phase image from a different patient shows focal area of increased signal (*arrow*). **D** Axial opposed-phase image shows signal loss consistent with focal fatty infiltration (*arrow*)

80 Focal Fatty Sparing Mimicking Liver Lesions

Occasionally, focal areas of normal parenchyma in an otherwise diffuse fatty liver may mimic mass lesions. Focally decreased blood flow from the main portal vein associated with aberrant venous drainage is a likely cause of the focal fatty sparing. These areas may be seen in the posterior edges of segments II and IV, and around the gallbladder fossa. One of the most common sites of focal fatty sparing is the posterior edge of segment IV (aberrant left gastric vein). To some extent sonographic features may facilitate identification of focal fatty sparing based on (1) characteristic location within the liver, (2) non-displaced blood vessels and (3) geometric pattern with straight edges. These findings, however, are non-specific. In addition, other benign or malignant lesions may concur. MR imaging should be applied if further characterization is necessary, for instance in patients with an underlying malignancy.

MR Imaging Findings

At MR imaging, focal fatty sparing appears as an area with high signal intensity on the opposed-phase images because the remainder of the liver shows signal loss due to fatty infiltration. Depending on the extent of the diffuse steatosis, focal fatty sparing may appear iso- or slightly hyperintense on the fat suppressed T2-weighted images. Focal fatty sparing may show some persistent enhancement; the enhancement pattern however should resemble the normal liver tissue. Other focal liver lesions such as small hemangiomas may concur (Figs. 80.1 – 80.3). In doubtful cases, follow-up with MR imaging may be considered or specific MR imaging contrast media may be applied to demonstrate the hepatic nature of the focal fatty sparing.

Differential Diagnosis

The differential diagnosis for liver lesions with high signal intensity on T1-weighted images may include melanoma metastases (visible on in-phase as well as opposed-phase images; highly vascular lesions); hemorrhage (often very bright rim of methemoglobin surrounds the lesion; no enhancement); and mucinous- or protein-rich metastases (lesions have solid component with completely different enhancement pattern).

Literature

1. Mitchell DG, Kim I, Chang TS, et al. (1991) Fatty liver. Chemical shift phase-difference and suppression magnetic resonance imaging techniques in animals, phantoms, and humans. Invest Radiol 26:1041–52
2. Chong VF, Fan YF (1994) Ultrasonographic hepatic pseudolesions: normal parenchyma mimicking mass lesions in fatty liver. Clin Radiol 49:326–329
3. Matsui O, Kadoya M, Takahashi S, et al. (1995) Focal sparing of segment IV in fatty livers shown by sonography and CT: correlation with aberrant gastric venous drainage. AJR 164:1137–1140

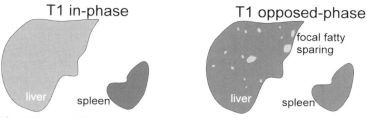

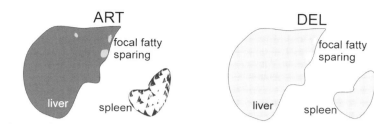

Fig. 80.1. Focal fatty sparing mimicking malignant liver lesions, drawings.
T1 in-phase: the liver shows a normal homogeneous signal without lesions;
T1 opposed-phase: the liver shows signal loss due to diffuse fatty infiltra-

tion, and areas with persistent high signal due to focal fatty sparing;
ART: some of the areas with focal fatty sparing show faint enhancement;
DEL: focal fatty sparing shows persistent enhancement

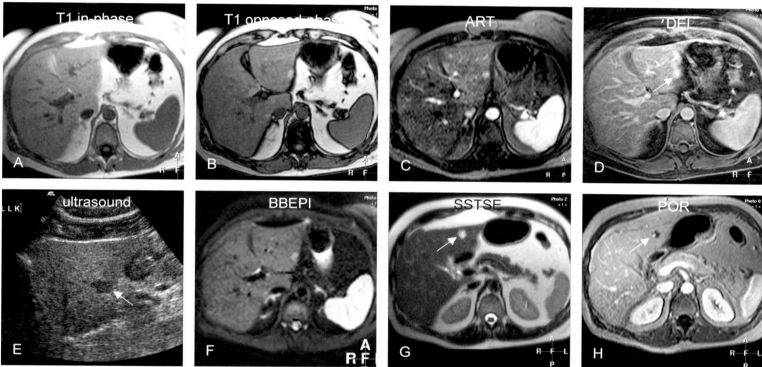

Fig. 80.2. Focal fatty sparing mimicking malignant liver lesions, MRI findings.
A Axial in-phase image (T1 in-phase) shows a normal liver with homogeneous signal without lesions. **B** Axial opposed-phase image (T1 opposed-
phase): The liver shows signal loss due to diffuse fatty infiltration, and areas
with persistent high signal due to focal fatty sparing. **C** Axial arterial phase
image (ART) shows faint enhancement in some of the areas with focal fatty
sparing. **D** Axial delayed phase image (DEL) shows persistent enhancement
in one or two areas (*arrow*). **E** Ultrasound (prior to MRI) shows a hypoecho-

ic lesion with suspicion of a metastasis (*arrow*). **F** Axial black-blood echoplanar imaging (BBEPI) shows unusually high signal in one of the focal fatty
sparing areas (*arrow*). Based on this and the enhancement, a follow-up MRI
was advised in 3–6 months. **G** Axial single-shot turbo spin echo image
(SSTSE) at a different anatomic level shows a bright lesion (*arrow*). **H** Axial
portal phase image (POR) shows peripheral nodular enhancement consistent with a small hemangioma

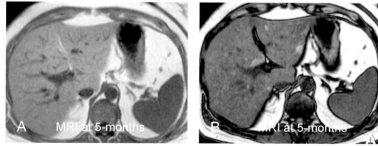

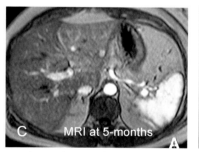

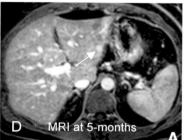

**Fig. 80.3. Focal fatty sparing mimicking malignant liver lesions, MRI findings at
5 months follow-up. A** Axial in-phase image (T1 in-phase) shows a normal
liver with homogeneous signal without lesions. **B** Axial opposed-phase image (T1 opposed-phase): The areas with focal fatty sparing are completely

unchanged. **C** Axial arterial phase image (ART) shows similar enhancement
to the previous MRI. **D** Axial delayed phase image (DEL) shows unchanged
persistent enhancement in one or two areas (*arrow*)

81 Hemosiderosis – Iron Deposition, Acquired Type

Iron is a paramagnetic substance and the intracellular iron that can be present in the form of deoxyhemoglobin, methemoglobin, ferritin, or hemosiderin behaves like tiny magnets within a strong magnetic field. Therefore, intracellular iron particles cause local field inhomogeneities and accelerate the $T2^*$ of tissues. This effect of iron can be visualized on MR imaging sequences that are sensitive to magnetic field inhomogeneities, including spin-echo as well as gradient-echo sequences. $T2^*$-weighted gradient echo (GRE) sequences are considered more sensitive than the T2-weighted spin-echo or fast spin-echo sequences. GRE sequences lack the refocusing pulses and are therefore more sensitive to field inhomogeneities and susceptibility artifacts. In hemosiderosis (transfusional iron overload), the excess iron is accumulated in the reticuloendothelial cells (Kupffer cells). Therefore, the signal intensity of both the liver and the spleen decreases on MR imaging with increasing TE values. Iron overload cannot be assessed on other imaging modalities.

MR Imaging Findings

At MR imaging, iron overload can be assessed with a breath-hold GRE sequence (at 1.5T) with a TR of 100–300 ms, a TE of 7–15 ms and a flip angle of less than 30° to minimize the influence of T1-weighting. For MR machines with lower and higher field strengths than 1.5T, the TE should be increased and decreased respectively. In our experience, a GRE sequence with a flip angle of 70–90° and a TE of around 12 ms works well. Such a sequence can be an adjunct to the dual-echo GRE sequence performed in a single breath hold with TEs of 2.3 and 4.6 ms at 1.5T, which is often a standard part of the liver protocol in many centers. The signal intensity of the skeletal muscle is used as the internal reference to compare the change in the signal intensities of other organs. In hemosiderosis, both the liver and spleen will typically show signal loss on sequences with longer TE values (Figs. 81.1–81.3). The extent of signal loss will depend on the severity of the iron deposition and can be expressed in a semiquantitative manner.

Literature

1. Pomerantz S, Siegelman ES (2002) MR imaging of iron depositional disease. Magn Reson Imaging Clin North Am 10:105–120
2. Siegelman ES, Mitchell DG, Rubin R, et al. (1991) Parenchymal versus reticuloendothelial iron overload in the liver: distinction with MR imaging [see comments]. Radiology 179:361–366
3. Siegelman ES, Mitchell DG, Semelka RC (1996) Abdominal iron deposition: metabolism, MR findings, and clinical importance. Radiology 199:13–22

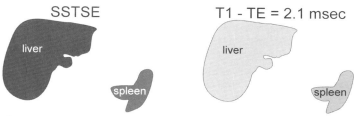 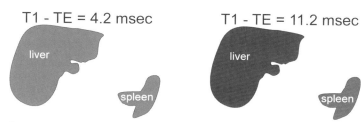

Fig. 81.1. Hemosiderosis, moderate to severe. SSTSE: the liver appears darker than usual; **T1 – TE = 2.1 ms**: the liver is brighter than the spleen; **T1 – TE = 4.2 ms**: the liver as well as the spleen has become darker; **T1 – TE = 11.2 ms**: the liver and the spleen further lose their signal, the liver more than the spleen

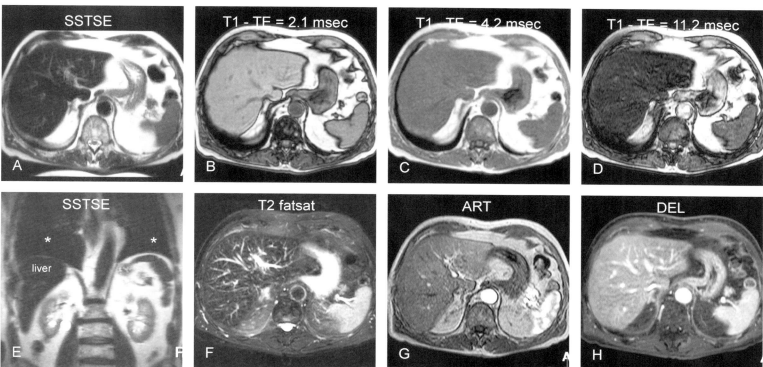

Fig. 81.2. Hemosiderosis, moderate to severe, MRI findings. A Axial SSTSE image (SSTSE): The liver is darker than usual (e.g., compared to muscle). **B** Axial T1 GRE image with a short TE (TE = 2.1 ms): The liver is brighter than the spleen, which is normal. **C** Axial T1 GRE image with a longer TE (TE = 4.2 ms): Both the liver and the spleen have become darker due to iron deposition. **D** Axial T1 GRE with a TE value of 11.2 ms: The liver and the spleen show further loss of signal, the liver more than the spleen, which confirms the iron deposition in both organs. **E** Coronal SSTSE image (SSTSE): The liver is almost as dark as the air in the lungs (*). **F** Axial fat-suppressed TSE image (T2 fatsat): The spleen appears much brighter than the liver; therefore, this sequence is less sensitive than the T1 GRE with a long TE of 11.2 ms. **G** Axial arterial phase image shows normal enhancement of the liver and the spleen without enhancing focal liver lesion. **H** Axial delayed phase image (DEL) shows homogeneous enhancement of the liver and the spleen

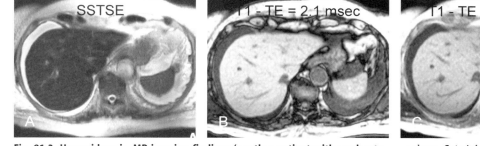 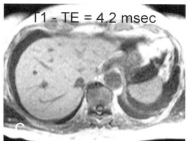 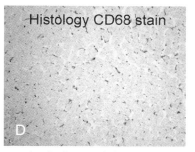

Fig. 81.3. Hemosiderosis, MR imaging findings (another patient with moderate iron deposition), and Kupffer cells at histology. A Axial SSTSE image (SSTSE): The liver is slightly darker than the spleen. The organs are surrounded by ascites. **B** Axial T1 image (TE = 2.1 ms): The liver is slightly brighter than the spleen. **C** Axial T1 GRE image (TE = 4.2 ms): The liver and the spleen have comparable signal intensity. **D** Photomicrograph shows the Kupffer cells aligned along the sinusoids. Kupffer cells store iron in hemosiderosis. CD68 stain, ×200

82 Hemochromatosis – Severe Type

Hereditary hemochromatosis (non-transfusional iron overload) is a common autosomal recessive disease that is characterized by an increase in the gastrointestinal absorption of iron, which can lead to deposits of iron in the liver, pancreas, heart, skin, and joints. Vital risks of hemochromatosis, such as cirrhosis and hepatocellular carcinoma, can be reduced by an early treatment which consists of repeated phlebotomies. Iron overload is often discovered at blood tests with an elevation of serum iron, transferrin saturation or ferritinemia or by doing family studies.

The diagnosis of hemochromatosis can be confirmed by genetic testing, with homozygosity for the Cys282Tyr mutation. MR imaging provides specific information concerning the presence of hemochromatosis and is very sensitive for any nodules in the liver. CT can demonstrate a non-specific increase in the density of the liver of >80 HU but cannot be used to assess or (semi)quantify the amount of iron in tissues. Many centers still consider liver biopsy and quantification of liver iron concentration by biochemical analysis as their gold standard for assessment of iron overload. Nevertheless, hepatic biopsy has associated risks as well as sampling variability, especially in cases of hepatic cirrhosis. MR imaging is a non-invasive method and may replace liver biopsy as a diagnostic test for the assessment of iron overload.

MR Imaging Findings

At MR imaging, primary hemochromatosis can be demonstrated with decreased signal intensity of the liver, pancreas, and the heart muscle on T2*-weighted fast spin-echo or GRE sequences with increasing values of TE. Because of the accumulation of iron in the parenchymal cells, the signal intensity of the spleen in hemochromatosis remains unchanged. In hemochromatosis, the amount of iron deposition is assessed qualitatively (mild, moderate, severe) by comparing the decrease of the signal intensity with increasing TE values as well as the involvement of the pancreas and myocardium. In mild to moderate cases, the pancreas and myocardium are less likely to be involved. Recent publications have shown that MR imaging is a very useful and non-invasive diagnostic tool that allows quantification of hepatic iron concentration at all possible levels of iron overload. Reproducibility of the technique however needs further assessment.

Literature

1. Siegelman ES, Mitchell DG, Outwater EK, et al. (1993) Idiopathic hemochromatosis: MR imaging findings in cirrhotic and precirrhotic patients. Radiology 188:637–641
2. Gandon Y, Guyader D, Heautot JF, et al. (1994) Hemochromatosis: diagnosis and quantification of liver iron with gradient-echo MR imaging. Radiology 193:533–538
3. Clark PR, St. Pierre TG (2000) Quantitative mapping of transverse relaxivity (1/T(2)) in hepatic iron overload: a single spin-echo imaging methodology. Magn Reson Imaging 18:431–438
4. Alustiza JM, Artetxe J, Castiella A, et al. (2004) MR quantification of hepatic iron concentration. Radiology 230:479–484

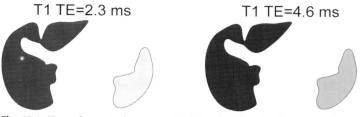

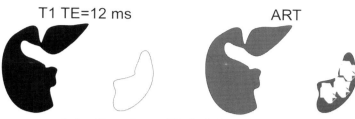

Fig. 82.1. Hemochromatosis, severe. T1 TE = 2.3 ms: the liver has abnormal low signal intensity; **T1 – TE = 4.6 ms:** the liver shows further decrease in signal without any decrease in signal of the spleen; **T1 – TE = 12 ms:** the liver becomes even darker. Due to longer TE, the inflow of unsaturated blood in the vessels causes high signal with pulsation artifacts. **ART:** the liver appears less darker (the TE of this sequence is set to a minimum of about 1.2 ms)

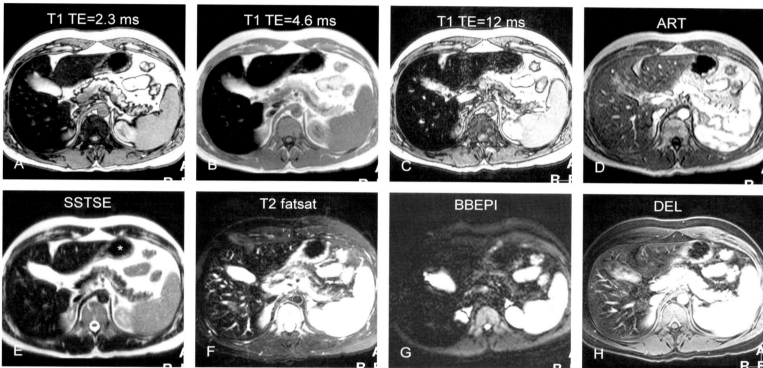

Fig. 82.2. Hemochromatosis, MRI findings. A Axial T1 with the short TE (T1 TE = 2.3 ms): The liver is abnormally dark (much darker than the spleen and the muscle) due to iron deposition within hepatocytes. **B** Axial T1 GRE with a longer TE (T1 TE = 4.6 ms): The liver becomes even darker. **C** Axial T1 GRE with a further increase in TE value (T1 TE = 12 ms): The liver shows further decrease in signal with high signal in the vessels caused by the inflow phenomenon which occurs with a longer TE. **D** Axial arterial T1 GRE image (ART): The liver is less dark due to a shorter TE (TE is set to a minimum to minimize susceptibility and inflow effects). **E** Axial SSTSE image (SSTSE): The liver is darker than normal [similar to the air in the stomach (*)]. **F** Axial fat-suppressed TSE image (T2 fatsat): The liver shows more susceptibility due to less refocusing pulses than in SSTSE. **G** Axial fat-suppressed black-blood EPI image (BBEPI): This sequence is extremely sensitive to the susceptibility of the iron and hence almost complete loss of signal in the liver. **H** Axial delayed phase image (DEL): This shows homogeneous enhancement

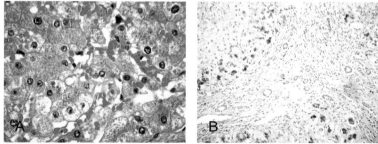

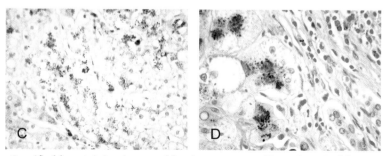

Fig. 82.3. Hemochromatosis, histology findings from different patients. A Photomicrograph shows a non-specific granular appearance of the cytoplasm of the hepatocytes due to iron deposition. H&E, ×400. **B** Photomicrograph: Specific blue staining is caused by the presence of iron. Iron Perls', ×40. **C, D** Photomicrographs: The blue staining within the cells suggests parenchymal iron deposition (hemochromatosis). Iron Perls', ×100 and ×200

83 Hemochromatosis with Solitary HCC

Hepatocellular carcinoma (HCC) is a well-known risk of hemochromatosis with or without cirrhosis. The presence of cirrhosis is not a prerequisite for the occurrence of HCC. Several reports indicate that iron may be involved in the pathogenesis of HCC. The risk of HCC appears to be related to the amount and duration of iron overload. Iron, which has been demonstrated to facilitate persistent hepatitis B or C infection, could also act as a co-factor in the pathogenesis of HCC in patients with hepatitis B or C and subsequent cirrhosis. Among the possible mechanisms by which iron could exert its carcinogenic potential, free radicals production responsible for heritable genetic alterations appears to be one of the most important, although the fibrogenic capability of iron, potentially leading to cirrhosis, cannot be underestimated. Iron overload is often discovered at blood tests with an elevation of serum iron, transferrin saturation or ferritinemia or by doing family studies.

MR Imaging Findings

The presence of the parenchymal iron basically reduces the signal intensity of the liver on T2- and T2*-weighted sequences, which makes the MR imaging an ideal imaging modality to detect HCC in the setting of hemochromatosis. Compared to the livers without iron deposition, HCC nodule appears much brighter on T2-weighted images. In addition, the effect of enhancement on the gradient echo images, which contain T2*-weighting, is much more obvious (Figs. 83.1, 83.2).

Pathology

On gross pathology, the liver with iron deposition appears brown and the HCC appears as a yellowish nodule. At histology, the presence of iron can be shown with Iron Perls staining. HCC may show glandular formation (Fig. 83.3).

Management

The risk for both cirrhosis as well as HCC can be reduced by repeated phlebotomies. The patients with HCC may receive palliative chemotherapy.

Literature

1. Lwakatare F, Hayashida Y, Yamashita Y. (2003) MR imaging of hepatocellular carcinoma arising in genetic hemochromatosis. Med Reson Med Sci 2:57–59
2. Fargion S, Mandelli C, Piperno A, et al. (1992) Survival and prognostic factors in 212 Italian patients with genetic hemochromatosis. Hepatology 15:655–659
3. Fargion S, Piperno A, Fracanzani AL, et al. (1991) Iron in the pathogenesis of hepatocellular carcinoma.Ital J Gastroenterol 23:584–588
4. Ito K, Mitchell DG, Gabata T, et al. (1999) Hepatocellular carcinoma: association with increased iron deposition in the cirrhotic liver at MR imaging. Radiology 212:235–240

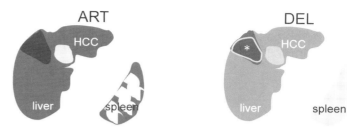

T2 fatsat   T1 in-phase   ART   DEL

Fig. 83.1. HCC, hemochromatosis, cirrhosis. T2 fatsat: HCC appears as a bright nodule within a dark liver due to iron deposition; the spleen has normal signal. The empty gallbladder fossa is caused by the atrophy of segment IV (*).

T1 in-phase: HCC appears bright due to unusually dark liver; **ART:** HCC shows heterogeneous enhancement; **DEL:** HCC remains visible due to the unusually dark liver. Gallbladder (*)

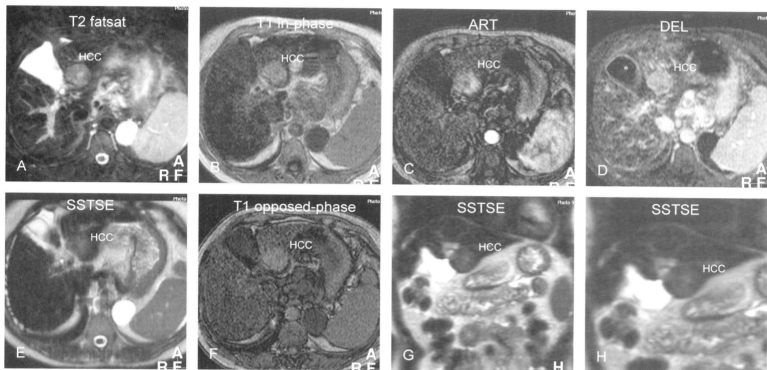

Fig. 83.2. HCC, hemochromatosis, cirrhotic liver, MRI findings. A Axial fat-suppressed TSE image (T2 fatsat): HCC appears as a bright nodule in an unusually dark liver due to the T2* effect of the iron within hepatocytes (hemochromatosis). The cirrhotic liver is irregular with atrophy of segment IV. The spleen has a normal signal intensity. **B** Axial in-phase image (T1 in-phase): HCC is bright in an unusually dark liver due to iron deposition. **C** Axial arterial phase image (ART): HCC shows heterogeneous enhance-

ment. **D** Axial delayed phase image (DEL): HCC shows some washout but remains visible due to the darker liver. Gallbladder (*). **E** Axial SSTSE image with a TE of 120 ms (T2 axial): HCC is slightly hyperintense to the liver. **F** Axial T1 opposed-phase image (T1 opposed-phase): HCC is slightly brighter than the liver. **G** Coronal SSTSE image (SSTSE): HCC is slightly brighter than the unusually dark liver. **H** A detailed view of the coronal SSTSE image (SSTSE): HCC is slightly brighter than the liver

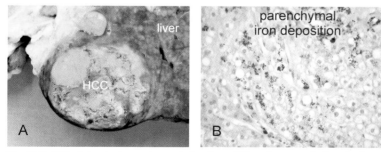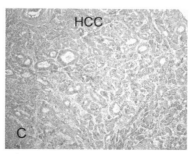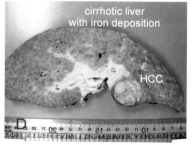

Fig. 83.3. HCC, cirrhosis, hemochromatosis, direct MR-explant correlation. A Photograph shows brown, cirrhotic liver with HCC. **B** Photomicrograph of another patient shows blue staining iron particles within hepatocytes (hemo-

chromatosis). Iron Perls', ×200. **C** Photomicrograph of the HCC shown above: large glandular structures indicate cholangiolar type of HCC, hence the bright T2 appearance. H&E, ×100. **D** Photograph of the explant with HCC

84 Hemochromatosis with Multiple HCC

Multiple hepatocellular carcinoma (HCC) may occur in the setting of hemochromatosis. Familiarity with this entity is important for radiologists because the lesions may mimic secondary liver lesions, especially if the signs of cirrhosis such as changed morphology of the liver include irregular contours, atrophy of certain segments (usually segment IV), central atrophy, and hypertrophy of other segments. Also the signal intensity on T2-weighted sequences as well as the enhancement patterns may be deceptive.

MR Imaging Findings

The presence of parenchymal as well as intralesional iron on T2*-weighted gradient echo [for instance, opposed- (short TE) and in-phase (long TE)] sequences is essential for the diagnosis of multiple HCC in the setting of hemochromatosis. Due to the longer TE value, the signal intensity of the lesions as well as the lesions on the in-phase images drops. Relatively high signal intensity of lesions on T2-weighted images and intense heterogeneous enhancement on the arterial phase images may resemble hypervascular liver metastases of, for instance, neuroendocrine origin (pancreatic as well as carcinoid) (Figs. 84.1, 84.2). Metastases do not show signal loss because they will be composed of non-hepatic tissue which will not contain iron.

Pathology

On gross pathology, the liver with iron deposition appears brown and the HCC appears as a yellowish nodule. At histology, HCC may show glandular formation (Fig. 84.3).

Literature

1. Lwakatare F, Hayashida Y, Yamashita Y (2003) MR imaging of hepatocellular carcinoma arising in genetic hemochromatosis. Med Reson Med Sci 2:57–59
2. Fargion S, Mandelli C, Piperno A, et al. (1992) Survival and prognostic factors in 212 Italian patients with genetic hemochromatosis. Hepatology 15:655–659
3. Fargion S, Piperno A, Fracanzani AL, et al. (1991) Iron in the pathogenesis of hepatocellular carcinoma. Ital J Gastroenterol 23:584–588
4. Ito K, Mitchell DG, Gabata T, et al. (1999) Hepatocellular carcinoma: association with increased iron deposition in the cirrhotic liver at MR imaging. Radiology 212:235–240

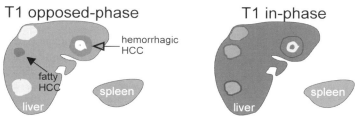
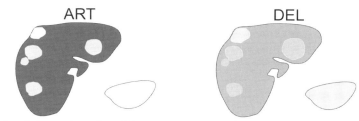

Fig. 84.1. HCC, hemochromatosis, cirrhosis. T1 opposed phase: HCCs predominantly appear brighter to the liver, though one is fatty (*solid arrow*) and another is hemorrhagic (*open arrow*); **T1 in-phase:** the liver has decreased in signal due to iron deposition; **ART:** HCCs predominantly show intense heterogeneous enhancement; **DEL:** HCCs show washout and become more heterogeneous with faint capsular enhancement

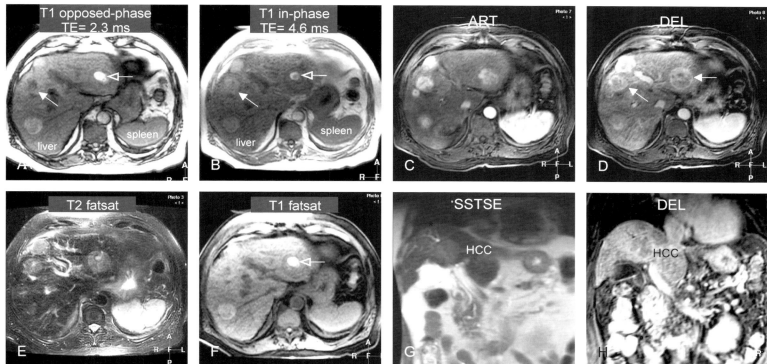

Fig. 84.2. HCC, hemochromatosis, cirrhosis, multiple lesions, MRI findings. A Axial T1 opposed-phase image (T1 opposed-phase): The liver is iso- to hypointense to the spleen. HCCs predominantly appear brighter, though one is fatty (*solid arrow*) and another hemorrhagic (*open arrow*). **B** Axial in-phase image (T1 in-phase): The liver becomes slightly darker with the longer TE with numerous small dark siderotic nodules (hemochromatosis). **C** Axial arterial phase image (ART): HCCs show intense heterogeneous enhancement. **D** Axial delayed phase image (DEL): HCCs show washout and become more heterogeneous with faint capsular enhancement. **E** Axial fat-suppressed T2-w image (T2 fatsat): HCCs are brighter in a dark liver. The spleen has normal size and signal. **F** Axial fat suppressed T1-w image (T1 fatsat): The hemorrhage within one of the HCCs (*open arrow*) remains bright, indicating that the high signal is not caused by a large amount of fat. **G** Axial SSTSE image (SSTSE): One of the HCCs is just visible. **H** Coronal delayed phase image (DEL): One of the HCCs is visible with washout

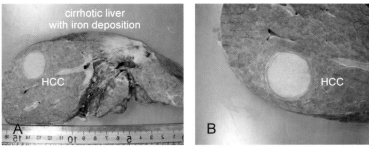
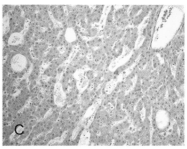
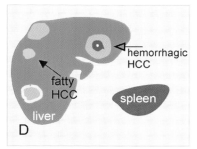

Fig. 84.3. HCC, hemochromatosis, cirrhosis, histopathology (from a different patient). A Photograph shows a siderotic and cirrhotic liver containing a large HCC. **B** A detailed photograph shows sharp margination of HCC to the liver. **C** Photomicrograph: large glandular structures indicate cholangiolar type of HCC, which appear bright on T2-weighted images. H&E, ×100. **D** Drawing explains the findings of MRI above

85 Thalassemia with Iron Deposition

Thalassemia major is one of the most prevalent diseases caused by an abnormality in a single gene (monogenic), which results in defects in hemoglobin production of alpha- or beta-chain and affects multiple organs. The worldwide birth rate of symptomatic globin disorders, including thalassemias, is no less than 240 per 100,000 births, of which 196 have sickle cell disease and 44 have thalassemias. Currently, over 2 million patients are transfusion-dependent worldwide, with the majority in Southeast Asia. Children with thalassemia usually become symptomatic between 6 and 12 months of age with symptoms of anemia and enlargement of the liver and spleen due to extramedullary hematopoiesis. Without iron chelation, iron-mediated free radical damage may cause hemosiderosis with liver fibrosis, myocardial damage with cardiac hypertrophy and dilatation (cardiomyopathy), skin pigmentation and endocrine failure including (bronze) diabetes mellitus, growth failure and delayed onset of puberty.

MR Imaging Findings

In thalassemia, as a result of blood transfusions, excessive iron deposition within Kupffer cells (hemosiderosis) may lead to secondary hemochromatosis (parenchymal) iron overload. Parenchymal iron deposition may also result from associated genetic hemochromatosis. At MR imaging signal loss may be observed both in organs with Kupffer cell (liver, spleen, bone marrow) and in parenchymal (pancreas and myocardium) compartments (Figs. 85.1 – 85.3).

Management

Management of the resulting anemia is through blood transfusions. Repeated transfusions result in excessive iron overload, removal of which is achieved through iron chelation therapy. Without blood transfusion, patients may develop massive bone marrow or extramedullary hematopoiesis, resulting in deformities of the facial bones, spinal cord compression and pathologic fractures. Desferrioxamine is the most widely used iron chelator.

Literature

1. Tyler PA, Madani G, Chaudhuri R, et al. (2006) The radiological appearances of thalassemia. Clin Radiol 61:40 – 52
2. Mazza P, Giua R, De Marco S, et al. (1995) Iron overload in thalassemia: comparative analysis of magnetic resonance imaging, serum ferritin and iron content of the liver. Haematologica 80:398 – 404
3. Papakonstantinou O, Kostaridou S, Maris T, et al. (1999) Quantification of liver iron overload by T2 quantitative magnetic resonance imaging in thalassemia: impact of chronic hepatitis C on measurements. J Pediatr Hematol Oncol 21:142 – 148
4. Rund D, Rachmilewitz E (2005) Beta-thalassemia. NEJM 353:1135 – 1146

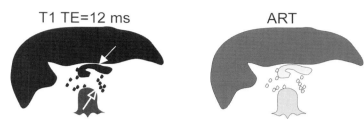
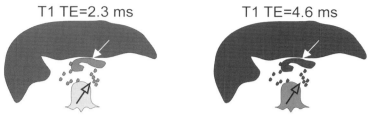

Fig. 85.1. Thalassemia with severe iron deposition. T1 TE = 2.3 ms: liver, pancreas (*solid arrow*) and lymph nodes (*open arrow*) have abnormally low signal intensity; T1 TE = 4.6 ms: note the loss of signal in the previously mentioned structures as well as in one of the vertebrae; T1 TE = 12 ms: there is further loss of signal; ART: the liver appears less dark (TE of this sequence is set to a minimum of about 1.2 ms) (patient had undergone splenectomy)

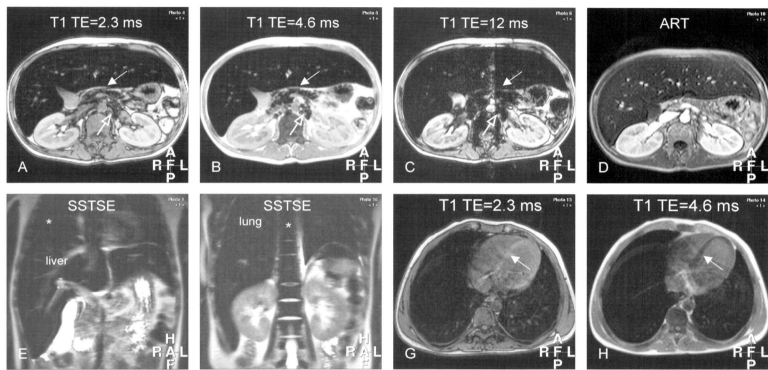

Fig. 85.2. Thalassemia with parenchymal and Kupffer cell iron deposition, severe, MRI findings. A Axial T1 with the short TE (T1 TE = 2.3 ms): The liver, pancreas (*solid arrow*), and lymph nodes (*open arrow*) are much darker than the muscle due to parenchymal and Kupffer cell iron deposition. **B** Axial T1 GRE with a longer TE (T1 TE = 4.6 ms): Also one of the vertebrae is darkened indicating involvement. **C** Axial T1 GRE with a longer TE (T1 TE = 12 ms) shows further decrease in signal. **D** Axial arterial image (ART): No enhancing nodules are present. **E** Coronal SSTSE image (SSTSE): The liver is as dark as the lung (*). **F** Coronal SSTSE image (SSTSE): The vertebra (*) is as dark as the lung. **G** and **H** Axial T1 with respectively the short (2.3 ms) and long TEs (4.6 ms) at the level of the heart: The myocardium shows loss of signal due to iron deposition (*arrows*)

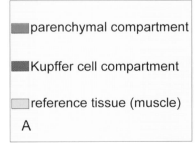
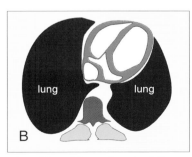
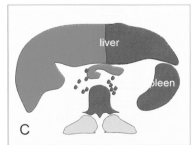
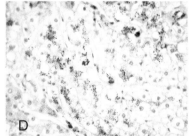

Fig. 85.3. Various compartments with iron deposition. A Legend to the following two drawings. **B** The drawing shows the myocardium (parenchymal) and the vertebra (Kupffer cells) compartments. **C** The drawing shows the liver (parenchyma as well as Kupffer cells), the vertebra, the lymph nodes, and the spleen (Kupffer cells), and the pancreas (parenchymal) compartments. **D** Photomicrograph of a different patient shows the parenchymal iron deposition in the liver. Iron Perls', ×100

Part IV

Vascular Liver Lesions

IV

86 Arterioportal Shunt I – Early Enhancing Lesion in a Cirrhotic Liver

Cirrhotic livers may contain various types of enhancing lesions and pseudolesions. In clinical practice with cirrhotic patients, however, we have sometimes encountered small nodular early enhancing hepatic lesions on arterial phase contrast-enhanced dynamic computed tomography (CT) or MRI that resembled hepatocellular carcinomas but disappeared or decreased in size during the clinical follow-up examinations. These lesions are considered to be nonneoplastic hypervascular pseudolesions caused by small arterioportal or other shunts including unknown causes and are often difficult to differentiate from hypervascular hepatocellular carcinomas (HCCs). Some reports indicate that single-level dynamic CT during hepatic arteriography and less invasive contrast-enhanced dynamic MRI with higher temporal resolution from early to late arterial phase may be helpful for differentiating the early enhancing lesions from HCC.

MR Imaging Findings

At MR imaging, the early enhancing lesions are typically small (a few millimeters) and visible in the arterial phase of the dynamic gadolinium-enhanced imaging, fading to isointensity in the delayed phase in most cases. On the maximum-intensity projection images, an enhanced arterial vessel may be seen coursing toward the area of an arterioportal shunt (Figs. 86.1–81.3A, B). Although delayed persistent enhancement has been described in the literature, any heterogeneity and signal abnormality on T2-weighted images as well as chemical shift imaging should be considered suspicious and warranting follow-up (Fig. 86.3C, D).

Differential Diagnosis

Dysplastic nodules and small HCCs may be distinguished from arterioportal shunt and pseudolesions (i.e., areas with non-specific transient increased enhancement) based on the appearance on the delayed phase as well as findings on other sequences. In ambiguous cases, follow-up MR imaging may facilitate distinction.

Literature

1. Ito K, Fujita T, Shimizu A, et al. (2004) Multiarterial phase dynamic MRI of small early enhancing hepatic lesions in cirrhosis or chronic hepatitis: differentiating between hypervascular hepatocellular carcinomas and pseudolesions AJR 183:699–705
2. Van den Bos IC, Hussain SM, Terkivatan T, et al. (2006) Step-wise carcinogenesis of hepatocellular carcinoma in the cirrhotic liver: demonstration on serial MR imaging. JMRI (in press)
3. Yu JS, Kim KW, Jeong MG, Lee JT, Yoo HS (2000) Nontumorous hepatic arterial-portal venous shunts: MR imaging findings. Radiology 217: 750–756
4. Ueda K, Matsui O, Kawamori Y, et al. (1998) Differentiation of hypervascular hepatic pseudolesions from hepatocellular carcinoma: value of single level dynamic CT during hepatic arteriography. JCAT 22:703–708

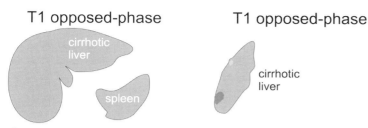

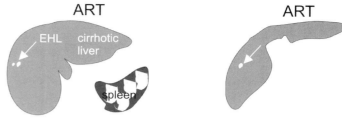

Fig. 86.1. Early enhancing lesion (EHL) in a cirrhotic liver, drawings. T1 opposed-phase: The liver shows morphologic signs of cirrhosis with enlarged spleen; **T1 opposed-phase:** (lower anatomic level) The liver shows signs of cirrhosis;

ART: at least two EHL's (*arrow*) are visible; **ART:** another EHL is visible at a lower anatomic level (*arrow*). (Follow-up MRI did not show any change or other signs of malignancy)

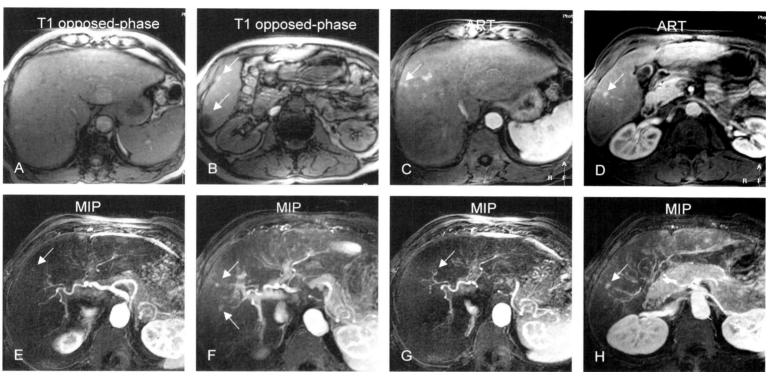

Fig. 86.2. Early enhancing lesion (EHL) in a cirrhotic liver, MRI findings. A Axial opposed-phase image (T1 opposed-phase): The liver shows several nodules and morphology of cirrhosis. **B** Axial opposed-phase image (T1 opposed-phase) at a lower anatomic level: The liver contains several nodules with variable signal intensity (*arrows*). **C** Axial arterial phase image (ART) shows the intensely enhancing EHLs (*arrow*). **D** Axial arterial phase image (ART) at a

lower anatomic level shows another EHL (*arrow*). **E–H** Maximum intensity projections (MIPs) based on the subtractions of the arterial and portal phases show several EHLs (*arrows*) with suggestion of arterioportal shunts. (Follow-up MR imaging during several months did not show any change or signs of malignancy)

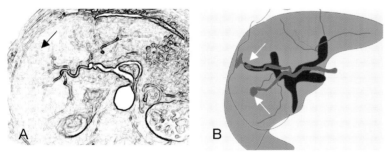

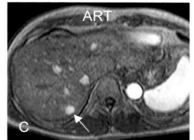

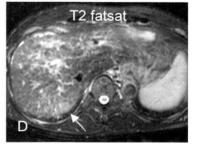

Fig. 86.3. EHLs in a cirrhotic liver, drawings (A, B); C, D show dysplastic nodule in another patient. A, B Drawings show the connection between the arteries and portal veins, suggesting arterioportal shunts. **C** Axial arterial phase (ART)

and **D** turbo spin echo (TSE) (T2 fatsat) images show an enhancing area (*arrow*) that is faintly hyperintense to the liver on the T2-weighted image (*arrow*). At follow-up MRI, this area developed into an HCC

87 Arterioportal Shunt II – Early Enhancing Lesion in a Non-Cirrhotic Liver

According to some authors, arterioportal (A-P) shunt is commonly associated with hepatocellular carcinoma and intrahepatic cholangiocarcinomas. However, congenital or acquired A-P shunt without any associated hepatic tumor may occur and cause difficulty in diagnosis on ultrasound (US) and CT. Particularly, on CT images the enhancing area of the liver may mimic a lesion. State-of-the-art MR imaging of the liver combines the information concerning the vascularity and soft tissue characteristics of the lesions, and can make a more confident diagnosis.

MR Imaging Findings

At MR imaging, A-P shunt is not visible on the T2-weighted and in-phase T1-weighted images. In a fatty liver, however, the area with the shunt may show fatty sparing on the opposed-phase images. After injection of gadolinium, the shunt may be visible as a small intensely enhancing lesion in the arterial phase, followed by a wedge-shaped enhancement of the surrounding parenchyma. In the delayed phase, the enhancing lesion and area fade to isointensity. In addition, other concurrent benign liver lesions may be seen (Figs. 87.1 – 87.3).

Differential Diagnosis

Any underlying or associated liver tumor such as cholangiocarcinomas or HCCs can be distinguished on MR imaging based on the tissue characteristics and enhancement patterns.

Literature

1. Routh WD, Keller FS, Cain WS, et al. (1992) Transcatheter embolization of a high-flow congenital intrahepatic arterial-portal venous malformation in an infant. J Pediatr Surg 27:511 – 514
2. Kitade M, Yoshiji H, Yarnao J, et al. (2005) Intrahepatic cholangiocarcinoma associated with central calcification and arterioportal shunt. Intern Med 44:825 – 828

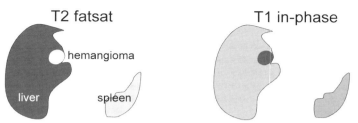 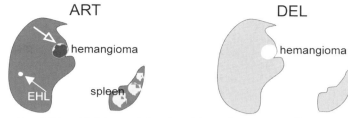

Fig. 87.1. Early enhancing lesion (EHL) and an hemangioma, drawings. T2 fatsat: at the site of EHL, no abnormality is visible; note an incidental bright hemangioma; **T1 in-phase**: the liver shows normal signal intensity; **ART**: EHL (*arrow*) is visible with faint peripheral nodular enhancement of hemangioma (*open arrow*); **DEL**: EHL is no longer visible; hemangioma shows homogeneous enhancement

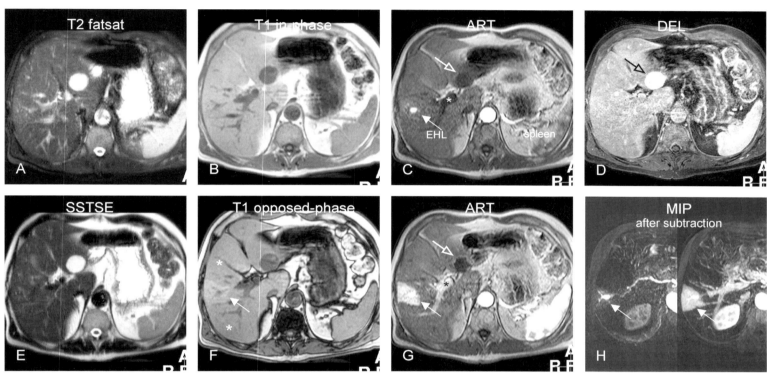

Fig. 87.2. Early enhancing lesion (EHL) and an hemangioma, MRI findings. A Axial fat-suppressed T2-w TSE image (T2 fatsat): the liver parenchyma is normal at the site of EHL. Hemangioma is hyperintense to the liver. **B** Axial in-phase GRE (T1 in-phase): The liver shows normal signal. **C** Axial early arterial phase image (ART) shows the intensely enhancing EHL (*arrow*) and faint peripheral nodular enhancement within hemangioma (*open arrow*); note that the portal vein has not yet enhanced (*). **D** Axial delayed phase image (DEL): EHL has disappeared and hemangioma shows homogeneous enhancement (*open arrow*). **E** Axial single-shot turbo spin echo image (SSTSE): hemangioma remains bright. **F** Axial opposed-phase image (T1 opposed-phase): Fatty infiltration (*) is present except around the area of the EHL. **G** Axial late arterial phase image (ART), with enhanced portal vein (*), shows wedge-shaped enhancement of the liver surrounding EHL. **H** MIP based on the subtractions of the early and late arterial phases strongly suggests an arterioportal shunt (*arrows*)

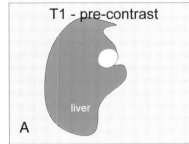 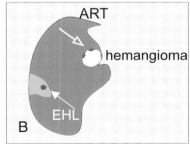 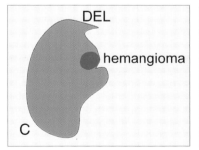 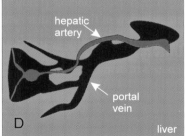

Fig. 87.3. EHL caused by arterioportal shunt and hemangioma, drawings. A Before contrast normal liver with an hemangioma is visible. **B** Arterial phase shows the EHL surrounded by an enhancing wedge-shaped area. **C** Delayed phase shows the enhanced hemangioma. **D** A composite drawing based on the subtraction images shows the connection between the arteries and portal veins, the most likely cause of the EHL (A-P shunt)

88 Budd-Chiari Syndrome I – Abnormal Enhancement and Intrahepatic Collaterals

Budd-Chiari syndrome (BCS) is a rare and potentially lethal condition related to the obstruction of the hepatic venous outflow tract. Women about 35 years of age are the most affected group. Heart failure and sinusoidal obstruction syndrome (formerly known as veno-occlusive disease) also impair hepatic venous outflow and share many features with BCS, but these are separate entities as causes and treatments differ. Thrombosis is the cause of primary BCS. As compared with pure hepatic vein thrombosis, inferior vena cava (IVC) thrombosis is more common in the Far East; it is more indolent and is complicated more commonly by hepatocellular carcinoma. Thus, the recently proposed distinction of primary hepatic vein thrombosis (true BCS) from primary IVC thrombosis (obliterative hepatocavopathy) is well suited for clinical and therapeutic objectives. However, etiologies are similar. In most studies, primary myeloproliferative disorders are found to be the leading cause of BCS. The blood outflow obstruction of the liver may result in liver congestion, portal hypertension, ischemic necrosis caused by sudden interruption of hepatic perfusion followed by fibrosis and liver failure, and ascites. Imaging evaluation of patients with suspected BCS may be critical, since the clinical presentation of this potentially fatal disease is often non-specific. The overall accuracy of US and CT for detecting hepatic venous thrombosis has been reported as approximately 70 % and 50 %, respectively.

MR Imaging Findings

Diagnostic percutaneous venography (may show spider web network pattern formed by the intrahepatic collaterals with incomplete occlusion of the hepatic veins) is invasive and obsolete in the era of state-of-the-art MR imaging. The diagnosis of primary BCS can be established when an obstructed hepatic outflow tract is shown in the absence of tumoral invasion or compression. MR imaging can show the parenchymal changes, the enhancement patterns in the arterial and delayed phases, and the intrahepatic collaterals, and can exclude any tumors with a high level of confidence (Figs. 88.1, 88.2). Ultrasound is an excellent modality for the evaluation of blood flow within hepatic vessels as well as after transjugular intrahepatic portosystemic shunt (TIPS) but does not provide an overview of the (vascular) anatomy (Fig. 88.3).

Differential Diagnosis and Management

These are discussed in the following two chapters.

Literature

1. Valla DC (2003) The diagnosis and management of the Budd-Chiari syndrome: consensus and controversies. Hepatology 38:793–803
2. Menon KV, Shah V, Karnath PS (2004) The Budd Chiari syndrome. NEJM 350:578–85
3. Noone TC, Semelka RC, Siegelman ES, Balci NC, Hussain SM, Mitchell DG (2000) Budd Chiari syndrome: spectrum of appearance of acute, subacute, and chronic magnetic resonance imaging. JMRI 11:44–50

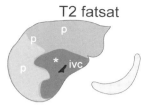

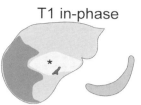

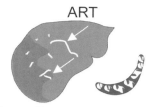

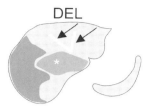

Fig. 88.1. Budd-Chiari syndrome, drawings. T2 fatsat: the liver shows peripheral atrophy (*p*) with high signal and central hypertrophy (*) with normal low signal (*ivc* = inferior vena cava); **T1 in-phase:** note almost normal high signal centrally (*); **ART:** intrahepatic abnormal arteries (intrahepatic collaterals) are visible (*arrows*); **DEL:** intrahepatic abnormal veins (intrahepatic collaterals) are visible (*arrows*); note peripheral increased enhancement

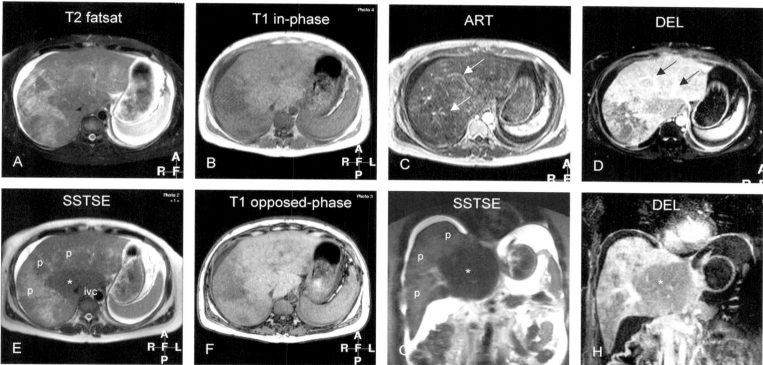

Fig. 88.2. Budd-Chiari syndrome, MRI findings. A Axial fat-saturated TSE image (T2 fatsat): The liver shows central hypertrophy with normal low signal and atrophy with abnormally high signal. Note the ascites. **B** Axial in-phase image (T1 fatsat): Central part shows normal signal. **C** Axial arterial phase 2D GRE image (ART): Multiple intrahepatic arterial collaterals are visible (*arrows*) with heterogeneous parenchymal enhancement. **D** Axial delayed phase image (DEL): Multiple intrahepatic venous collaterals are visible (*arrows*) with peripheral heterogeneous enhancement. **E** Axial SSTSE (SSTSE): The liver shows central hypertrophy with normal low signal (*) and peripheral atrophy with abnormally high signal (*p*) (*ivc* = inferior vena cava). **F** Axial opposed-phase image (T1 opposed-phase): There is no fatty infiltration. **G** Coronal SSTSE (SSTSE): Note the central hypertrophy with low signal (*) and peripheral atrophy with abnormal signal (*p*). **H** Coronal delayed phase image (DEL): The central part shows less enhancement (*) than the periphery

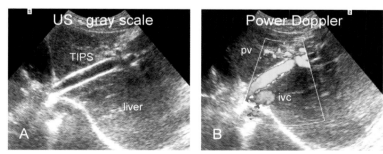

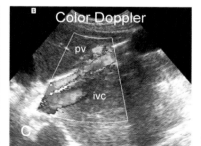

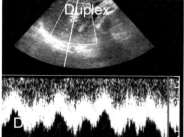

Fig. 88.3. Budd-Chiari syndrome, TIPS evaluation with US in a different patient. A Ultrasound (*gray scale*) shows the TIPS with flow void indicating its patency. **B** Power Doppler shows flow within the TIPS, inferior vena cava (*ivc*), and the portal vein (*pv*). **C** Color Doppler shows flow within the TIPS that connects the *ivc* and *pv*. **D** Duplex measures the flow within TIPS (4 – 6 cm/s). The variability is caused by the respiration and the changing intrathoracic pressure

89 Budd-Chiari Syndrome II – Gradual Deformation of the Liver

The natural history of Budd-Chiari syndrome (BCS) is poorly understood as most patients have received some form of treatment. On anticoagulation alone, some patients with an acute presentation may recover spontaneously, at least partially, as judged from improved liver function tests, disappearance or easy control of ascites, and improvement of the appearance of the liver at imaging. However, aggravation may occur unpredictably in the form of ascites becoming refractory, wasting, recurrent gastrointestinal bleeding, or development of liver failure. The risk for aggravation and death generally has been described as highest within the first 1–2 years after diagnosis, whereas patients surviving beyond 2 years have an excellent 10-year survival rate. The extent of fibrosis, congestion, or necrosis is associated with a poor outcome and indicates severity of the disease. Due to the persistent chronic and superimposed acute changes, the liver may show complex findings at imaging. Eventually, these changes may be reflected in the peculiar morphology of the liver that is often observed in patients with longstanding BCS.

MR Imaging Findings

At MR imaging, acute, subacute, and chronic changes may be seen concurrently. In acute BCS, T1-weighted imaging reveals decreased signal intensity within the liver periphery and preservation of more normal, higher signal intensity within the caudate lobe. On T2-weighted images, the liver periphery is heterogeneously increased in signal intensity, and the caudate lobe is more homogeneous, and of normal, lower signal intensity. Dynamic post-gadolinium imaging reveals increased enhancement within the caudate lobe on the immediate post-gadolinium images, which persists on delayed images. Caudate lobe may be enlarged. In subacute and chronic BCS, caudate lobe may show further increase in size with preserved signal intensity (Figs. 89.1, 89.2). Over time, gradual deformation of the liver often occurs (Fig. 89.3).

Differential Diagnosis

Similar morphologic changes of the liver with underlying fibrosis and cirrhosis with the development of (regenerative) nodules may result from other etiologies.

Management

See next chapter.

Literature

1. Valla DC (2003) The diagnosis and management of the Budd-Chiari syndrome: consensus and controversies. Hepatology 38:793–803
2. Menon KV, Shah V, Karnath PS (2004) The Budd Chiari syndrome. NEJM 350:578–85
3. Noone TC, Semelka RC, Siegelman ES, Balci NC, Hussain SM, Mitchell DG (2000) Budd Chiari syndrome: spectrum of appearance of acute, subacute, and chronic magnetic resonance imaging. JMRI 11:44–50

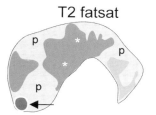

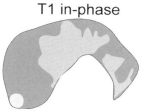

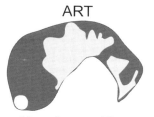

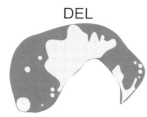

Fig. 89.1. Budd-Chiari syndrome, drawings. T2 fatsat: The liver (with abnormal shape) shows peripheral atrophy (*p*) with heterogeneous signal, central hypertrophy (*), and a dark nodule (*arrow*); **T1 in-phase:** the nodule is bright, comparable to the central liver; **ART:** the nodule shows increased enhancement; **DEL:** the central liver and several nodules remain homogeneously enhanced without any washout

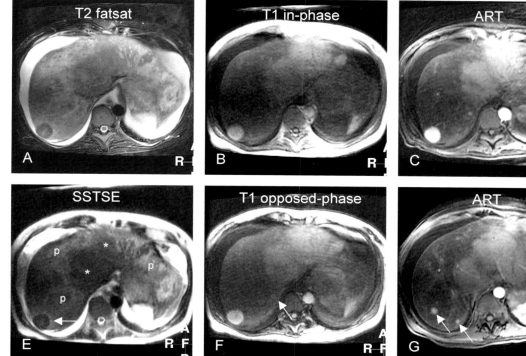

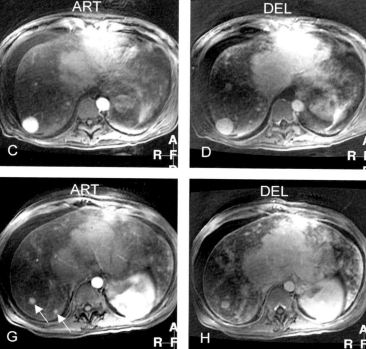

Fig. 89.2. Budd-Chiari syndrome, MRI findings. A Axial fat-saturated TSE image (T2 fatsat): The liver shows central hypertrophy and a nodule with lower signal, and peripheral atrophy with abnormally high signal. Note the ascites. **B** Axial in-phase image (T1 in-phase): The central part and the nodule show almost normal signal. **C** Axial arterial phase GRE image (ART): The nodule shows intense homogeneous enhancement. **D** Axial delayed phase GRE image (DEL): The enhanced structures show no washout of contrast indicating their benign nature. **E** Axial SSTSE (SSTSE): The liver shows central hypertrophy with lower signal (*) and peripheral atrophy with abnormally high signal (*p*). Note that the nodule (*arrow*) is similar in signal to the central liver. **F** Axial opposed-phase image (T1 opposed-phase): An additional smaller nodule is visible (*arrow*). **G** Axial arterial phase image at a lower level (ART): More enhancing areas and nodules are visible (*arrows*). **H** Axial delayed phase image at a lower level (DEL): The enhanced nodules and areas retain their contrast

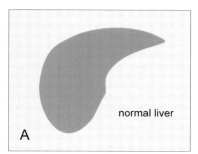

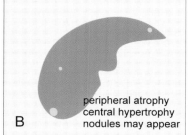

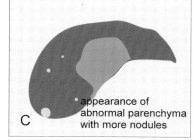

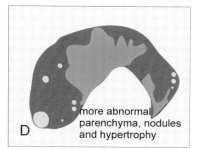

Fig. 89.3. Budd-Chiari syndrome, changing liver morphology. A Drawing illustrates a normal liver. **B** Drawing shows the early changes of Budd-Chiari with peripheral atrophy and central (mainly segment I and a part of segments VI and VII) hypertrophy. Nodules may also appear. **C** Drawing illustrates progressive changes most likely due to persistent vascular abnormalities. **D** Drawing illustrates further hypertrophy, increased abnormal parenchyma and appearance of more (regenerative) nodules

90 Budd-Chiari Syndrome III – Nodules Mimicking Malignancy

Hepatocellular carcinoma (HCC) has been described occasionally in patients with Budd-Chiari syndrome, mostly in those with long-standing obstruction of the IVC. Differential diagnosis of regenerative nodules from HCC at imaging is almost impossible at US and CT. Therefore, MR imaging should be performed including T2-weighted and dynamic contrast-enhanced sequences to distinguish Budd-Chiari nodules from HCC.

MR Imaging Findings

The nodules are isointense to the liver on T1- and T2-weighted images and show homogeneous intense arterial enhancement with fading to isointensity on later phases (Figs. 90.1, 90.2). Unlike multifocal HCC, the lesions do not have high signal on T2 or show washout or capsular enhancement on the delayed phase images.

Differential Diagnosis

Budd-Chiari nodules are currently considered as nodular parenchymal hyperplasia likely caused by local circulatory disturbances; histologically, nodules show similarities with focal nodular hyperplasia, regenerative nodules and hepatocellular adenoma. Budd-Chiari nodules may easily be recognized based on their appearance in the presence of multiple intrahepatic collaterals and typical hepatic morphologic changes (Fig. 90.3).

Management of Budd-Chiari syndrome

TIPS and liver transplantation (LTX) are recognized methods of treatment. TIPS is recommended in patients with preserved hepatic function and architecture. In the presence of fulminant forms, cirrhosis, or defined hepatic metabolic defects (e.g., protein C or protein S deficiency), LTX is the treatment of choice. In most cases of BCS, a thrombophilic disorder can be identified. However, it is important to note that postoperative vascular thrombosis has been identified in patients with BCS who do not have a definable hypercoagulable predisposition. Therefore, initiate intravenous heparin therapy in all patients with BCS immediately after surgery, and continue lifelong anticoagulation with coumadin.

Literature

1. Brancatelli G, Federle MP, Grazioli L, et al. (2002) Benign regenerative nodules in Budd Chiari syndrome and other vascular disorders of the liver: radiologic-pathologic and clinical correlation. Radiographics 22:847–62
2. Klein AS, Molmenti EP (2003) Surgical treatment of Budd-Chiari syndrome. Liver Transpl 9:891–896
3. Wanless IR (1994) Regenerative nodules in Budd-Chiari syndrome. Hepatology 19:1391
4. Ibarrola C, Castellano VM, Colina F (2004) Focal hyperplastic hepatocellular nodules in hepatic venous outflow obstruction: a clinicopathological study of four patients and 24 nodules. Histopathology 44:172–179

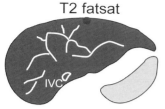
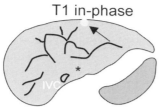
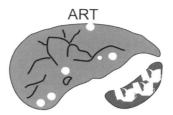
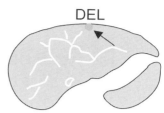

T2 fatsat   T1 in-phase   ART   DEL

Fig. 90.1. Budd-Chiari syndrome, drawings. T2 fatsat: multiple intrahepatic collaterals are visible that make no connection to the inferior vena cava (*IVC*); **T1 in-phase**: note slight hypertrophy of the left liver including seg-

ment I (*) as well as a bright nodule (*arrow*); **ART**: multiple nodules show intense homogeneous enhancement; **DEL**: the nodules fade to isointensity, except the nodule visible before contrast (*arrow*)

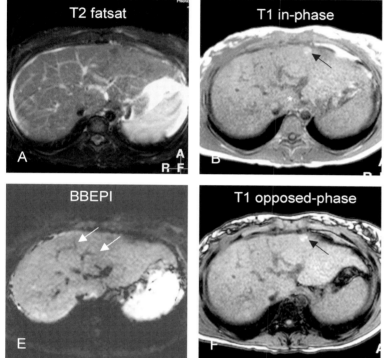
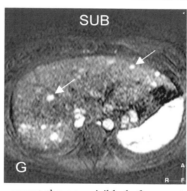
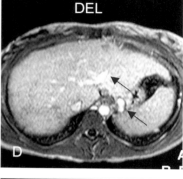
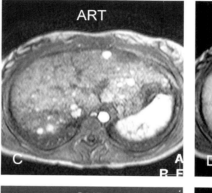
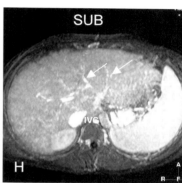

Fig. 90.2. Budd-Chiari syndrome with nodules, MRI findings. A Axial fat-saturated T2-w TSE image (T2 fatsat): The liver shows increased signal with multiple abnormal vessels (collaterals) and ascites. **B** Axial in-phase GRE image (T1 in-phase): Note a bright nodule (*arrow*), and the slight hypertrophy of the left liver and segment I (*). **C** Axial arterial phase post-Gd GRE image (ART): Multiple nodules show intense homogeneous enhancement throughout the liver. **D** Axial delayed phase GRE image (DEL): All nodules,

except the one visible before contrast, fade to isointensity. Note the enhanced intra- and extrahepatic collaterals (*arrows*). **E** Axial T2-w black-blood echoplanar image (BBEPI): The intrahepatic collaterals show signal void indicating flow (*arrows*). **F** Axial opposed-phase image (T1 opposed-phase): The nodule contains no fat (*arrow*). **G** A subtraction of the arterial phase (SUB) shows the enhanced nodules (*arrows*). **H** A subtraction of the venous phase (SUB) shows the intrahepatic collaterals (*arrows*)

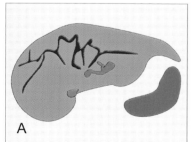
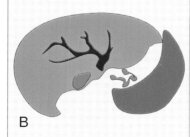
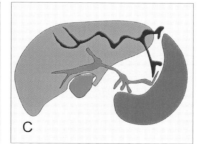
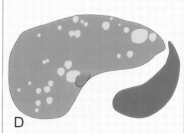

Fig. 90.3. Budd-Chiari syndrome, a spectrum of findings. A Drawing illustrates abnormal intrahepatic venous (*dark blue*) and portal (*pink*) vessels. **B** Drawing at a different level shows venous (*dark blue*) collaterals that make no connection to the inferior vena cava (*light blue*). Note also the extrahepatic

collaterals (*green*). **C** Drawing shows that the intrahepatic vessels connect to extrahepatic vessels to facilitate drainage and to lower the portal pressure. **D** Multiple Budd-Chiari nodules (most likely a form of regenerative nodules)

91 Hereditary Hemorrhagic Telangiectasia or Rendu-Osler-Weber Disease

Hereditary hemorrhagic telangiectasia (HHT) is an autosomal dominant disorder characterized by angiodysplastic lesions [telangiectases and arteriovenous (AV) malformations] that affect many organs. Liver involvement in patients with this disease has not been fully characterized and may occur in up to 30%. However, a few patients with liver abnormalities may be symptomatic with high-output heart failure (elevated cardiac output and an elevated pulmonary-capillary wedge pressure), portal hypertension (elevated hepatic sinusoidal pressure, gastroesophageal varices, with or without ascites), and biliary disease. The liver has a unique vascular supply. Blood enters the liver from two sources, the portal vein and the hepatic artery, merging at the level of the hepatic sinusoids and exiting through the hepatic veins. In patients with HHT, liver involvement predominantly results in shunting from the hepatic artery to the hepatic veins. Patients may eventually develop cirrhosis. The biliary tree obtains its blood supply from the peribiliary plexus that arises from the hepatic artery. AV shunts may cause hypoperfusion of the peribiliary plexus and ischemic necrosis of bile ducts, or both, with the subsequent development of a biliary stricture.

MR Imaging Findings

At MR imaging, saccular dilatations of the intrahepatic bile ducts can be evaluated using magnetic resonance cholangiopancreatography (MRCP).

Typical telangiectases and AV malformations are particularly visible on the dynamic contrast-enhanced images as numerous curvilinear subcapsular and parenchymal vessels which form connections between the arteries and the veins (Figs. 91.1, 91.2). Some of these vessels may be large. US can show abnormal vessels. CT and particularly digital subtraction angiography (DSA) can be used to visualize the hepatic abnormalities including the AV shunts (Fig. 91.3).

Differential Diagnosis

Saccular dilatations and stenoses of the bile ducts may mimic Caroli's disease and primary sclerosing cholangitis.

Management

Liver biopsy should be avoided because it is risky and does not contribute to the management. *Hepatic artery embolization* or ligation has been performed and may relieve some symptoms but it may also cause hepatic or biliary necrosis, or both, and should therefore be used only under special circumstances. *Liver transplantation* has been performed by some with good results.

Literature

1. Garcia-Tsao G, Korzenik JR, Young L, et al. (2000) Liver disease in patients with hereditary hemorrhagic telangiectasia. NEJM 343:931–936
2. Stabile Ianora AA, Memeo M, Sabba C, et al. (2004) Hereditary hemorrhagic telangiectasia: MDCT assessment of hepatic involvement. Radiology 230:250–259
3. Chavan A, Caselitz M, Gratz KF, et al. (2004) Hepatic artery embolization for treatment of patients with HHT and symptomatic hepatic vascular malformations. Eur Radiol 14:2079–2085

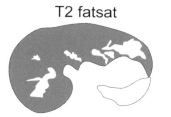

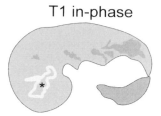

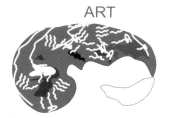

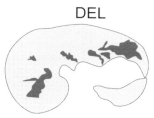

T2 fatsat   T1 in-phase   ART   DEL

Fig. 91.1. Hereditary hemorrhagic teleangiectasia (HHT) of the liver, drawings. T2 fatsat: saccular dilatations of the intrahepatic bile ducts are present; T1 in-phase: dilated ducts (*) with high signal indicate cholestasis; ART: mul-

tiple intrahepatic and subcapsular angioplastic lesions, including arteriovenous malformations and angiectasia, are enhanced; DEL: the liver shows homogeneous enhancement

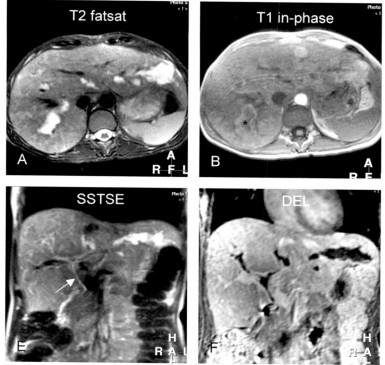

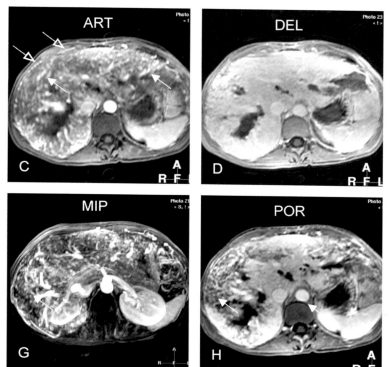

Fig. 91.2. Hereditary hemorrhagic teleangiectasia (HHT; also called Rendu-Osler-Weber disease) of the liver, MRI findings. A Axial TSE image (T2 fatsat): irregular and saccular dilatations of the intrahepatic bile ducts are most likely caused by ischemia. **B** Axial in-phase image (T1 in-phase): one of the dilated ducts shows high signal due to cholestasis (*). **C** Axial arterial phase image (ART): Multiple intrahepatic (*solid arrow*) and subcapsular (*open arrows*) angioplastic lesions, including arteriovenous malformations and angiecta-

sia, are enhanced. **D** Axial delayed phase image (DEL): The liver shows homogeneous enhancement. **E** Coronal SSTSE image (SSTSE): The common bile duct is normal (*arrow*). **F** Coronal delayed phase image (DEL): Unenhanced bile ducts correlate well with the previous image. **G** MIP of the arterial phase shows an overview of the vascular abnormalities. **H** Axial portal phase image (POR) shows large areas of the liver with incomplete enhancement due to shunting

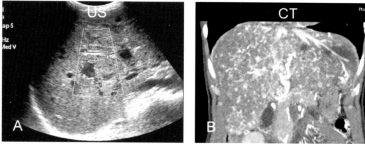

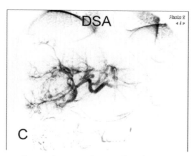

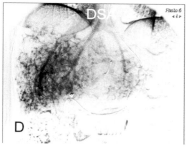

Fig. 91.3. Hereditary hemorrhagic teleangiectasia (HHT; also called Rendu-Osler-Weber disease) of the liver, US, CT, and DSA correlation. A US showed non-specific dilated bile ducts and increased color Doppler signal. **B** CT (coronal reformat) shows patchy enhancement of the vascular abnormalities. **C** Digital

subtraction angiography (DSA) in the early phase shows the angiectasia. **D** DSA in the later phase shows patchy enhancement caused by numerous arteriovenous shunts

Part V

Biliary Tree Abnormalities

92 Caroli's Disease I – Intrahepatic with Segmental Changes

Caroli's disease is an autosomal recessive disorder comprising communicating cavernous ectasia of the intrahepatic bile ducts. The disease is considered among the ductal plate abnormalities that occur at different levels in the developing biliary tree, leading to several clinicopathologic entities. The abnormalities can be present at the level of the large ducts (Caroli's disease), small ducts (congenital hepatic fibrosis), or both (congenital hepatic fibrosis with Caroli's disease, also called Caroli's syndrome). Clinically, the entity is divided as follows: type I (Caroli's disease) that is rare and is characterized by recurrent episodes of cholangitis, and type II (Caroli's disease associated with fibrosis) that is more frequent and is characterized by fibrosis and portal hypertension. Ultrasound (US) and computed tomography (CT) can show the multiple intrahepatic cysts in close relation to the biliary system. They fail however to actually demonstrate the communication between the two, which is important in distinguishing Caroli's disease from polycystic liver disease or multiple abscesses. Also at endoscopic retrograde cholangiopancreatography (ERCP) and cholangiography, it may difficult to get an overview of the entire biliary tree. MR imaging provides a better view of the biliary as well as the parenchymal system non-invasively.

MR Imaging Findings

T2-weighted and magnetic resonance cholangiopancreatography (MRCP) sequences show multiple saccular dilatations of the intrahepatic bile ducts. The abnormalities may be segmental with increased signal of the parenchyma on the pre-contrast T1-weighted sequences, likely due to biliary stasis. The abnormal parenchyma may show diffuse increased periportal enhancement in the arterial phase, fading to isointensity in the delayed phase. This may indicate inflammation. On the delayed phase imaging, the unenhanced bile ducts provide another possibility to assess for communicating cysts (Figs. 92.1, 92.2).

Pathology

Gross pathology and histology of Caroli's disease are characterized by the saccular dilatation of the biliary tree with or without fibrosis, and stasis of bile duct. Periductal inflammation and fibrosis are often present in long-standing disease (Fig. 92.3).

Literature

1. Levy AD, Rohrmann CA Jr, Murakata LA, et al. (2002) Caroli's disease. AJR 179:1053–1057
2. Desmet VJ (1992) Congenital diseases of intrahepatic bile ducts: variations on the theme „ductal plate malformation." Hepatology 16:1069–1083
3. Caroli J, Soupault R, Kossakowski J, Plocker L, Paradowska M (1958) La dilatation polykystique congénitale des voies biliaires intrahépatiques: essai de classification. Sem Hop Paris 34:128–135

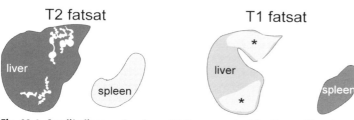
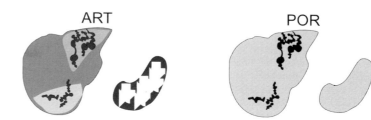

Fig. 92.1. Caroli's disease, drawings. T2 fatsat: typical fusiform dilatations are present in the left and right liver; **T1 fatsat:** (at a different anatomic level) affected areas show increased signal due to cholestasis (*); **ART:** increased enhancement around the dilated ducts is probably caused by cholangitis; **POR:** the enhanced areas become isointense confirming the benign nature of the increased arterial enhancement

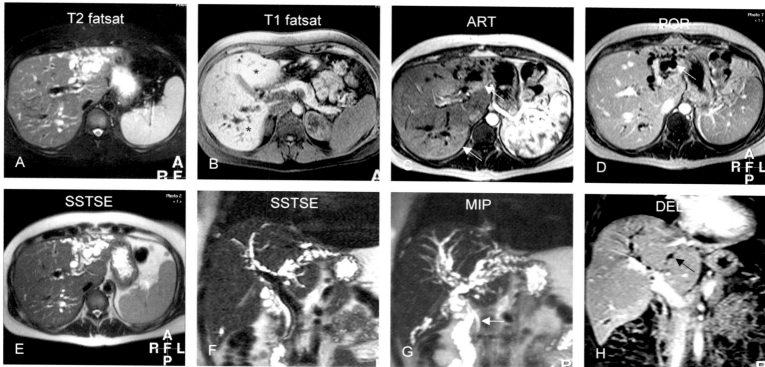

Fig. 92.2. Caroli's disease, typical MRI findings. A Axial fat-suppressed T2-w TSE image (T2 fatsat): Typical fusiform dilatations of the bile ducts are visible in the left and the right liver, with atrophy on the left side. **B** Axial fat-suppressed T1-w image at a lower anatomic level (T1 fatsat): Increased signal of the liver parenchyma is probably caused by cholestasis (*). **C** Axial arterial phase image (ART): Increased enhancement around the dilated ducts is most likely caused by cholangitis (*arrows*). **D** Axial portal phase image (POR): The enhanced areas become isointense indicating their benign na-

ture. Note the non-enhancing dilated bile ducts (*arrow*). **E** Axial single-shot turbo spin echo image (SSTSE): The dilated ducts can be followed up to the subcapsular region of the liver. **F** Coronal SSTSE image (SSTSE): Typical dilatations of the bile ducts are visible. **G** Maximum intensity projection of the SSTSE (MIP): The full extent of the affected bile ducts is visible with sparing of the common bile duct (*arrow*). **H** Coronal delayed phase image (DEL): The fusiform dilated ducts are well visible (*arrow*)

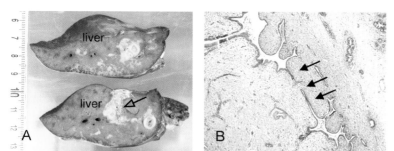
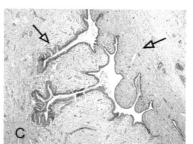
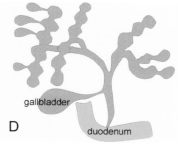

Fig. 92.3. Caroli's disease, pathology (explant of another patient with long-standing disease). A Photograph of the explant shows a greenish liver due to cholestasis. The bile ducts are surrounded by fibrosis (*open arrow*). **B, C** Photomicrographs show typical fusiform dilatations and narrowing of the bile ducts (*arrows*), which are surrounded by inflammatory cells (*open arrows*). H&E, × 100. **D** A drawing (based on a Caroli's original drawing) shows typical fusiform dilatations of the biliary tree

93 Caroli's Disease II – Involvement of the Liver and Kidneys

Caroli's disease is a form of congenital (with likely autosomal recessive inheritance) dilatation of intrahepatic bile ducts. It usually manifests in childhood. The association of Caroli's disease with extrahepatic bile duct dilatation may be present in up to 21 % of patients. Repeated bouts of cholangitis, stone formation, and stone passage may explain extrahepatic duct dilatation in some patients with Caroli's disease or Caroli's syndrome. Caroli's disease may also occur in association with cysts in the kidneys. In such cases, Caroli's disease should be distinguished from adult polycystic liver and kidney disease. Cholangiocarcinoma is a well-known complication of long-standing Caroli's disease. Since the original description by Caroli et al. in 1958, a number of case reports and small series have appeared in the radiology literature describing the cholangiographic, sonographic, CT, and MR imaging features of the disease.

MR Imaging Findings

On T2-weighted images, isolated hyperintense cystic lesions may be present as part of Caroli's disease. Occasionally, the comma-shaped appearance of such cystic liver lesions may suggest biliary connection. MRCP, however, allows the evaluation of the full extent of the disease. In addition, both kidneys may show cystic lesions as well. Compared to pathology, MR imaging allows the assessment of multiple organs in a single study (Figs. 93.1–93.3).

Differential Diagnosis

This includes primary sclerosing cholangitis (long stenoses and dilatations; 70 % have ulcerative colitis), recurrent pyogenic cholangitis, polycystic liver disease, a choledochal cyst, biliary papillomatosis, and (occasionally) obstructive biliary dilatation.

Management

This form has a very unfavorable prognosis and treatment consists of segmental liver resection or liver transplantation.

Literature

1. Mortele et al. (2001) Cystic focal liver lesions in the adult. Radiographics 21:895–910
2. Krause et al. (2002) MRI for evaluation of congenital bile duct abnormalities. JCAT 26:541–552
3. Desmet VJ (1992) Congenital diseases of intrahepatic bile ducts: variations on the theme „ductal plate malformation." Hepatology 16:1069–1083
4. Caroli J, Soupault R, Kossakowski J, Plocker L, Paradowska M (1958) La dilatation polykystique congénitale des voies biliaires intrahépatiques: essai de classification. Sem Hop Paris 34:128–135
5. Todani T, Watanabe Y, Narusue M, et al. (1977) Congenital bile duct cysts: classification, operative procedures, and review of thirty-seven cases including cancer arising from choledochal cyst. Am J Surg 134:263–269

T2 fatsat   T1 opposed-phase   ART   DEL

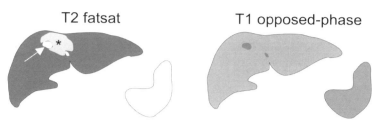

Fig. 93.1. Caroli's disease, drawings. T2 fatsat: cyst-like abnormality (*arrow*) is surrounded by tissue with high signal (*); **T1 opposed-phase:** no tissue abnormalities are visible; **ART:** local increased enhancement around the dilat-

ed ducts is probably caused by cholangitis (*); **DEL:** the enhanced area remains visible without getting heterogeneous, suggesting a benign lesion (*)

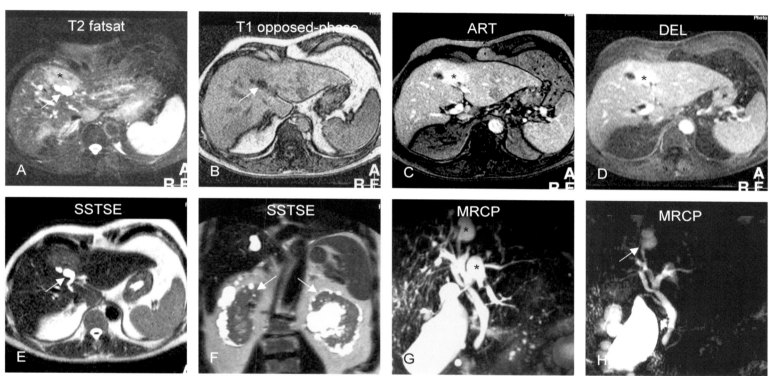

Fig. 93.2. Caroli's disease, liver and kidney involvement, MRI findings. A Axial fat-suppressed T2-w TSE image (T2 fatsat): Cyst-like dilated bile ducts (*arrow*) are surrounded by an area of the liver with increased signal intensity (*). **B** Axial opposed-phase T1-w image (T1 opposed-phase): Dilated bile duct (*arrow*) is visible without parenchymal abnormalities. The area with high signal on T2 has almost normal signal on T1. **C** Axial arterial phase image (ART): Increased enhancement around the dilated ducts is most likely

caused by cholangitis (*). **D** Axial delayed phase image (DEL) shows persistent enhancement without signs of washout of contrast (*). **E** Axial single-shot turbo spin-echo (SSTSE) shows typical comma-shaped dilated bile duct (*arrow*). **F** Coronal SSTSE image (SSTSE) shows cystic changes in both kidneys (*arrows*). **G** MRCP provides an overview of the dilated intrahepatic bile ducts (*) as well as the gallbladder (GB). **H** MRCP from another angle shows the cyst-like structures connected to the bile ducts (*arrow*)

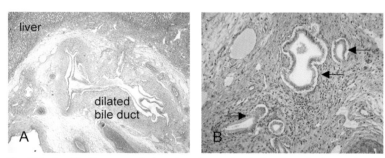
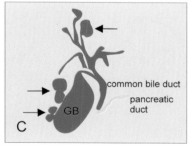
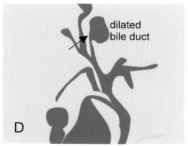

Fig. 93.3. Caroli's disease, pathology (another patient), drawings. A Photomicrograph shows dilated intrahepatic bile ducts surrounded by fibrosis and inflammation. H&E, × 100. **B** Photomicrograph shows typical fusiform dilatations of several bile ducts (*arrows*). H&E, × 200. **C** Drawing (based on

MRCP) shows typical dilated intrahepatic bile ducts (*arrows*) (*GB* = gallbladder). **D** A detailed view of the drawing shows the cyst-like dilatation with its narrow connection to the biliary tree (*arrow*)

94 Cholelithiasis (Gallstones)

Cholelithiasis (gallstone disease) remains one of the most common medical problems leading to surgical intervention. Gallstones represent a polygenic disorder that affects more than 30,000,000 (10%) Americans and results in more than 750,000 cholecystectomies in the United States annually. Risk factors include age, gender, race, parity, obesity, and diabetes. A family history of gallstones also has been identified as a risk factor, suggesting that genetics play a role in gallstone formation. Genetic factors are responsible in at least 30% of cases of symptomatic gallstone disease. Approximately three-fourths of the patients with gallstones in the United States have stones that are composed primarily of cholesterol. The pathogenesis of cholesterol gallstones is known to be multifactorial. Approximately 35% of patients with gallstones develop complications or recurrent symptoms leading to cholecystectomy. The sensitivity of abdominal US for cholelithiasis or gallbladder stones is in excess of 95%. The sensitivity of conventional CT in the setting of suspected choledocholithiasis ranges from 76% to 90%. Because up to 15–25% of patients with acute calculous cholecystitis have choledocholithiasis, MRCP may play a role in gallstone disease, particularly in patients with gallstone pancreatitis, and cystic duct and gallbladder neck calculi.

MR Imaging Findings

At MR imaging, the gallstones are visible as a signal void within the bright fluid of the gallbladder on MRCP and heavily T2-weighted sequences. A combination of thin-slice, single-shot turbo or fast spin-echo and two-dimensional thick-slab MRCP sequences are essential components of the MR imaging protocol. On T1-weighted images the cholesterol stones often have high signal intensity (Figs. 94.1–94.3). MRCP should be performed in combination with gadolinium-enhanced imaging to demonstrate any unexpected soft tissue abnormalities such as cholecystitis or gallbladder tumors.

Management

Laparoscopic cholecystectomy is currently the standard operation for gallstone disease.

Literature

1. Cooperberg PL, Burhenne HJ (1980) Real-time ultrasonography diagnostic technique of choice in calculous gallbladder disease. N Engl J Med 302:1277–1279
2. Kelekis NL, Semelka RC (1996) MR imaging of the gallbladder. TMRI 8:312–320
3. Park MS, Yu JS, Kim YH, et al. (1998) Acute cholecystitis: comparison of MR cholangiography and US. Radiology 209:781–785
4. Vitellas KM, Keogan MT, Spritzer CE, et al. (2000) MR cholangiopancreatography of bile and pancreatic duct abnormalities with emphasis on the single-shot fast spin-echo technique. Radiographics 20:939–957
5. Shamiyeh A, Wayant W (2005) Current status of laparoscopic therapy of cholecystolithiasis and common bile duct stones. Dig Dis 23:119–126

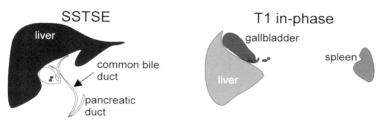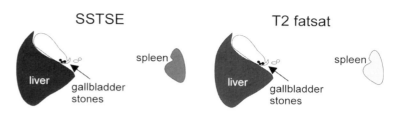

Fig. 94.1. Cholelithiasis (gallstones), drawings. SSTSE: coronal image shows two small stones in the gallbladder. Normal appearance of the common bile duct and the pancreatic duct. **T1 in-phase:** the stones are not visible in the gallbladder; **SSTSE:** dark stones are present within the bright gallbladder; **T2 fatsat:** the stones show improved visibility due to fat suppression and higher signal-to-noise ratio

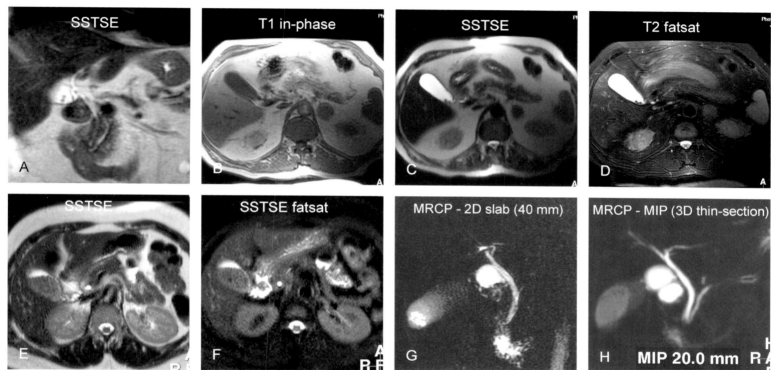

Fig. 94.2. Cholelithiasis (gallstones; two different patients), typical MRI findings. A Coronal SSTSE image (SSTSE) shows two small stones in the gallbladder. Note the normal appearance of the common bile duct and the pancreatic duct. **B** Axial in-phase image (T1 in-phase): The stones are not visible in the gallbladder due to their similar signal intensity. **C** Axial SSTSE image (SSTSE): Stones are visible as signal void within the bright gallbladder. **D** Axial TSE (T2 fatsat): The stones show improved visibility due to fat sup-pression and higher signal-to-noise ratio. **E–H** Another patient with multi-ple gallstones, which are better visible on the cross-sectional SSTSE and SSTSE fatsat images than on the MRCP images due to partial volume and other issues. 2D slab MRCP (acquisition time: 2 s) is a direct imaging with sharper definition of the gallbladder and the biliary tree. 3D MRCP is a MIP of the individual thin-sections acquired during free-breathing and respira-tory-triggering (acquisition time: 5–10 min!)

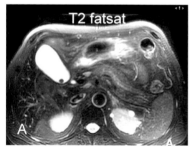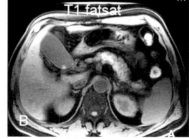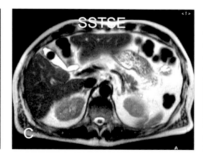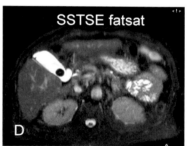

Fig. 94.3. Cholelithiasis, bright T1 and moving stones (two different patients), MRI findings. A Axial TSE image (T2 fatsat) shows a small stone as a signal void. **B** Axial T1 image (T1 fatsat): Parts of the small stone are bright, likely due to the presence of cholesterol. **C** Axial SSTSE image (SSTSE) shows a large stone in the fundus of the gallbladder. **D** Axial SSTSE image (SSTSE fat-sat) (10 min later) shows the stone in another location with more filling of the gallbladder

95 Choledocholithiasis (Bile Duct Stones)

Choledocholithiasis (bile duct stones) has been reported to occur in up to 15 % of patients with symptomatic gallstones. The sensitivities of US for common duct stones range from 18 % to 74 %. This variable sensitivity is related in part to the operator-dependent nature of US and the obscuration of stones by bowel gas. Many centers still perform diagnostic endoscopic retrograde cholangiopancreatography (ERCP) in patients with suspected bile duct stones. Recent data show that ERCP is associated with major complications in 4.0 % of cases, including pancreatitis (1.3 %), cholangitis (0.87 %), hemorrhage (0.76 %), duodenal perforation (0.58 %), and others (0.51 %). Diagnostic ERCPs show a major complication rate of 1.38 % and a death rate of 0.21 %, whereas therapeutic ERCPs show a significantly higher rate for major complications (5.4 %) and deaths (0.49 %). Sensitivity and specificity of MRCP for choledocholithiasis exceeds 90 %. Negative predictive values of MRCP are also quite high, ranging from 96 % to 100 %. Thus, perhaps more important than the ability of MRCP to detect common bile duct stones is its ability to exclude stones because the absence of common bile duct stones at MRCP may result in avoidance of diagnostic ERCP along with its potential complications. Excellent performance of MRCP can result in the avoidance of ERCP in 52 % and 80 % of patients with high and low risk for common bile duct stones, respectively.

MR Imaging Findings

At MR imaging, the bile duct stones are visible as signal void within the bright fluid of the bile duct on MRCP and heavily T2-weighted sequences. Two-dimensional thick-slab MRCP sequences provide an overview of the anatomy and a road map for any therapeutic procedures. The exact number and location of stones can be visualized. In addition, intrahepatic bile duct stones with or without any underlying biliary disease or pneumobilia can also be visualized non-invasively (Figs. 95.1–95.3). MRCP should be performed in combination with gadolinium-enhanced imaging to demonstrate any unexpected soft tissue abnormalities such as cholangitis and tumors causing biliary obstruction.

Literature

1. Soto JA, Barish MA, Alvarez O, et al. (2000) Detection of choledocholithiasis with MR cholangiography: comparison of three-dimensional fast spin-echo and single- and multisection half-Fourier rapid acquisition with relaxation enhancement sequences. Radiology 215:737–45
2. Reinhold C, Taourel P, Bret PM, et al. (1998) Choledocholithiasis: evaluation of MR cholangiography for diagnosis. Radiology 209:435–442
3. Fulcher AS, Turner MA, Capps GW, et al. (1998) Half-Fourier RARE MR cholangiopancreatography in 300 subjects. Radiology 207:21–32
4. Loperfido S, Angelini G, Benedetti G, et al. (1998) Major early complications from diagnostic and therapeutic ERCP: a prospective multicenter study. Gastrointest Endosc 48:1–10
5. Fulcher AS (2002) MRCP and ERCP in the diagnosis of common bile duct stones. Gastroint Endosc 56:S178–182

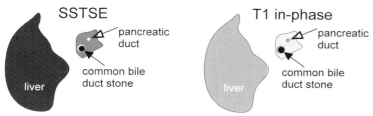

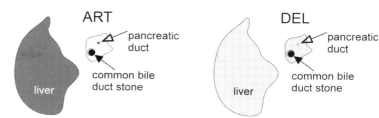

Fig. 95.1. Choledocholithiasis (bile duct stones), drawings. SSTSE: a stone appears as signal void (*arrow*) and almost completely fills the common bile duct; note a thin film of bright fluid surrounds the stone; **T1 in-phase**: the stone appears larger because the surrounding fluid is also dark; **ART**: obviously, the stone does not show enhancement and remains dark; **DEL**: the stone is the darkest structure in the image

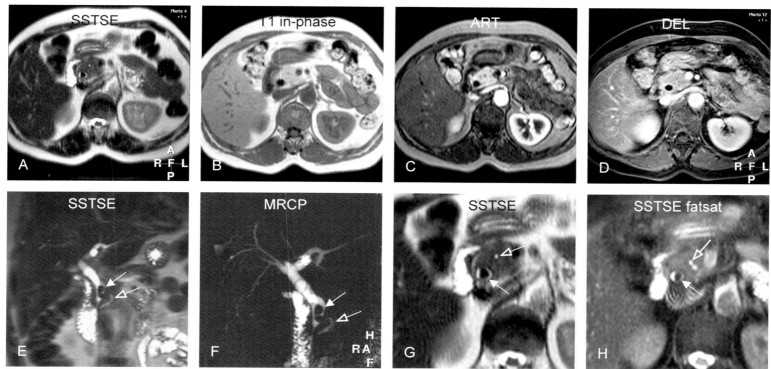

Fig. 95.2. Choledocholithiasis (bile duct stones), typical MRI findings. A Axial SSTSE image (SSTSE) shows a stone as a signal void (*arrow*) and almost completely fills the common bile duct (CBD). **B** Axial in-phase image (T1 in-phase): The stones appear larger because the fluid is also dark. **C** Axial arterial phase image (ART): No enhancement is present. **D** Axial delayed phase image (DEL): The stone is the darkest structure in the image. **E** Coronal SSTSE image (SSTSE) shows in fact two large stones within the distal, slightly dilated CBD (*solid arrow*). Normal pancreatic duct (*open arrow*). **F** MRCP (thick slab of 40 mm) provides an overview of the biliary tree with the two stones in the CBD (*solid arrow*). Note the normal pancreatic duct (*open arrow*). **G** Axial SSTSE image (SSTSE) shows bile duct stone (*solid arrow*). Pancreatic duct (*open arrow*). **H** A detailed view of the axial fat-suppressed SSTSE image (SSTSE fatsat) shows similar findings of the CBD stone (*solid arrow*) and the pancreatic duct (*open arrow*) but the anatomic detail is less obvious due to fat suppression

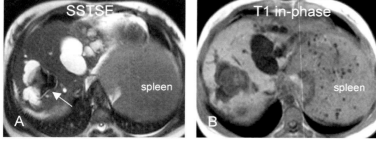

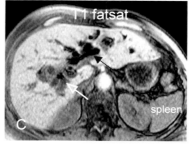

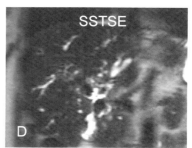

Fig. 95.3. Choledocholithiasis – intrahepatic stones (two different patients), MRI findings. A Axial TSE image (T2 fatsat) shows large dilated ducts in a patient with Caroli's disease, containing a large calculus (*arrow*). **B** Axial T1 in-phase image (T1 in-phase) shows – in part bright – calculus (cholesterol stone). **C** Axial T1 image (T1 fatsat) (another patient) shows dilated bile ducts with pneumobilia (*solid arrow*) and cholelithiasis (*open arrow*). **D** Coronal SSTSE image (SSTSE) shows the biliary tree with typical appearance of PSC

96 Gallbladder Carcinoma I – Versus Gallbladder Wall Edema

Primary carcinoma of the gallbladder is the sixth most common gastrointestinal malignancy, following cancer of the colon, pancreas, stomach, liver, and esophagus. Annually, about 7000 new cases are diagnosed. Risk factors may include chronic *Salmonella typhi* infection, exposure to chemicals used in the rubber, automobile, wood finishing, and metal fabricating industries, and cholelithiasis. The symptoms at presentation are vague and are most often related to adjacent organ invasion. Therefore, despite advances in cross-sectional imaging, early-stage tumors are not often encountered. The vast majority of gallbladder carcinomas are adenocarcinomas. Because most patients present with advanced disease, the prognosis is poor, with a reported 5-year survival rate of less than 5% in most large series. Imaging studies may reveal a mass replacing the normal gallbladder (up to 65%), diffuse or focal thickening of the gallbladder wall (up to 30%), or a polypoid mass within the gallbladder lumen (up to 25%). The liver may be involved by direct contiguous spread in up to 90% of cases, followed by the colon, duodenum, and pancreas.

MR Imaging Findings

At MR imaging, gallbladder carcinoma may be visible with irregular wall thickening as well as a mass at the level of the gallbladder fossa due to direct contiguous spread. Gallstones may be present. Concurrent liver metastases often have a similar T2 appearance and enhancement pattern to the primary lesion. Wall thickening due to edema can easily be distinguished from neoplastic lesions based on morphology and enhancement pattern (Figs. 96.1–96.3).

Differential Diagnosis

Smooth gallbladder wall thickening may be caused by heart failure, cirrhosis, hepatitis, hypoalbuminemia, renal failure, and cholecystitis (xanthogranulomatous cholecystitis with irregular wall thickening mimics carcinoma). Smoothly delineated enhancement is reported to be present in chronic cholecystitis, and irregular progressive enhancement in carcinomas. Transient increased pericholecystic hepatic enhancement can be seen in acute cholecystitis. Other causes of wall abnormality can be adenomyomatosis.

Literature

1. Levin B (1999) Gallbladder carcinoma. Ann Oncol 10:129–130
2. Yoshimitsu K, Honda H, Jimi M, et al. (1999) MR diagnosis of adenomyomatosis of the gallbladder and differentiation from gallbladder carcinoma: importance of showing Rokitansky-Aschoff sinuses. AJR 172:1535–1540
3. Demachi H, Matsui O, Hoshiba K, et al. (1997) Dynamic MRI using a surface coil in chronic cholecystitis and gallbladder carcinoma: radiologic and histopathologic correlation. JCAT 21:643–651
4. Loud PA, Semelka RC, Kettritz U, et al. (1996) MRI of acute cholecystitis: comparison with the normal gallbladder and other entities. MRI 14:349–355
5. Chun KA, Ha HK, Yu ES, et al. (1997) Xanthogranulomatous cholecystitis: CT features with emphasis on differentiation from gallbladder carcinoma. Radiology 203:93–97

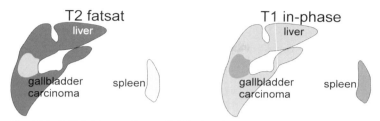

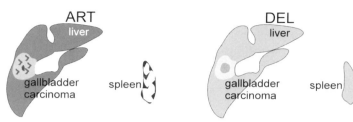

Fig. 96.1. Gallbladder carcinoma (GBC), drawings. T2 fatsat: GBC is hyperintense to the liver and represents a cranial intrahepatic extension within the gallbladder fossa; T1 in-phase: GBC is hypointense to the liver; ART: GBC shows heterogeneous enhancement; DEL: GBC shows in part washout and in part persistent enhancement

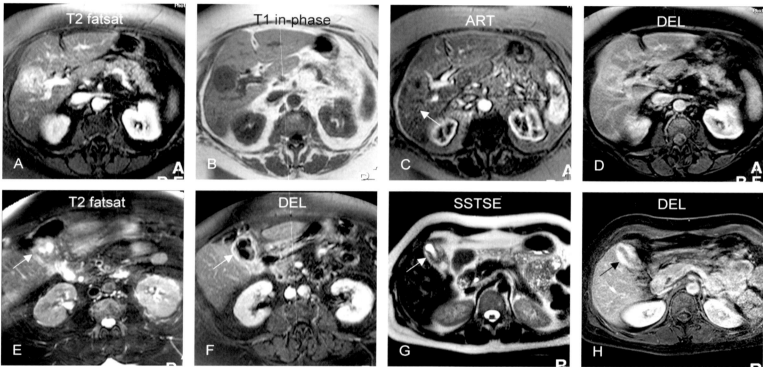

Fig. 96.2. Gallbladder carcinoma (GBC), MRI findings (G and H show another patient). A Axial TSE image (T2 fatsat): GBC is hyperintense to the liver and represents a cranial intrahepatic extension within the gallbladder fossa. **B** Axial in-phase image (T1 in-phase): GBC is hypointense to the liver. **C** Axial arterial phase image (ART): GBC shows heterogeneous enhancement. **D** Axial delayed phase image (DEL): GBC shows in part washout and in part persistent enhancement. **E** Axial TSE image at a lower anatomic level (T2 fatsat): Gallbladder shows irregular wall thickening consistent with the GBC, which extends into the liver and presents as a mass shown in the previous images (*arrow*). **F** Axial delayed phase image (DEL): Thickened gallbladder wall shows heterogeneous enhancement (*arrow*). **G** Axial SSTSE image (SSTSE) and **H** axial delayed phase image (DEL) from another patient show another example of gallbladder carcinoma (*arrow*)

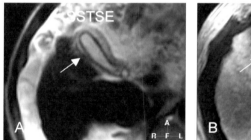

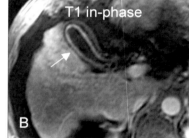

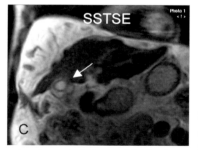

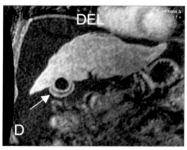

Fig. 96.3. Gallbladder wall thickening (with cirrhosis, portal hypertension and ascites). A Axial SSTSE image (SSTSE) shows smooth and evenly thickened gallbladder wall caused by edema (*arrow*). **B** Axial delayed phase image (DEL) shows thin mucosal and serosal enhancement, excluding a solid lesion (*arrow*). **C** Coronal SSTSE image (SSTSE) shows the cirrhotic liver with edematous gallbladder wall (*arrow*). **D** Coronal delayed phase image (DEL) shows clearly the two smooth and enhanced layers of the gallbladder wall (*arrow*)

97 Gallbladder Carcinoma II – Hepatoid Type of Adenocarcinoma

Hepatoid adenocarcinoma (HAC) is a rare variant of extrahepatic adenocarcinoma, consisting of foci of both adenomatous and hepatocellular differentiations which behave like hepatocellular carcinoma (HCC) in morphology and functionality. It occurs in a multitude of organs, most frequently in the stomach, but it has been reported to occur rarely in other areas as well, including the lung, kidney, female reproductive tract, pancreas, and gallbladder. Typically, an elevated level of serum alpha-fetoprotein (AFP) is detected, although normal levels have also been reported. At imaging the tumor in combination with elevated AFP may mimic HCC.

MR Imaging Findings

At T2-weighted MR imaging the tumor has a typical morphology of an intrahepatic cholangiocarcinoma (low signal centrally due to desmoplasia with a thick rim of high signal peripherally). Also the enhancement pattern is similar to intrahepatic cholangiocarcinomas. Specific contrast media such as superparamagnetic iron oxide (SPIO) may show lack of Kupffer cells (Figs. 97.1 – 97.3).

Differential Diagnosis

Especially with involvement of the gallbladder wall, differentiation from HCC or combined HCC and cholangiocarcinoma is challenging. At immunohistochemistry, CD10 may be positive indicating canalicular differentiation, and positive CD7 and CD19 indicate bile duct adenocarcinoma, since HCC is generally not positive for CD10, CD7 and CD19. In addition, the staining for cytoplasmic AFP may be positive. This combination with the morphology and anatomic location are suggestive for HAC.

Literature

1. Ishikura H, Kishimoto T, Andachi H, et al. (1997) Gastrointestinal hepatoid adenocarcinoma: venous permeation and mimicry of hepatocellular carcinoma, a report of four cases. Histopathology 31:47 – 54
2. Terracciano LM, Glatz K, Mhawech P, et al. (2003) Hepatoid adenocarcinoma with liver metastasis mimicking hepatocellular carcinoma: an immunohistochemical and molecular study of eight cases. Am J Surg Pathol 27:1302 – 1312
3. Sakamoto K, Monobe Y, Kouno M, et al. (2004) Hepatoid adenocarcinoma of the gallbladder: case report and review of the literature. Pathol Int 54:52 – 56
4. Van den Bos IC, Hussain SM, Dwarkasing RS, et al. Hepatoid adenocarcinoma of the gallbladder: a mimicker of hepatocellular carcinoma. BJR (in press)

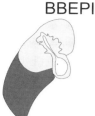 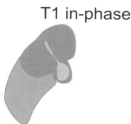 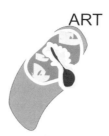 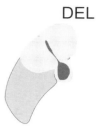

BBEPI T1 in-phase ART DEL

Fig. 97.1. Gallbladder hepatoid adenocarcinoma (HAC), drawings. BBEPI: HAC is hyperintense to the liver and arises from the gallbladder; **T1 in-phase**: HAC is hypointense to the liver; **ART**: HAC shows heterogeneous enhancement; **DEL**: HAC shows enhancement of the more fibrotic central part of the tumor

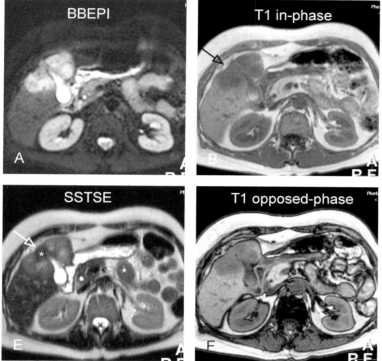 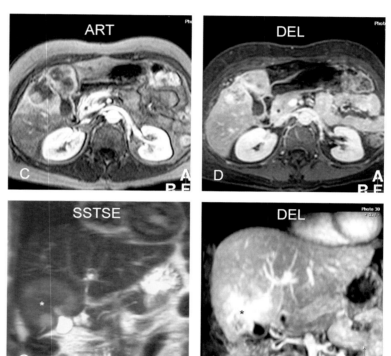

Fig. 97.2. Gallbladder hepatoid adenocarcinoma (HAC), MRI findings. A Axial black-blood echoplanar imaging (BBEPI): HAC is hyperintense to the liver with a hypointense center due to desmoplasia that is a typical feature of cholangiocarcinomas. **B** Axial in-phase image (T1 in-phase): HAC is hypointense to the liver with umbilication caused by central desmoplasia (*open arrow*). **C** Axial arterial phase image (ART): HAC shows heterogeneous enhancement with some perilesional enhancement. **D** Axial delayed phase image (DEL): HAC shows enhancement of more fibrotic areas. **E** Axial SSTSE image with longer TE (SSTSE): HAC is brighter in the periphery and darker in the center (*) with an umbilication (*open arrow*). **F** Axial opposed-phase image (T1 opposed-phase): HAC is hypointense to the liver. **G** Coronal SSTSE image (SSTSE): HAC is brighter in the periphery and darker in the center (*). **H** Coronal delayed phase image (DEL): HAC shows enhancement of more fibrotic central areas (*)

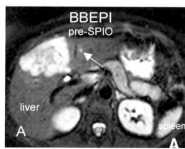 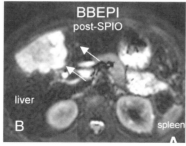 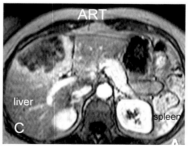 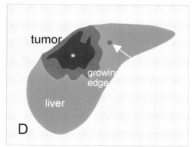

Fig. 97.3. Gallbladder hepatoid adenocarcinoma at a different anatomic level. A Axial black-blood EPI (BBEPI): HAC is hyperintense to the liver with a small intrahepatic metastasis (*arrow*). **B** Axial BBEPI after the uptake of SPIO: the liver and spleen show signal loss, whereas the metastasis (*arrows*) remains bright. **C** Axial arterial phase image (ART): HAC shows enhancement of mainly the growing edge of the tumor. **D** Drawing illustrates the tumor anatomy: tumor center (*). Metastasis (*arrow*)

98 Hilar Cholangiocarcinoma I – Typical

Cholangiocarcinoma (CC) represents less than 1% of all newly diagnosed cancers in North America. Hilar CC (Klatskin tumor) is an adenocarcinoma arising from the hepatic duct or near its bifurcation. Hilar CC accounts for 10–25% of all CC. This tumor is generally divided into three types: infiltrative (spread along the wall of the duct), nodular (tending to obliterate the duct), and papillary (rare intraductal variant). Overall 5-year survival rate is 1%. Even after so-called curative resection, the 5-year survival rate is only 20% because of the locally invasive nature of the tumor. The tumor may be associated with primary sclerosing cholangitis, Caroli's disease, biliary lithiasis, clonorchiasis, and recurrent pyogenic cholangitis. MR imaging with MRCP is a non-invasive technique which can play an important role in the workup of these lesions. MR imaging provides an overview of the biliary anatomy and facilitates the delineation of the tumor from the surrounding liver parenchyma.

MR Imaging Findings

At MR imaging, hilar cholangiocarcinoma may only be visible indirectly by the dilated intrahepatic bile ducts that end abruptly at the hilum, causing a negative impression of the mass. At T2-weighted images, the mass may have subtle increased signal compared to the surrounding liver and on T1-weighted images. The findings may be unremarkable. After injection of gadolinium, the tumors may show ring-shaped or heterogeneous enhancement with persistent (heterogeneous) enhancement in the later phases (Figs. 98.1, 98.2). Other tumors may show little or no enhancement. The exact delineation of the tumor (Bismuth classification), which is essential for any curative surgery, may be challenging on state-of-the-art MR imaging. In our experience, such aspects are even more challenging on US and CT.

Pathology

Most cholangiocarcinomas are mainly composed of desmoplastic matrix, which contains islands of tumor cells. The tumor typically infiltrates the adjacent tissues in finger-like extensions. Often a few vessels will be present. The combination of extensive desmoplastic matrix (relatively low signal on T2), infiltrative growth pattern, and hypovascularity makes it difficult to delineate the tumor from the surroundings on imaging (Fig. 98.3).

Literature

1. Lee WJ, Lim HK, Jang KM, et al. (2001) Radiologic spectrum of cholangiocarcinoma: emphasis on unusual manifestation and differential diagnoses. Radiographics 21:S97–S116
2. Klatskin G (1965) Adenocarcinoma of the hepatic duct at its bifurcation within the porta hepatis: an unusual tumor with distinctive clinical and pathological features. Am J Med 38:241–256
3. Bismuth H, Corlette MB (1975) Intrahepatic cholangioenteric anastomosis in carcinoma of the hilus of the liver. Surg Gynecol Obstet 140:170–178

T2 fatsat

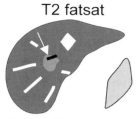

T1 fatsat

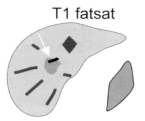

ART

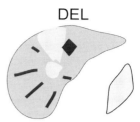

DEL

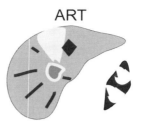

Fig. 98.1. Hilar cholangiocarcinoma (CC), drawings. T2 fatsat: CC is slightly hyperintense to the surrounding liver with dilated bile ducts (*arrow*). T1 fatsat: CC is slightly hypointense to the surrounding liver (*arrow*). ART: CC shows irregular ring-shaped enhancement with an enhancing wedge-shaped area due to the portal compression. DEL: CC shows faint heterogeneous enhancement with some residual wedge-shaped enhancement of the liver

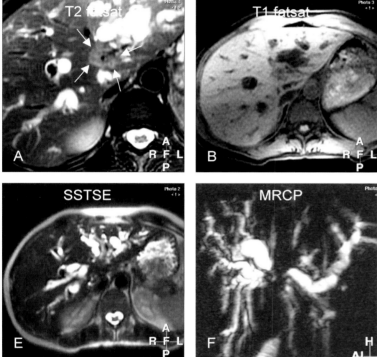

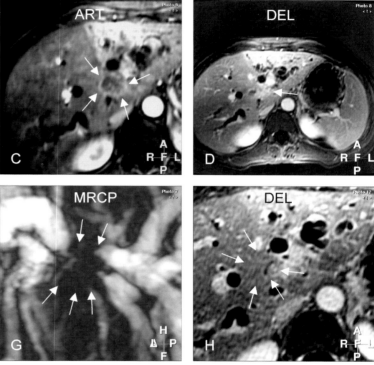

Fig. 98.2. Hilar cholangiocarcinoma (CC), MR findings. A Axial fat-suppressed TSE image (T2 fatsat): CC is slightly higher in signal intensity than the surrounding liver (*arrows*). **B** Axial fat suppressed T1-w GRE (T1fatsat): CC is slightly hypointense. **C** Axial arterial phase 3D gradient recalled echo (GRE) image (ART): CC shows irregular ring-shaped enhancement (*arrows*) with a wedge-shaped enhancement of a part of the liver due to portal compression. **D** Axial delayed phase image (DEL): CC shows faint heterogeneous enhancement of the CC with some residual wedge-shaped enhancement. **E** Axial SSTSE image (SSTSE) shows the bright (fluid-containing) dilated bile ducts that end abruptly, suggesting a lesion at the hilum of the liver. **F** A 2D 20-mm-thick-slab MRCP (MRCP) shows the dilated bile ducts with a central area of sudden caliber change. **G** A detailed view of MRCP shows the dilated ducts with caliber change in more detail (*arrows*). **H** A detailed view from the axial delayed phase image (DEL) indirectly suggests a mass (*arrows*)

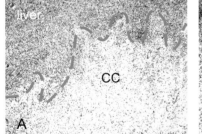

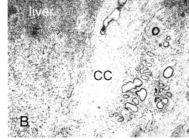

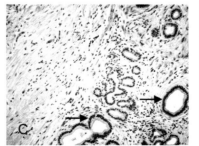

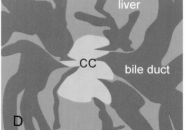

Fig. 98.3. Hilar cholangiocarcinoma (CC), histology (another patient), drawings. A Photomicrograph shows the demarcation (*dashed blue line*) between the CC and the liver with finger-like ingrowth of the tumor. H&E, ×40. **B** Photomicrograph shows CC composed of tumor matrix of desmoplasia with scattered glandular structures. H&E, ×100. **C** Photomicrograph shows epithelium of the glands (*arrows*). H&E, ×200. **D** Drawing based on the MRCP above

99 Hilar Cholangiocarcinoma II – Intrahepatic Mass

Klatskin described the hilar cholangiocarcinoma (CC) in 1965. CC can cause malignant obstruction at the hilum which can extend into multiple biliary radices. To describe the most common situations, Bismuth and colleagues typed the abnormalities: tumors below the confluence of the left and right hepatic ducts (type I), tumors reaching the confluence (type II), tumors occluding the common hepatic duct and either the right or the left hepatic duct (types IIIa and IIIb, respectively), and tumors that are multicentric or that involve the confluence and both the right and left hepatic ducts (type IV). Most cholangiocarcinomas involve the perihilar and distal extrahepatic bile ducts. This classification is used as the basis for management of hilar CC.

MR Imaging Findings

At MR imaging, hilar cholangiocarcinoma may show extension into the liver parenchyma. Some of the hilar CC may comprise glandular tissue with mucin production and hence higher fluid content than the desmoplastic types of tumor. On the T2-weighted images, the tumors may appear brighter and easier to detect. These tumors show little enhancement in either the arterial or the delayed phase (Figs. 99.1 – 99.3).

Management

The Bismuth classification is often used for surgical planning: Surgery may be attempted with or without subsequent radiation. Palliation includes biliary drainage with endoprosthesis or stenting. Metallic self-expanding stents are commonly used for hilar malignancies. Stent placement in the right and left biliary ducts is performed with a bilateral transhepatic approach. Due to debris or tumor overgrowth, stent occlusion can occur in up to 27 % of cases 2.5 months after the initial insertion. The key to successful long-term treatment is to „overstent" to ensure adequate purchase above hilar tumors and insertion in a balanced position.

Literature

1. Lee MJ, Dawson SL, Mueller PR, et al. (1993) Percutaneous management of hilar biliary malignancies with metallic endoprostheses: results, technical problems, and causes of failure. Radiographics 13:1249–1263
2. Klatskin G (1965) Adenocarcinoma of the hepatic duct at its bifurcation within the porta hepatis: an unusual tumor with distinctive clinical and pathological features. Am J Med 38:241–256
3. Bismuth H, Corlette MB (1975) Intrahepatic cholangioenteric anastomosis in carcinoma of the hilus of the liver. Surg Gynecol Obstet 140:170–178
4. De Groen, Gores GJ, LaRusso NF, et al. (1999) Biliary tract cancers. NEJM 341:1368–1378

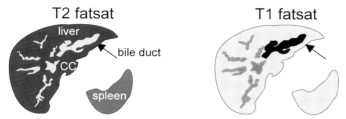
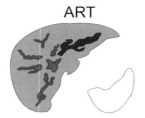
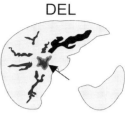

Fig. 99.1. Hilar cholangiocarcinoma (CC), drawings. T2 fatsat: CC has a similar appearance to the dilated bile ducts; **T1 fatsat:** one of the ducts in the left liver contains air (most likely introduced by an earlier intervention) and

appears much darker (*arrow*); **ART:** CC does not show much enhancement; **DEL:** CC (*arrow*) shows better delineation due to the homogeneous enhancement of the surrounding liver

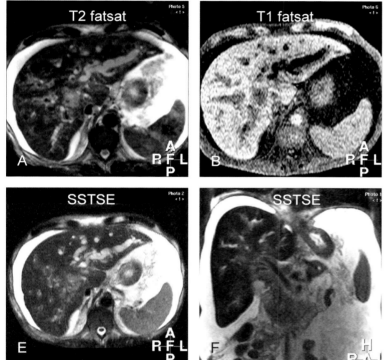
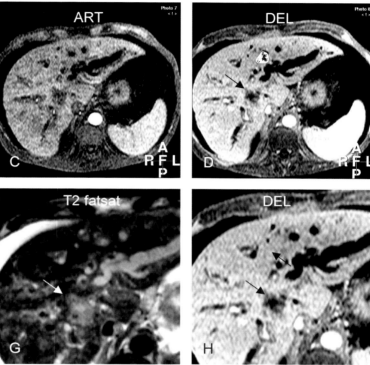
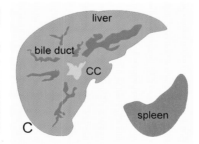
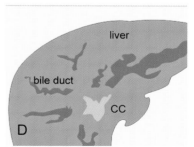

Fig. 99.2. Hilar cholangiocarcinoma (CC), MR findings. A Axial fat-suppressed TSE image (T2 fatsat): CC has a similar appearance to the dilated bile duct, suggesting its high fluid content. **B** Axial fat suppressed T1-w GRE image (T1 fatsat): One of the bile ducts in the left liver appears dark because of the air (most likely introduced by an earlier intervention). **C** Axial arterial phase image (ART): CC does not show much enhancement. **D** Axial delayed phase image (DEL): CC shows better delineation due to homogeneous enhancement of the surrounding liver (*arrow*). **E** Axial SSTSE image (SSTSE) shows

mainly the dilated ducts in the left liver. **F** Coronal SSTSE image (SSTSE) shows ascites that surrounds the liver and the normal-sized spleen. **G** A detailed view of the axial fat-suppressed TSE image (T2 fatsat): Most likely due to its high fluid content, CC shows good delineation from the surrounding liver (*arrow*). **H** A detailed axial delayed phase image (DEL): The periphery of the CC is enhanced and becomes isointense with the liver; CC therefore appears smaller compared to the previous image (*arrow*)

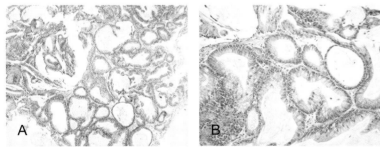

Fig. 99.3. Hilar cholangiocarcinoma (CC), drawings and direct MR-biopsy correlation. A Photomicrograph of an endoscopic biopsy shows glands and little stroma of CC, which explains its high signal on T2 images. H&E, ×200. **B** Photomicrograph shows the glands in detail that have cylindrical epitheli-

um. H&E, ×400. **C** Drawing based on the axial images above shows the dilated bile ducts with sudden caliber change at a certain distance from the CC. **D** A detailed view of the drawing shows the CC surrounding the dilated bile ducts

100 Hilar Cholangiocarcinoma III – Partially Extrahepatic Tumor

In patients with hilar cholangiocarcinoma (CC), early detection and accurate evaluation of tumor extent are necessary for proper treatment. Endoscopic retrograde cholangiopancreatography (ERCP) and percutaneous transhepatic cholangiography (PTC) have been used to detect and classify hilar CC. These imaging modalities provide only information about the intraluminal components (wall irregularity or filling defect). In the past, digital subtraction angiography (DSA) has been helpful in determining vascular involvement. The ability of CT to detect and accurately delineate the hilar CC is limited, mainly because of the lack of tissue contrast. MR imaging can provide a comprehensive workup of the lesions including the vascularity, the extent within the liver as well as extrahepatic extension.

MR Imaging Findings

At MR imaging, the extrahepatic extension is even easier to evaluate than the intrahepatic component because the tumor forms excellent contrast with the background bright fat on non-fat suppressed images. On magnetic resonance cholangiopancreatography (MRCP) images, which are equivalent to ERCP images, the extraluminal extent cannot be evaluated. MRCP, unlike ERCP, can however visualize the entire biliary tree including the obstructed segments because it does not rely on injection of any contrast media. MR imaging can also provide information about the exact location for any biopsy for histological proof (Figs. 100.1 – 100.3).

Management

MR imaging, including MRCP sequences, can be used as a road map for any interventional procedure. Hilar CC may involve the main hepatic duct, both hepatic ducts, on segmental ducts. When a tumor obstructs the right and left hepatic ducts, palliation with transhepatic stent placement can be achieved by (a) draining only one system through a single transhepatic track, (b) draining both systems through separate transhepatic tracks, or (c) draining both systems through a single transhepatic track. MR imaging can successfully be used for follow-up in the presence of a (metal) stent.

Literature

1. Lee MJ, Dawson SL, Mueller PR, et al. (1993) Percutaneous management of hilar biliary malignancies with metallic endoprostheses: results, technical problems, and causes of failure. Radiographics 13:1249 – 1263
2. Hanninen EL, Pech M, Jonas S, et al. (2005) Magnetic resonance imaging including magnetic resonance cholangiopancreatography for tumor localization and therapy planning in malignant hilar obstructions. Acta Radiol 46:462 – 70
3. Leyendecker JR, Elsayes KM, Gratz BI, et al. (2002) MR cholangiopancreatography: spectrum of pancreatic duct abnormalities. AJR 179:1465 – 1471
4. Reinhold C, Bret PM (1996) Current status of MR cholangiopancreatography. AJR 166:1285 – 1295

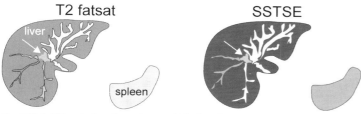 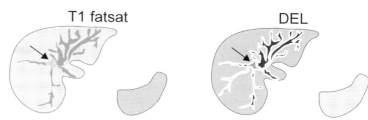

Fig. 100.1. Hilar cholangiocarcinoma (CC), drawings. T2 fatsat: CC is difficult to distinguish from the surrounding dilated bile ducts and the liver (*arrow*); **SSTSE:** the dilated bile ducts show sudden caliber change at the hilum (*arrow*); **T1 fatsat:** CC is slightly hypointense to the liver (*arrow*); **DEL:** CC (*arrow*) shows peripheral enhancement but the dilated bile ducts enhance in a similar fashion, making the distinction difficult

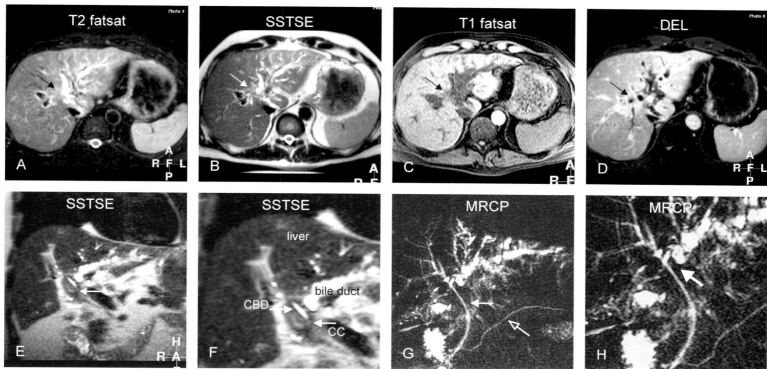

Fig. 100.2. Hilar cholangiocarcinoma (CC), MR findings. A Axial fat-suppressed TSE image (T2 fatsat): CC is suggested by the dilated bile ducts (*arrow*). **B** Axial SSTSE image (SSTSE): The dilated bile ducts show sudden caliber change at the hilum, suggesting a mass (*arrow*). **C** Axial fat suppressed T1-w image before contrast (T1 fatsat): CC is slightly hypointense to the liver (*arrow*). **D** Axial delayed phase image (DEL): CC shows faint ring-shaped enhancement like the dilated bile ducts, making it difficult to distinguish the two (*arrow*). **E** Coronal SSTSE image (SSTSE) shows the dilated bile ducts in the left liver and a mass at the hilum of the liver which is probably the extrahepatic part of the CC (*arrow*). **F** A detailed view of the coronal SSTSE (SSTSE) shows the CC that surrounds the common bile duct (CBD) with an endoprosthesis in situ. **G** MRCP (MRCP) shows mainly the dilated ducts in the left liver because the endoprosthesis (*solid arrow*) drains the right side. Pancreatic duct (*open arrow*). **H** A detailed view (MRCP) indirectly suggests a hilar mass (*arrow*)

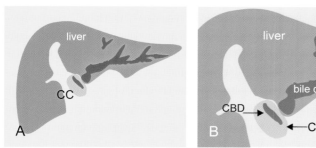 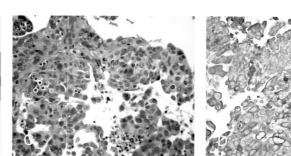

Fig. 100.3. Hilar cholangiocarcinoma (CC), drawings and direct MR-biopsy correlation. A Drawing shows the dilated bile ducts with sudden caliber change caused by a mass (CC) at the liver hilum. **B** Detailed drawing shows the cholangiocarcinoma (CC) that surrounds the common bile duct (CBD). **C** Photomicrograph from endoscopic biopsy material shows findings compatible with CC. H&E, × 400. **D** Photomicrograph shows the presence of abundant connective (fibrotic) tissue which is a characteristic component of cholangiocarcinomas. Keratin-20, × 400

101 Hilar Cholangiocarcinoma IV – Metal Stent with Interval Growth

Most patients with hilar cholangiocarcinoma (CC) clinically present with painless jaundice; however, other common symptoms include pruritus, weight loss, and abdominal pain. Although surgical resection offers the only hope for cure, most patients are found to have unresectable disease on initial presentation and have an extremely grim prognosis. This has led to an emphasis on the role of palliative care, with relief of biliary obstruction, in the management of these patients. Surgery of cholangiocarcinoma has been replaced by percutaneous biliary stent placement. After several months, stents may become occluded by debris or tumor growth. MR imaging can reliably demonstrate tumor growth in the presence of the stent.

MR Imaging Findings

At MR imaging, stent causes susceptibility artifacts mainly on the gradient echo sequences. Despite these artifacts, the tumor detection and delineation is very reliable at MR imaging. The tumor as well as any liver metastases have moderately high signal compared to the liver. The lesions show irregular rim enhancement with transient wedge-shaped enhancement in the arterial phase. In the delayed phase, parts of the tumor show persistent enhancement. On MRCP sequences, the increase in the distance between the right and the left biliary system indicates indirect interval tumor growth (Figs. 101.1 – 101.3).

Management

Reobstruction is the most common late complication after stent placement for hilar CC. In such cases, reintervention should be considered.

Literature

1. Lee MJ, Dawson SL, Mueller PR, et al. (1993) Percutaneous management of hilar biliary malignancies with metallic endoprostheses: results, technical problems, and causes of failure. Radiographics 13:1249–1263
2. Hanninen EL, Pech M, Jonas S, et al. (2005) Magnetic resonance imaging including magnetic resonance cholangiopancreatography for tumor localization and therapy planning in malignant hilar obstructions. Acta Radiol 46:462–70
3. Freeman ML, Oyerby C (2003) Selective MRCP and CT-targeted drainage of malignant hilar biliary obstruction with self-expanding metallic stents. Gastrointest Endosc 58:41–9
4. Reinhold C, Bret PM (1996) Current status of MR cholangiopancreatography. AJR 166:1285–1295
5. Inal M, Akgul E, Aksungur E, et al. (2003) Percutaneous self-expandable uncovered metallic stents in malignant biliary obstruction. Complications, follow-up and reintervention in 154 patients. Acta Radiol 44:139–146

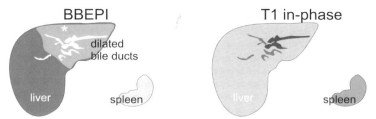
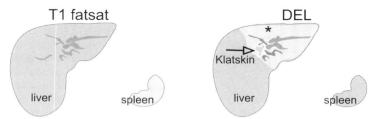

Fig. 101.1. Hilar cholangiocarcinoma, drawings. BBEPI: dilated left-sided bile ducts surrounded by edema (*); no mass is visible; **T1 in-phase**: pneumobilia rendering dark signal within bile ducts after placement of an endopros- thesis; **T1 fatsat**: no mass is visible; **DEL**: Klatskin tumor is slightly less enhanced than the surrounding liver. Note also the slightly increased parenchymal enhancement (*)

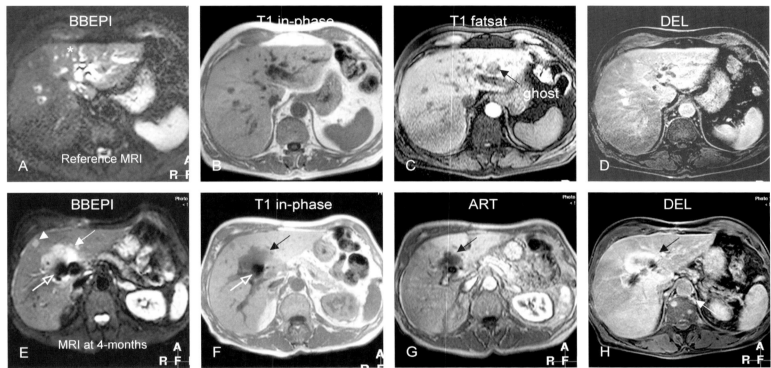

Fig. 101.2. Hilar cholangiocarcinoma (CC), interval growth, MRI findings. A Axial TSE image (T2 fatsat): Dilated left-sided bile ducts with edema (*); no mass is visible. **B** Axial in-phase image (T1 in-phase): Status post endoprosthesis with pneumobilia rendering some of the bile ducts very dark. **C** Axial GRE image (T1 fatsat): No mass is visible. **D** Axial delayed phase image (DEL): CC is slightly less enhanced than the surrounding liver. Note also slightly increased parenchymal enhancement. **E** Axial TSE image (T2 fatsat) at 4 months follow-up shows considerable increase in the hilar mass (*solid*

arrow) that appears hyperintense to the liver with encasement of the metal- lic stent (*open arrow*), placed after removal of the endoprosthesis. Note also a metastasis (*arrowhead*). **F** Axial in-phase image (T1 in-phase): note the stent (*open arrow*) in the center of the mass (*solid arrow*). **G** Axial arterial phase image (ART) shows heterogeneous enhancement. **H** Axial delayed phase image (DEL): CC is better delineated from the surrounding liver (*arrow*)

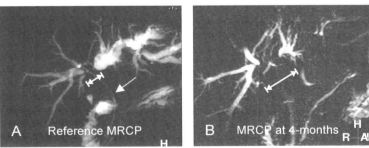
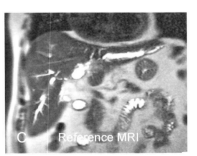
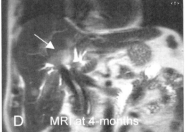

Fig. 101.3. Hilar cholangiocarcinoma, interval growth, MRCP versus MRI findings. A MRCP shows mainly the dilated bile ducts in the left liver with a plastic stent in situ (*arrow*) with indirect suggestion of a hilar mass (*double arrow*).

B MRCP (at 4 months) suggests an increased size of the hilar mass (*double-headed arrow*). **C** Coronal SSTSE image shows dilated bile ducts. **D** Coronal SSTSE image at 4 months shows the hilar mass (*arrow*)

102 Hilar Cholangiocarcinoma V – Biliary Dilatation Mimicking Klatskin Tumor at CT

The appearance of most liver lesions is well established at imaging. However, considerable overlap may be present among the appearance of various lesions. Computed tomography (CT) is well known for the occurrence of pseudolesions and pitfalls. Particularly, some cystic lesions may contain fluid with higher density than simple fluid and mimic solid lesions. Most CT examinations are performed as single (portal) phase contrast-enhanced examinations, and lack the dynamic enhancement pattern information which might facilitate distinction between benign and malignant lesions. In addition, the low intrinsic soft tissue contrast does not allow distinction between high fluid-content and solid liver lesions.

MR Imaging Findings

At MR imaging, lesions or structures with high fluid content, such as dilated bile ducts, display very high signal intensity on heavily T2-weighted sequences and hence allow easy distinction from solid lesions. In addition, many centers perform routine dynamic gadolinium-enhanced imaging, which provides additional information concerning the benign versus malignant nature of the lesions. Therefore, cystic dilatation of the bile ducts which may mimic a solid lesion at CT can be correctly identified as a benign lesion at MR imaging (Figs. 102.1 – 102.3).

Management

MR imaging may prevent unnecessary surgery and can be used for follow-up of lesions causing pitfalls at CT.

Literature

1. Ito K, Honjo K, Fujita T, et al. (1996) Liver neoplasms: diagnostic pitfalls in cross-sectional imaging. Radiographics 16:273 – 293
2. Yoshimitsu K, Honda H, Kuroiwa T, et al. (2001) Unusual hemodynamics and pseudolesions of the noncirrhotic liver at CT. Radiographics 21:S81 – S96
3. Hanninen EL, Pech M, Jonas S, et al. (2005) Magnetic resonance imaging including magnetic resonance cholangiopancreatography for tumor localization and therapy planning in malignant hilar obstructions. Acta Radiol 46:462 – 70
4. Reinhold C, Bret PM (1996) Current status of MR cholangiopancreatography. AJR 166:1285 – 1295

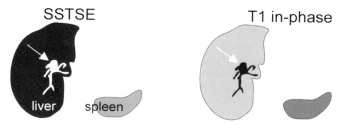

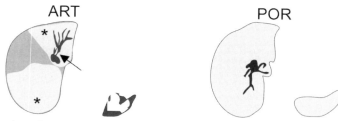

Fig. 102.1. Biliary dilatation mimicking cholangiocarcinoma at CT, drawings. SSTSE: local fusiform dilatation of the bile ducts (*arrow*), without a mass. T1 in-phase: dilated bile ducts (*arrow*); ART (**slightly different anatomic level**): wedge-shaped areas suggest biliary compression or cholangitis (*). Note a local biliary stenosis (*arrow*); POR: homogeneous enhancement of the liver surrounding the dilated bile ducts

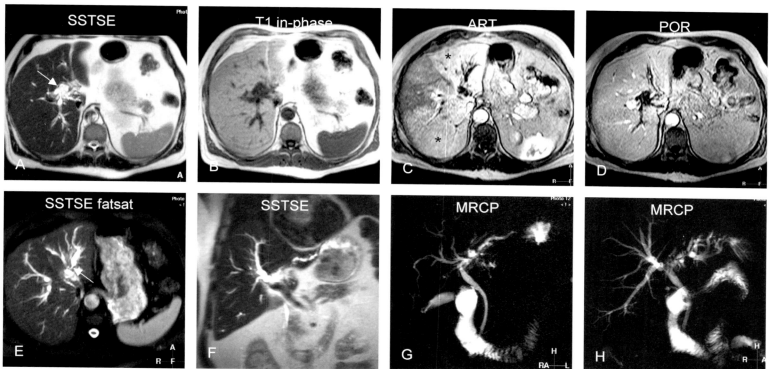

Fig. 102.2. Biliary dilatation mimicking cholangiocarcinoma at CT, MR findings.
A Axial SSTSE image (SSTSE): dilated bile ducts without a mass (*arrow*).
B Axial in-phase image (T1 in-phase): Dilated bile ducts are hypointense (*arrow*). **C** Axial arterial phase image (ART): Wedge-shaped enhancement (*) suggests compression of the bile ducts and/or cholangitis. **D** Axial portal phase image (POR): The liver parenchyma surrounding the dilated bile ducts shows homogeneous enhancement. **E** Axial fat-suppressed SSTSE im-
age (SSTSE fatsat) at a different anatomic level shows dilated bile ducts as well as a stenosis (*arrow*); no mass is seen. **F** Coronal SSTSE image (SSTSE): Again dilated bile ducts are present on both sides of the liver. **G** A 2D 40-mm-thick-slab MRCP (MRCP) shows the dilated intrahepatic bile ducts as well as the common bile duct. **H** MRCP from another angle provides an overview of the abnormal bile ducts. Based on MR imaging, CT diagnosis of CC was questioned; subsequent biopsies were negative for malignancy

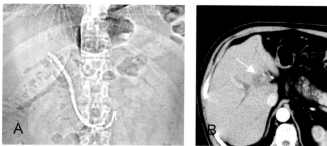
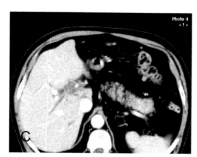
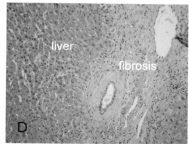

Fig. 102.3. Biliary dilatation mimicking cholangiocarcinoma at CT. A Scout view shows the endoprosthesis in-situ. **B** CT in the arterial phase: One of the dilated bile ducts was mistaken for a hilar mass (*arrow*). **C** CT in the portal phase shows homogeneous enhancement of the liver. **D** Photomicrograph
taken from one of the several biopsies performed after MRI shows fibrosis and normal liver tissue without any evidence for malignancy. H&E stain, ×100

103 Primary Sclerosing Cholangitis I – Cholangitis and Segmental Atrophy

Primary sclerosing cholangitis (PSC) is a chronic cholestatic liver disease commonly associated with inflammatory bowel disease (IBD), which is present in two-thirds of patients. It is characterized by fibrosing inflammatory destruction of intrahepatic and extrahepatic bile ducts, ultimately leading to death by liver failure and cholangiocarcinoma (10–30%). PSC is considered to be an immune-mediated liver disease of multifactorial and multigenetic etiology. The annual incidence is reported to be 0.91 per 100,000. Symptoms and signs of liver or biliary disease may be present. Patients have biochemical cholestasis from the time of diagnosis. Association with autoimmune hepatitis and pancreatitis has been described.

MR Imaging Findings

At MR imaging, in patients with PSC abnormal findings can be seen including (1) intrahepatic bile duct dilatation; (2) intrahepatic bile duct stenosis; (3) intrahepatic bile duct beading; (4) periportal high signal intensity on T2-weighted images with increased enhancement of the liver parenchyma on dynamic arterial-phase images, predominantly in the peripheral areas of the liver; (5) extrahepatic bile duct wall thickening and enhancement; (6) extrahepatic bile duct stenosis; (7) hypertrophy of certain segments, for instance caudate lobe and atrophy of other segments; (8) periportal lymphadenopathy; and (9) enlarged gallbladder. MR cholangiography and contrast-enhanced dynamic MR techniques are useful for revealing intra- and extrahepatic signs of primary sclerosing cholangitis. Atrophy of certain segments of the liver results from recurrent cholangitis and fibrosis (Figs. 103.1 – 103.3).

Management

Medical treatment consists of ursodeoxycholic acid and immunosuppressant agents. Repeat endoscopic dilatations for dominant strictures can be carried out. In most cases, the only treatment option for PSC accompanied by inflammatory intestinal disease is liver transplantation.

Literature

1. MacFaul GR, Chapman RW (2005) Sclerosing cholangitis. Curr Opin Gastroenterol 21:348–53
2. Vitellas KM, Enns RA, Keogan MT, et al. (2002) Comparison of MR cholangiopancreatographic techniques with contrast-enhanced cholangiography in the evaluation of sclerosing cholangitis. AJR 178:327–334
3. Revelon G, Rashid A, Kawamoto S, et al. (1999) Primary sclerosing cholangitis: MR imaging findings with pathologic correlation. AJR 173:1037–1042
4. Ito K, Mitchell DG, Outwater EK, et al. (1999) Primary sclerosing cholangitis: MR imaging features. AJR 172:1527–1533
5. Bader TR, Beavers KL, Semelka RC (2003) MR imaging features of primary sclerosing cholangitis: patterns of cirrhosis in relationship to clinical severity of the disease. Radiology 226:675–685

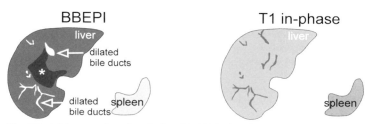
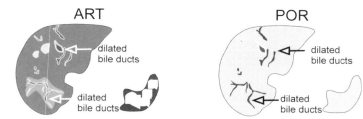

Fig. 103.1. Primary sclerosing cholangitis (PSC), drawings. BBEPI: bile ducts are dilated in the periphery of the liver with concomitant increased parenchymal signal intensity due to inflammation; normal parenchyma (*); T1 in-phase: the liver parenchyma appears normal; ART: increased enhancement around some of the dilated ducts indicates cholangitis; POR: the enhanced areas become isointense to the liver

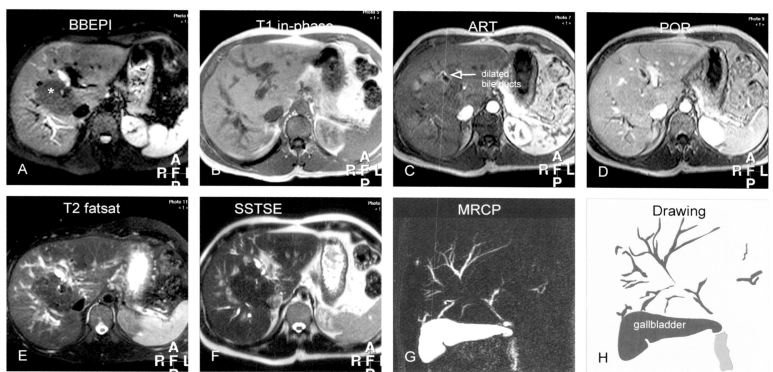

Fig. 103.2. Primary sclerosing cholangitis (PSC) with cholangitis, MRI findings. A Axial BBEPI image (BBEPI): Dilated bile ducts are located in the periphery of the liver with concomitant increased signal intensity due to inflammation. Central liver has a normal signal (*). B Axial in-phase image (T1 in-phase): The liver parenchyma appears quite normal. C Axial arterial phase image (ART): increased enhancement of the wall of the dilated ducts and in the parenchyma around some of the dilated ducts indicates moderate to severe cholangitis. D Axial portal phase image (POR): The enhanced areas become isointense to the liver. E Axial TSE image (T2 fatsat): The dilated bile ducts are difficult to distinguish from the intrahepatic in-plane vessels because of similar high signal intensity. F Axial SSTSE image (SSTSE): The dilated bile ducts can be followed onto the subcapsular region. G and H MRCP (MRCP) with the drawing shows typical appearance of the biliary tree with PSC. The large size of the gallbladder suggests impaired emptying, most likely due to narrowing of the common bile duct

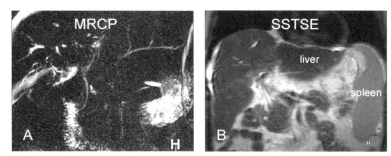
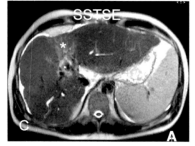
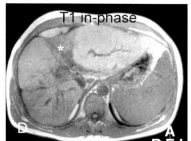

Fig. 103.3. PSC (another patient) complicated with a fibrosis or cirrhosis, splenomegaly, ascites, and segmental atrophy due to recurrent cholangitis, MR findings. A MRCP shows typical PSC appearance of the biliary tree. B Coronal SSTSE shows the liver with fibrosis or cirrhosis, ascites, and splenomegaly. C Axial SSTSE image shows high signal in segment IV with atrophy (*). D Axial in-phase image shows abnormally low signal in segment IV with atrophy (*)

104 Primary Sclerosing Cholangitis II – With Intrahepatic Cholestasis

Primary sclerosing cholangitis (PSC) is characterized by chronic inflammation and fibrosis of bile ducts. Progressive and obliterative fibrosis of small, medium, and large bile ducts causes secondary biliary cirrhosis and cholestasis, which results in hepatic insufficiency. Primary pigmented stones occur in 30 % of patients with PSC secondary to bile stasis. Endoscopic retrograde cholangiopancreatography (ERCP) has been replaced by MR imaging and magnetic resonance cholangiopancreatography (MRCP) as the standard reference for the evaluation of bile ducts. Currently, MR imaging is the modality of choice for the evaluation of asymptomatic patients and in the early diagnosis of complications, especially cholangiocellular carcinoma, which is highly likely to develop in patients who have PSC. Both morphological changes, which can be seen in the biliary system, and parenchymal changes, which are accompanied by PSC, can be evaluated by MR imaging non-invasively.

MR Imaging Findings

At MR imaging, MRCP has a high sensitivity (83–89 %) and specificity (92–99 %) for PSC. MRCP typically shows variable caliber of the intra- and extrahepatic bile ducts with signs of cholestasis (high signal within dilated bile ducts on T1-weighted images. Reactive periportal lymph nodes can be seen as a bright nodular structure on the T2-weighted images. At histology, sclerosis with narrowing, dilatations, and cholestasis confirm the MR imaging findings (Figs. 104.1–104.3).

Differential Diagnosis

Secondary causes such as stricture, stones, or bacterial cholangitis secondary to earlier surgery, parasitic infections, ischemia, or cholangitis secondary to chemotherapy should be eliminated before diagnosing PSC.

Literature

1. Fulcher AS, Turner MA, Franklin KJ, et al. (2000) Primary sclerosing cholangitis: evaluation with MR cholangiography. A case control study. Radiology 215:71–80
2. Vitellas KM, Enns RA, Keogan MT, et al. (2002) Comparison of MR cholangiopancreatographic techniques with contrast-enhanced cholangiography in the evaluation of sclerosing cholangitis. AJR 178:327–334
3. Revelon G, Rashid A, Kawamoto S, et al. (1999) Primary sclerosing cholangitis: MR imaging findings with pathologic correlation. AJR 173:1037–1042

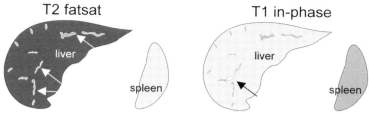
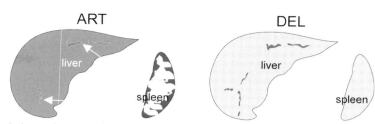

Fig. 104.1. Primary sclerosing cholangitis (PSC), drawings. T2 fatsat: typical bile ducts (*arrows*) with long segments of stenoses and dilatations, extending into the periphery of the liver; **T1 in-phase:** high signal is due to local cholesta-sis (*arrow*); **ART:** subtle increased enhancement around some of the dilated ducts indicates mild cholangitis (*arrows*); **DEL:** the enhanced areas become isointense to the liver

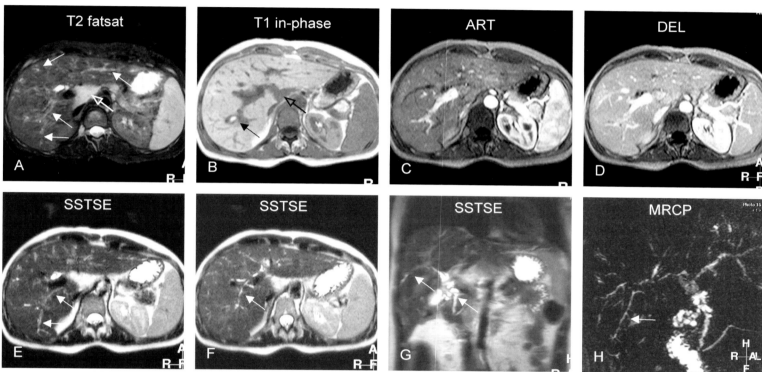

Fig. 104.2. Primary sclerosing cholangitis (PSC) in a patient with ulcerative colitis, typical MRI findings. A Axial TSE image (T2 fatsat): Bile ducts with long segments of stenoses and dilatations, extending into the periphery of the liver, are typical for PSC (*solid arrows*). Note also enlarged reactive periportal lymph nodes (*open arrow*). **B** Axial in-phase image (T1 in-phase): High signal indicates local cholestasis in one of the dilated ducts (*arrow*). **C** Axial arterial phase image (ART): Faintly increased enhancement around some of the dilated ducts indicates mild cholangitis. **D** Axial delayed phase image (DEL): The enhanced areas become isointense to the liver. **E–G** Intra- as well as extrahepatic abnormal bile ducts (*arrows*) indicate a systemic disease. **H** MRCP (MRCP) provides an overview of the biliary tree with typical appearance of PSC. Note the elongated bile ducts with variable diameter, extending into the sub-capsular region of the liver (*arrow*)

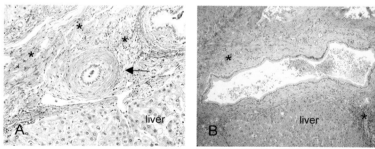
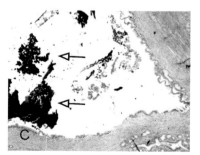
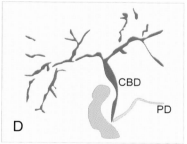

Fig. 104.3. PSC, pathology (another patient), drawing. A Photomicrograph (H&E stain, 200×) shows a bile duct with thickened wall (sclerosis) and narrow lumen (*arrow*). Note also cholestasis (*greenish*). **B** Photomicrograph (H&E, 100×) shows a dilated bile duct surrounded by fibrosis and debris. **C** Photomicrograph (H&E, 40×) shows a dilated duct with cholestasis (*open arrows*). **D** Drawing shows typical appearance of PSC (CBD = common bile duct; PD = pancreatic duct)

105 Primary Sclerosing Cholangitis III – With Intrahepatic Stones

Primary sclerosing cholangitis (PSC) causes progressive changes including irregularities, multifocal strictures, and dilatations in different levels of the biliary channels. Large bile duct dilatations cause secondary cholestasis, which may result in primary pigmented stones in up to 30% of patients. Other cholangiographic findings include webs and diverticula. A diverticulum is a focal, eccentric, saccular dilatation of the bile duct. Up to 27% of patients with PSC have diverticula. MR imaging with MRCP should be the modality of choice for evaluation of bile ducts with intrahepatic stones.

MR Imaging Findings

At MR imaging, intrahepatic stones are visible as filling defects on the T2-weighted and MRCP sequences, and as hyperintense signal within the dilated dark bile ducts on T1-weighted images. Occasionally, segmental PSC with intrahepatic stones may also be seen (Figs. 105.1 – 105.3).

Differential Diagnosis

Caroli's disease with intrahepatic stones should be excluded. *Clonorchis sinensis* and *Ascaris lumbricoides* can inhabit the bile ducts and induce ductal injury and strictures. Oriental cholangiohepatitis is uncommon in Western countries. Cholangiographic findings include multifocal strictures and dilatation of the intrahepatic bile ducts, stones, disproportionate dilatation of the extrahepatic bile duct unrelated to strictures or stones, a right-angle branching pattern, and decreased arborization. In rare instances, cholangiectasis or „bile lakes" can occur from ongoing obstruction and inflammation. Complications include primary pigmented stones (80% of cases), hepatic abscess, and cholangiocarcinoma (2.5 – 5.0%).

Literature

1. Vitellas KM, Keogan MT, Freed KS, Enns RA, Spritzer CE, Baillie JM, Nelson RC (2000) Radiologic manifestations of sclerosing cholangitis with emphasis on MR cholangiopancreatography. Radiographics 20:959 – 975
2. Cotton PB (1991) Bile duct diverticula and webs: nonspecific cholangiographic features of primary sclerosing cholangitis. AJR 157:281 – 285
3. Ito K, Mitchell DG, Outwater EK, et al. (1999) Primary sclerosing cholangitis: MR imaging features. AJR 172:1527 – 1533

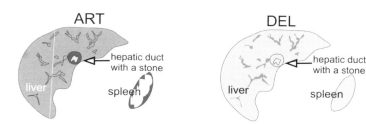
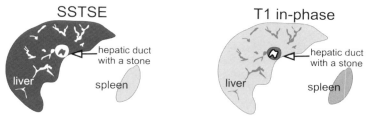

Fig. 105.1. Primary sclerosing cholangitis (PSC), drawings. SSTSE: bile ducts with long stenoses and dilatations; dilated hepatic duct with a large stone; **T1 in-phase:** the stone has a high signal, which suggests its high cholesterol content (cholesterol stone); **ART:** slight increased diffuse enhancement of the liver; **DEL:** the liver shows homogeneous enhancement

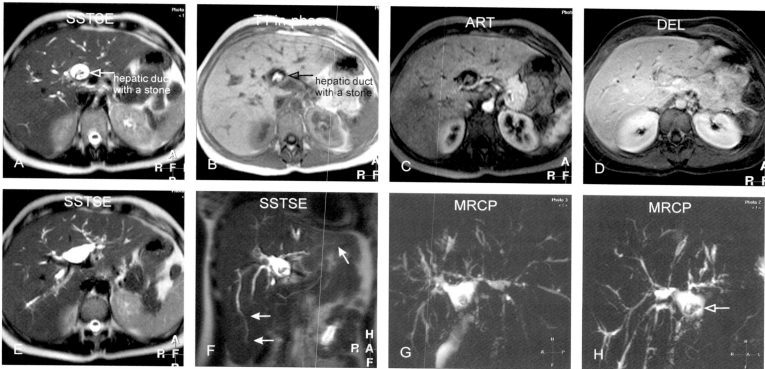

Fig. 105.2. Primary sclerosing cholangitis (PSC) with an intrahepatic stone, MRI findings. A Axial SSTSE image (SSTSE): bile ducts with long stenoses and dilatations, typical of PSC. Dilated hepatic duct contains a large stone (contrast sparing). **B** Axial in-phase image (T1 in-phase): The stone has a high signal (*open arrow*), which suggests high cholesterol content (cholesterol stone). **C** Axial arterial phase image (ART) shows slightly increased liver enhancement. **D** Axial delayed image (DEL): The liver shows homo-geneous enhancement. **E** Axial SSTSE image (SSTSE) at a slightly different anatomic level shows the dilated bile ducts at the bifurcation as well as intra-hepatic ducts. **F** Coronal SSTSE image (SSTSE) shows the elongated bile ducts, which are a common finding in PSC (*solid arrows*). **G** and **H** MRCP (MRCP) provides an overview of the biliary tree with the stone in the hepat-ic duct (*open arrow*)

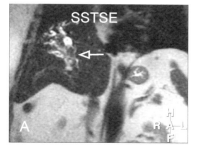
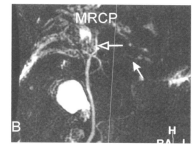
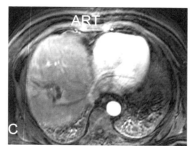
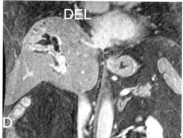

Fig. 105.3. PSC (another patient) complicated with a segmental PSC and intrahe-patic stones, MR findings. A Coronal SSTSE shows dilated bile ducts with stones in segment VIII (*open arrow*). **B** MRCP shows typical PSC findings in the liver (*solid arrow*) and severe segmental involvement with stones (*open arrow*). **C** Axial arterial phase image shows enhancement around the dilated ducts suggesting cholangitis. **D** Coronal delayed phase image shows homo-geneous enhancement of the liver with segmental dilated bile ducts

106 Primary Sclerosing Cholangitis IV – With Biliary Cirrhosis

Primary sclerosing cholangitis (PSC) can result in obliterative fibrosis of small, medium, and large bile ducts, which in turn results in cholestasis with progression to secondary biliary cirrhosis and hepatic failure. The spectrum of MR imaging appearances of PSC with fibrosis or cirrhosis can be diverse and may be present in a majority of patients with long-standing PSC. Large central regenerative nodules, hypertrophy of the caudate lobe, and peripheral atrophy are frequent findings in patients with PSC and cirrhosis. This constellation of findings may result from the peripheral small-duct PSC initially, and gradually progressing to the larger, more central bile ducts (large-duct PSC). The combination of the dilated and the irregular bile duct and large regenerative nodules is often not found in other types of cirrhosis. MRCP and serial gadolinium-enhanced MR images are essential in demonstrating the full spectrum of imaging findings of PSC and should be acquired for a full assessment of this disease. MR imaging is an excellent modality for the surveillance of any complication of the biliary cirrhosis such as hepatocellular and cholangiocarcinoma.

MR Imaging Findings

At MR imaging, increased peripheral parenchymal signal and atrophy can be seen on T2-weighted images. Hypertrophy with more normal parenchymal signal is present centrally on T1- and T2-weighted sequences. After injection of gadolinium, increased (heterogeneous) enhancement may be present in the peripheral and periportal regions due to the presence of cholangitis. This enhancement may fade or persist in the later phases. Heavily T2-weighted and MRCP sequences may show the abnormal bile ducts, ascites, splenomegaly, and collaterals (Figs. 106.1 – 106.3).

Literature

1. Vitellas KM, Keogan MT, Freed KS, Enns RA, Spritzer CE, Baillie JM, Nelson RC (2000) Radiologic manifestations of sclerosing cholangitis with emphasis on MR cholangiopancreatography. Radiographics 20:959 – 975
2. Ito K, Mitchell DG, Outwater EK, et al. (1999) Primary sclerosing cholangitis: MR imaging features. AJR 172:1527 – 1533
3. Bader TR, Beavers KL, Semelka RC (2003) MR imaging features of primary sclerosing cholangitis: patterns of cirrhosis in relationship to clinical severity of the disease. Radiology 226:675 – 685

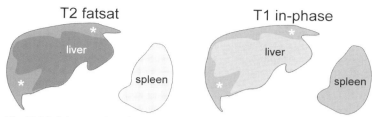

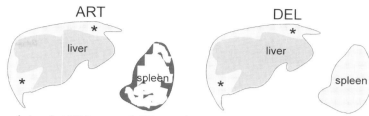

Fig. 106.1. Primary sclerosing cholangitis (PSC) with cirrhosis, drawings. T2 fatsat: peripheral atrophy with increased signal (*) and central hypertrophy is present; T1 in-phase: the central part with hypertrophy has a relatively normal signal; ART: increased diffuse enhancement is present in the periphery of the liver*; DEL: note persistent peripheral enhancement (*)

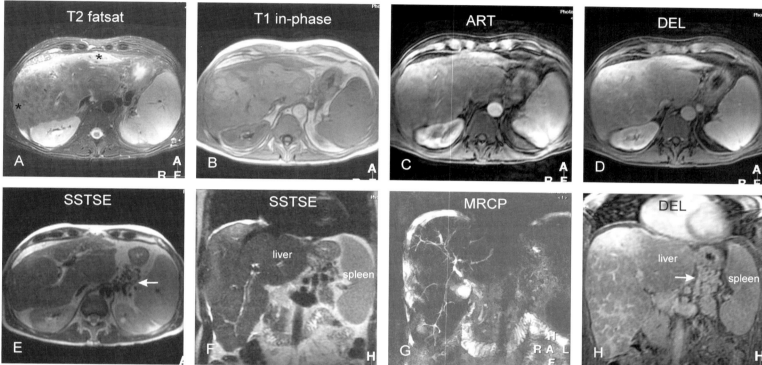

Fig. 106.2. Primary sclerosing cholangitis (PSC) with cirrhosis, MRI findings. A Axial TSE image (T2 fatsat): Peripheral atrophy with increased signal (*) and central hypertrophy is present. **B** Axial in-phase image (T1 in-phase): The central part with hypertrophy has a relatively normal signal. **C** Axial arterial phase image (ART) shows increased diffuse enhancement in the periphery of the liver. **D** Axial delayed image (DEL) shows persistent peripheral and septal enhancement, which indicates the presence of cirrhosis. **E** Axial SSTSE image (SSTSE) shows collaterals (*arrow*), which is a sign of portal hypertension. **F** Coronal SSTSE image (SSTSE) shows the cirrhotic liver with an enlarged spleen, surrounded by ascites. **G** MRCP (MRCP) shows the biliary tree with typical appearance of severe PSC. **H** Axial delayed image (DEL) shows the septal enhancement, which indicates the presence of cirrhosis and collaterals (*arrow*)

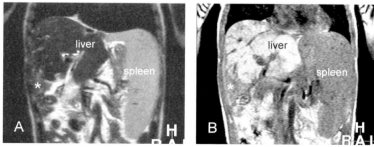

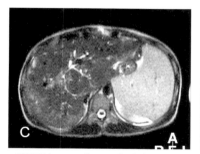

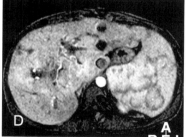

Fig. 106.3. PSC (another patient) with cirrhosis, MR findings. A Coronal SSTSE shows cirrhotic liver with an enlarged spleen. Note the increased signal in the periphery (*). **B** Coronal T1-weighted in-phase image shows decreased signal in the periphery, consistent with peripheral atrophy (*). **C** Axial SSTSE image shows the biliary tree with PSC. **D** Axial arterial phase image shows increased enhancement around the dilated ducts indicating cholangitis

107 Primary Sclerosing Cholangitis V – With Intrahepatic Cholangiocarcinoma

Primary sclerosing cholangitis (PSC) is a chronic liver disease, characterized by inflammation, destruction and fibrosis of the intrahepatic as well as extrahepatic bile ducts, which eventually results in biliary cirrhosis. The diagnosis is based on a combination of cholestatic liver tests, a characteristic appearance at MRCP – stenotic areas alternating with areas of dilatation – and if necessary a liver biopsy specimen showing periportal inflammation, bile duct destruction, cholestasis, and fibrosis. The disease is usually progressive and the only known treatment for advanced, decompensated disease is orthotopic liver transplantation. Cholangiocarcinoma is a well-known complication of PSC. Currently, there are no simple criteria that determine whether a stricture is benign or malignant in patients with PSC. Although lifetime risks in excess of 30% have been reported, the risk in most studies is around 10%. Cholangiocarcinoma may be the first sign of PSC; it can also be found within 2 years after PSC is diagnosed. Ultrasound, CT, and cholangiogram are ineffective in the detection of cholangiocarcinoma in the setting of PSC. We recommend surveillance with MRI/MRCP in combination with serum cancer antigen (CA 19–9).

MR Imaging Findings
State-of-the-art MR imaging, including MRCP and dynamic gadolinium-enhanced sequences, allows early detection of intrahepatic cholangiocarcinoma. Small lesions have predominantly high signal on the T2-weighted sequences. After injection of gadolinium, the lesion typically shows irregular ring-shaped heterogeneous enhancement and washout in the delayed phase. The lesions may show rapid interval growth with even more pronounced arterial enhancement and delayed washout (Figs. 107.1–107.3). Comprehensive MR imaging, including MRCP sequences, is essential for the surveillance of patients with PSC.

Literature
1. Ahrendt SA, Pitt HA, Nakeeb A, et al. (1999) Diagnosis and management of cholangiocarcinoma in primary sclerosing cholangitis. J Gastrointest Surg 3:357–367
2. Kaya M, de Groen PC, Angulo P, et al. (2001) Treatment of cholangiocarcinoma complicating primary sclerosing cholangitis: the Mayo Clinic experience. Am J Gastroenterol 96:1164–1169
3. Goss JA, Shackleton CR, Farmer DG, et al. (1997) Orthotopic liver transplantation for primary sclerosing cholangitis. A 12-year single center experience. Ann Surg 225:472–478
4. de Groen PC, Gores GJ, LaRusso NF, et al. (1999) Biliary tract cancers. NEJM 341:1368–1378

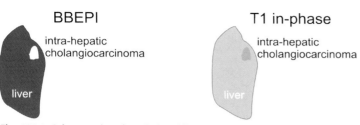

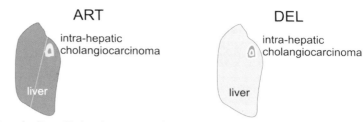

Fig. 107.1. Primary sclerosing cholangitis (PSC) complicated by cirrhosis and an intrahepatic cholangiocarcinoma (ICC), drawings. BBEPI: small ICC is brighter than the liver; **T1 in-phase:** ICC is hypointense to the liver; **ART:** ICC shows irregular ring-shaped enhancement; **DEL:** ICC becomes heterogeneous

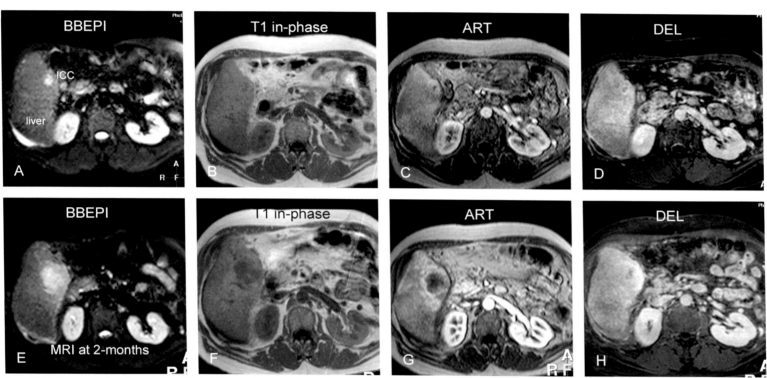

Fig. 107.2. Primary sclerosing cholangitis (PSC) complicated by cirrhosis and an intrahepatic cholangiocarcinoma (ICC), MRI findings. A Axial BBEPI image (BBEPI): ICC is hyperintense to the liver. **B** Axial in-phase image (T1 in-phase): ICC is hypointense to the liver. **C** Axial arterial phase image (ART): ICC shows irregular ring-shaped enhancement. **D** Axial delayed phase im-age (DEL): ICC becomes heterogeneous. **E–H** MRI at 2 months follow-up: ICC has increased in size and enhancement. Note also in the arterial phase image increased enhancement of the liver surrounding the larger lesion, suggesting more widespread disease

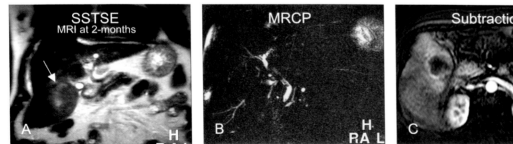

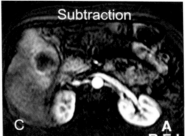

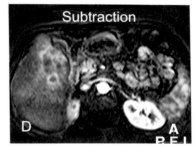

Fig. 107.3. PSC complicated by cirrhosis and an intrahepatic cholangiocarcinoma (ICC), MRI findings at 2 months follow-up (continued). A Coronal SSTSE image shows a cirrhotic liver with a large ICC that is slightly hyperintense to the liver (*arrow*). **B** MRCP shows typical appearance of the biliary tree with PSC. **C, D** Subtraction of the arterial phase images at two anatomic levels shows the ICC growing along the bile ducts toward the liver hilum

108 Primary Sclerosing Cholangitis VI – With Hilar Cholangiocarcinoma

Biliary tract cancer is the second most common primary hepatobiliary cancer, after hepatocellular cancer. Approximately 7500 new cases of biliary tract cancer are diagnosed per year; about 5000 of these are gallbladder cancer, and between 2000 and 3000 are bile-duct cancers. Currently, the term „cholangiocarcinoma" includes intrahepatic, perihilar, and distal extrahepatic tumors of the bile ducts. Perihilar tumors involving the bifurcation of the hepatic duct are also called Klatskin tumors, from Klatskin's original description in 1965. Clinical and biochemical presentation of PSC patients with and without CC does not differ during the year before cancer diagnosis. Liver transplantation is carried out, even in the presence of incidental CC. However, the presence of CC with PSC is associated with poor recipient survival. Recurrent PSC occurs in approximately 9% of cases after liver transplantation but does not affect patient survival. MR imaging with MRCP is the modality of choice in patients with PSC who need surveillance for hilar cholangiocarcinoma.

MR Imaging Findings

In the setting of PSC and CC, the intrahepatic biliary dilatation will be minimal, which hampers the diagnosis if only MRCP (fluid-sensitive) sequence is performed. MR imaging with multiple T1- and T2-weighted sequences, as well as dynamic gadolinium-enhanced imaging, is essential for diagnosis. At MR imaging, hilar CC may show a relatively low signal intensity mass surrounding the hilar region. The low signal is likely caused by desmoplasia within the tumor. The tumor will typically show minimal enhancement. MR imaging also allows the evaluation of liver metastases (Figs. 108.1 – 108.3).

Literature

1. Bergquist A, Glaumann H, Persson B, et al. (1998) Risk factors and clinical presentation of hepatobiliary carcinoma in patients with primary sclerosing cholangitis: a case-control study. Hepatology 27:311 – 316
2. Goss JA, Shackleton CR, Farmer DG, et al. (1997) Orthotopic liver transplantation for primary sclerosing cholangitis. A 12-year single center experience. Ann Surg 225:472 – 478
3. de Groen PC, Gores GJ, LaRusso NF, et al. (1999) Biliary tract cancers. NEJM 341:1368 – 1378

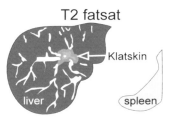
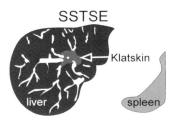
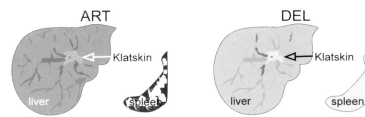

Fig. 108.1. Primary sclerosing cholangitis (PSC) complicated by a hilar cholangio-carcinoma (Klatskin), drawings. T2 fatsat: Klatskin is slightly hypointense to the liver; SSTSE: Klatskin tumor is hypointense to the liver and contains an endo-prosthesis (central dot of high signal); ART: Klatskin shows faint heterogeneous enhancement; DEL: Klatskin is slightly more enhanced than the liver

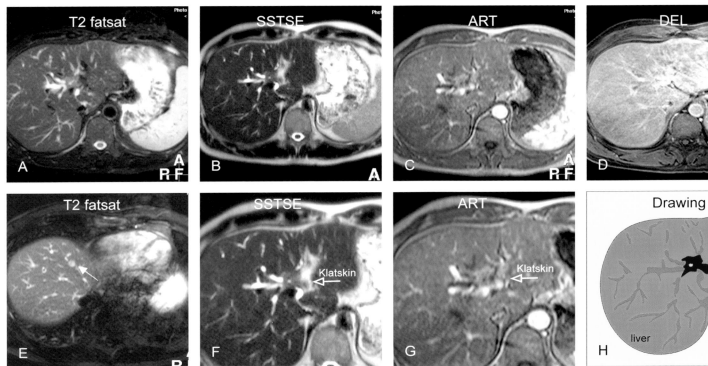

Fig. 108.2. Primary sclerosing cholangitis (PSC) complicated by a hilar cholangio-carcinoma (CC), MRI findings. A Axial TSE image (T2 fatsat): CC is slightly hypointense to the liver. **B** Axial SSTSE image (SSTSE): CC is hypointense to the liver and contains an endoprosthesis (central dot of high signal). **C** Axial arterial phase image (ART): CC shows faint heterogeneous enhancement. **D** Axial delayed phase image (DEL): CC is slightly more enhanced than the liver. **E** Axial TSE image (T2 fatsat) at a higher anatomic level shows a focal lesion consistent with a metastasis (*arrow*). **F** A detailed view of the axial SSTSE image (SSTSE): CC is clearly hypointense to the liver with abruptly ending bile ducts. **G** A detailed view of the axial arterial phase image (ART): CC shows faint heterogeneous enhancement. **H** Drawing shows typical appearance of the bile ducts with PSC that end abruptly due to the hilar cholangiocarcinoma

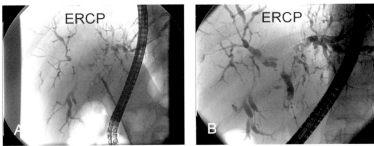
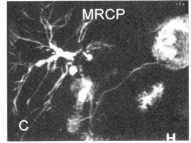
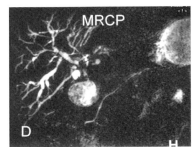

Fig. 108.3. PSC complicated by a hilar cholangiocarcinoma, ERCP versus MRCP. A, B Endoscopic retrograde cholangiopancreatography (ERCP) shows findings with suspicion of a hilar malignancy. **C, D** MRCP (as a part of the MRI examination shown above) confirms the ERCP findings. Additional MRI sequences are essential for a comprehensive evaluation

Part VI

Differential Diagnosis

VI

Differential Diagnosis

109 T2 Bright Liver Lesions

- Evaluation of the T2-weighted sequences (Figs. 109.1A–109.4A):
  - Lesions and the liver differ in appearance in all four examples. The first two types of lesions are however very bright, and multiple, in a non-cirrhotic liver. The third example shows a large moderately bright lesion with a non-cirrhotic liver, whereas in the final example a faintly bright nodule, cirrhotic liver, and ascites constitute the image.
- Evaluation of the T1-weighted sequences (Figs. 109.1B–109.4B):
  - The first two types of lesions are similar in appearance. The third example shows isointense lesions, whereas in the final example a faintly T1 bright nodule is visible.
- Evaluation of the arterial enhancement pattern (Figs. 109.1C – 109.4C):
  - The lesions in the four examples show peripheral nodular, ring-shaped, almost homogeneous, and heterogeneous enhancement patterns, respectively.
- Evaluation of the delayed enhancement pattern (Figs. 109.1D – 109.4D):
  - The lesions in the four examples show persistent, washout without a capsule, homogeneous without a capsule, and washout with a capsular enhancement within a cirrhotic liver, respectively.

Based on the following pertinent combination of findings the lesions can be characterized as:

1. Multiple hemangiomas (T2 bright with peripheral nodular enhancement)
2. Multiple metastases (ring-shaped enhancement and washout without a capsule)
3. Multiple hepatocellular adenomas (T1 isointense, almost homogeneous enhancement without washout or capsule)
4. Multiple hepatocellular carcinomas (cirrhotic liver, slightly T2 bright lesion, heterogeneous enhancement, and washout with capsular enhancement)

T2 very bright lesions T1 dark lesions Peripheral nodular enhancement Persistent enhancement	T2 very bright lesions T1 dark lesions Ring-shaped enhancement Washout	T2 bright-isointense lesions T1 isointense lesions Homogeneous enhancement Fade to isointensity	T2 slightly bright-isointense lesions T1 slightly bright-isointense Heterogeneous enhancement Washout with capsular enhancement
⇓	⇓	⇓	⇓

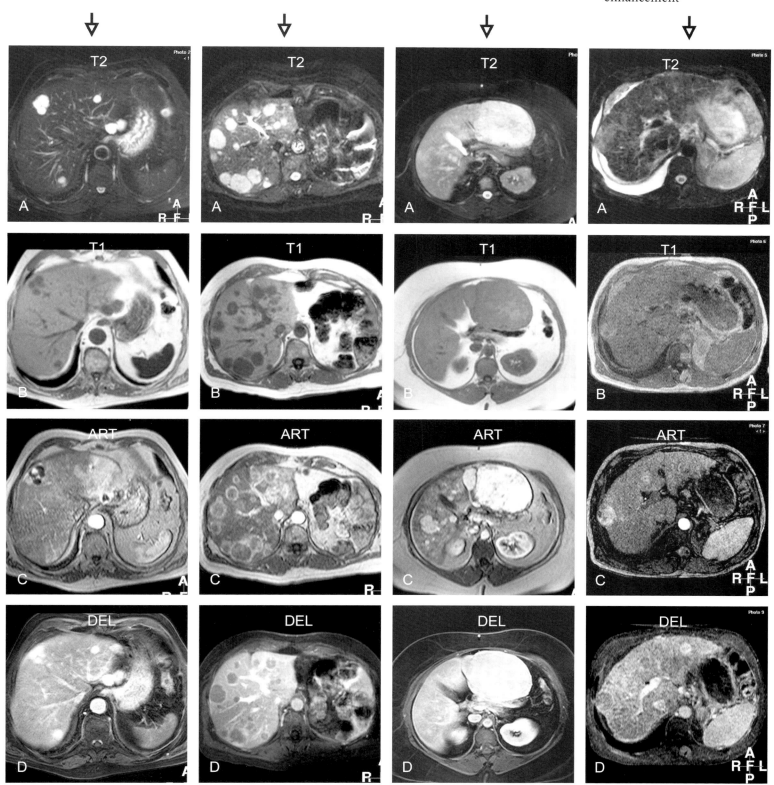

Fig. 109.1. Multiple hemangiomas   **Fig. 109.2.** Multiple metastases   **Fig. 109.3.** Hepatocellular adenomas   **Fig. 109.4.** Hepatocellular carcinomas

110 T1 Bright Liver Lesions

- Evaluation of the T1-weighted sequence (Figs. 110.1A – 110.4A):
  - All lesions have components with bright signal within a non-cirrhotic liver. In the first example, the lesion is surrounded by a dark rim. The second example shows a large lesion with a central bright area. The third example shows a cystic lesion with bright contents in the left liver. The fourth example shows multiple, predominantly bright lesions, including one with a ring-shaped appearance.
- Evaluation of the T2-weighted sequence (Figs. 110.1B – 110.4B):
  - In the first example, the lesion is surrounded by a dark rim with increased thickness. The second example shows a large lesion with a central dark area. The third example shows two bright lesions with cystic and solid components. The fourth example shows one large and small bright lesions.
- Evaluation of the arterial enhancement pattern (Figs. 110.1C – 110.4C):
  - In the first example, the lesion does not show any enhancement (bright signal was present prior to contrast injection). The second lesion shows some heterogeneous enhancement. The third example shows lesions with a thick rim of enhancement. In the fourth example, the lesions show intense enhancement.
- Evaluation of the delayed enhancement pattern (Figs. 110.1D – 110.4D):
  - In the first example, the lesion shows lack of enhancement (mimics washout). The second lesion shows washout with some persistent heterogeneous enhancement. The third example shows lesions with a persistent rim of enhancement. In the fourth example, the lesions show washout and become less intense.

Based on the following pertinent combination of findings the lesions can be characterized as:

1. Hematoma (T1 bright due to methemoglobin with a rim of hemosiderin)
2. Hemorrhagic carcinoid metastasis (suggests metastases; non-specific findings; recommend clinical and somatostatin-scintigraphy correlation)
3. Protein-producing carcinoid metastases (suggests metastases; non-specific findings; recommend clinical and somatostatin-scintigraphy correlation)
4. Melanoma metastasis (T1 bright lesions in a patient with a history of uveal melanoma; intense enhancement and washout are typical for melanin-containing liver metastases)

T1 bright with a dark rim
T2 bright with a dark rim
No enhancement
No enhancement

T1 very bright within a dark
   lesion
T2 dark with a bright lesion
Heterogeneous enhancement
   within the lesion
Washout within the solid lesion

T1 bright and dark lesions
T2 mixed signal intensity
Irregular ring-shaped
   enhancement
Heterogeneous and persistent
   enhancement

T1 (predominantly) bright
   lesions
T2 isointense to very bright
Enhancement of the T1-bright
   parts
Heterogeneous and persistent
   enhancement

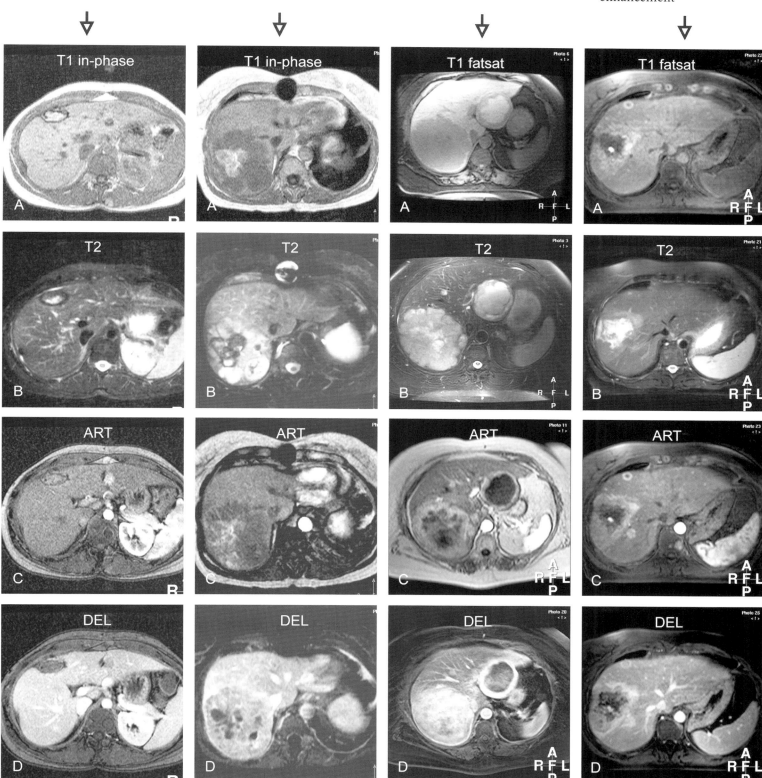

Fig. 110.1. Hematoma after surgery

Fig. 110.2. Hemorrhagic carcinoid metastasis

Fig. 110.3. Protein-producing carcinoid metastasis

Fig. 110.4. Melanoma metastases

111 T2 Bright Central Scar

- Evaluation of the T2-weighted sequence (Figs. 111.1A – 111.4A):
  - All lesions have a bright central scar in non-cirrhotic liver. In the first example, the lesion is bright with a brighter central scar. The second example shows only the bright central scar within an almost isointense lesion. The third and fourth examples show large course central scars within large solitary lesions.
- Evaluation of the arterial enhancement pattern (Figs. 111.1B – 111.4B):
  - In the first example, the lesion shows peripheral nodular enhancement. The second lesion shows very intense homogeneous enhancement with a central scar and septal sparing. The third and fourth lesions show heterogeneous enhancement.
- Evaluation of the portal enhancement pattern (Figs. 111.1C – 111.4C):
  - In the first example, the lesion shows more prominent peripheral nodular enhancement. The following lesion becomes almost isointense. The third and fourth lesions show washout with some capsular enhancement.
- Evaluation of the delayed enhancement pattern (Figs. 111.1D – 111.4D):
  - In the first example, the lesion shows persistent enhancement with central scar sparing. The second lesion became isointense with central scar and septal enhancement.

Based on the following pertinent combination of findings the lesions can be characterized as:

1. Giant hemangioma (T2 bright lesion with a brighter central scar and peripheral nodular enhancement)
2. Focal nodular hyperplasia (isointense on T2; bright well-formed central scar; intense homogeneous arterial enhancement, and enhanced central scar and septa)
3. Hepatocellular carcinoma (large solitary lesion; large coarse central scar; heterogeneous enhancement with washout and capsular enhancement in a non-cirrhotic liver)
4. Hepatocellular carcinoma (idem)

T2 bright lesion
T2 brighter scar
Peripheral nodular enhancement
Persistent enhancement

T2 isointense
T2 slightly brighter scar
Homogeneous enhancement
   fades to isointensity

T2 slightly bright lesion
T2 brighter scar
Heterogeneous enhancement
Washout with capsular
   enhancement

T2 slightly bright lesion
T2 brighter scar
Heterogeneous enhancement
Washout with capsular
   enhancement

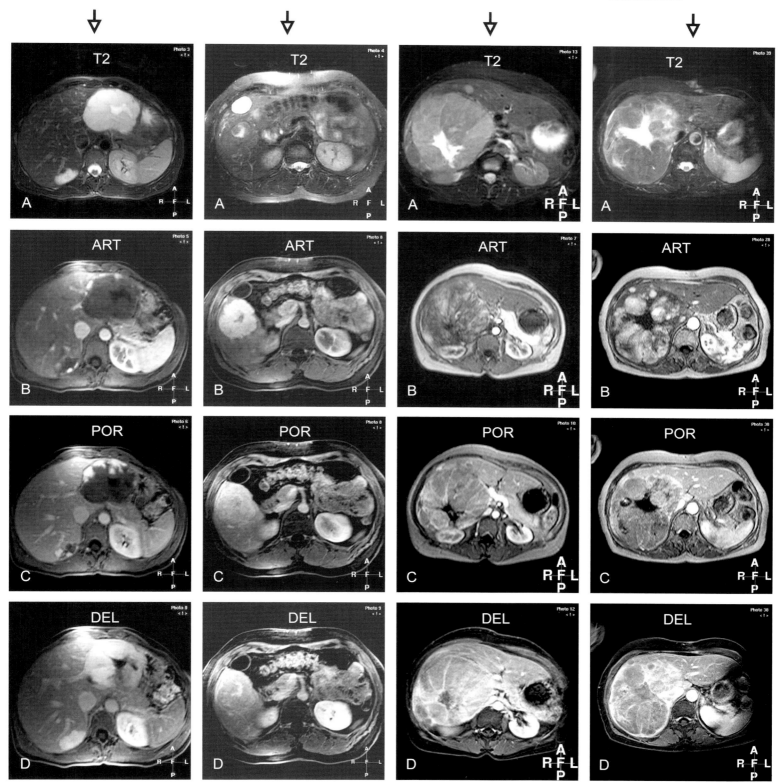

Fig. 111.1. Giant and a mid-size hemangioma

Fig. 111.2. Focal nodular hyperplasia

Fig. 111.3. Hepatocellular carcinoma

Fig. 111.4. Hepatocellular carcinoma

112 Lesions in Fatty Liver

- Evaluation of the opposed- and in-phase T1-weighted sequence (Figs. 112.1A, B – 112.4A, B):
  - All livers become dark on opposed-phase images consistent with fatty liver. The lesions in the first example are isointense and surrounded by a rim of fatty sparing. In the third and fourth examples, the liver is severely fatty infiltrated and the lesions appear bright on opposed-phase images.
- Evaluation of the T2-weighted sequences (Figs. 112.1C – 112.4C):
  - The lesions appear brighter than the liver. The third lesion contains a bright central scar.
- Evaluation of the delayed enhancement pattern (Figs. 112.1D – 112.4D):
  - In the first example, the lesions show some persistent perilesional enhancement. The lesions in the third example become almost isointense. The third lesion shows enhanced central scar and the lesion appears brighter within a strongly fatty liver after fat suppression. In the fourth example, the lesions appear brighter within a strongly fatty liver after fat suppression.

Based on the following pertinent combination of findings the lesions can be characterized as:

1. Colorectal carcinoma metastases (T2 bright lesions; persistent perifocal fatty sparing and enhancement)
2. Focal fatty sparing (isointense on in-phase T1; appear bright on fat-suppressed T2 and show faintly more enhancement)
3. Focal nodular hyperplasia (the appearance of this classical FNH is changed due to the severe fatty infiltration of the surrounding liver)
4. Hepatocellular adenoma (strong fatty infiltration of the liver is common in multiple adenomas)

T1 opposed-phase: lesions surrounded by persistent high signal of non-steatosis
T1 in-phase: hypointense lesions
T2: hyperintense lesions delayed phase: irregular ring-enhancement

T1 opposed-phase: lesions hyperintense
T1 in-phase: no lesions are visible; liver has normal signal
T2: some areas show high signal delayed phase; some lesions show faint persistent enhancement

T1 opposed-phase: lesion appears hyperintense to the dark liver
T1 in-phase: lesion is hypointense
T2: lesion is hyperintense to the liver with a bright central scar delayed phase: lesion shows enhanced central scar

T1 opposed-phase: lesions appear hyperintense to the dark liver
T1 in-phase: lesions are hypointense
T2: lesions are slightly hyperintense delayed phase: lesions show homogeneous enhancement

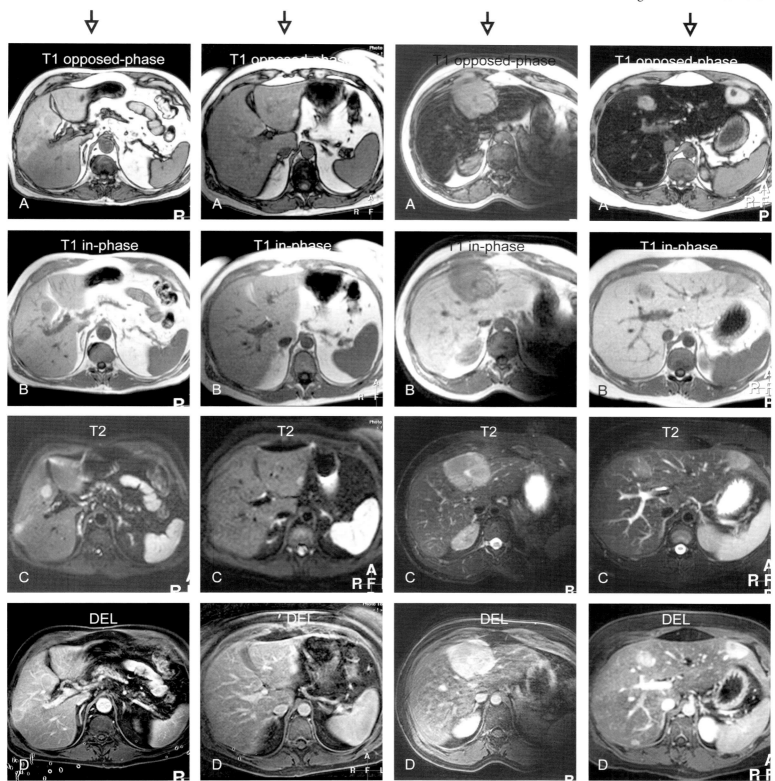

Fig. 112.1. Colorectal carcinoma metastases

Fig. 112.2. Focal fatty sparing

Fig. 112.3. Focal nodular hyperplasia

Fig. 112.4. Hepatocellular adenomas

Part VII

Appendices

113 Appendix I: MR Imaging Technique and Protocol

Typical MR imaging protocol (at 1.5T) for the liver should contain the following or similar types of sequences (**Fig. 113.1**):

1) *Coronal single-Shot turbo or fast spin-echo (SSTSE or SSFSE) or Half-Fourier Single-shot Turbo spin-Echo (HASTE)*: repetition time (TR), 8; echo time (TE), 120 msec; flip angle, 90°; acquisition time, 20 seconds (a single breath hold sequence) → serves as a localizer and provides an overview of the anatomy.

2) *Axial SSTSE with relatively short (80 msec) and longer (120–180 msec) TE*; acquisition time 20–25 seconds (two breath holds) → detection and characterization of fluid-containing liver lesions such as cysts, hemangiomas, and biliary hamartomas.

3) *Axial black-blood echo planar imaging (BBEPI)*: TR, 3400 ms (minimum); TE, 60 ms; frequency and phase matrix 144×256; filed-of-view, 310–350 cm with a rectangular FOV 80%; EPI factor, 109; sensitivity encoding (SENSE) factor, 2; half scan factor 60%; b-value 20; acquisition time 25 sec; Bandwidth per pixel in the phase encoding direction was 9.2 Hz and in the EPI readout direction 1387.1 Hz; and the polarity of the phase encoding gradient was set to posterior → provides T2-weighted images in breath hold with better liver-to-lesion contrast than the standard T2-weighted turbo spin-echo with fat suppression.

4) *Axial two-dimensional (2D) dual gradient echo (both in- and opposed-phase as one sequence in a single breath hold)*: TR, 150–170 msec; TE, 4.2/2.1 msec; flip angle 80–90°; acquisition time, 20 sec → provides T1-information and detects focal or diffuse fatty infiltration in tumors and tissues.

5) *Axial dynamic three-dimensional fat-suppressed gradient echo sequence (VIBE; THRIVE; LAVA)*: TR, minimum; TE, minimum; flip angle, 10–15°; slice thickness 4–8 mm, interpolated to about 60 overlapping reconstructed sections of 4–2 mm; bandwidth, 62 kHz; acquisition time, 20–25 sec in a single breath-hold → arterial phase is the single most important sequence and serves for the detection of liver lesions; all phases are utilized for the characterization based on the enhancement patterns of lesions.

6) *Coronal delayed three-dimensional fat-suppressed gradient echo sequence*: TR/TE, minimum; flip angle, 10–15°; slice thickness 4–6 mm, interpolated to about 40 overlapping reconstructed sections of 2–3 mm; bandwidth, 62 kHz; acquisition time, 20–25 sec in a single breath-hold → provides information about the persistent enhancement of lesions such as hemangiomas, capsular enhancement of hepatocellular carcinomas, and peritoneal spread of disease, and biliary tree abnormalities.

7) *Axial T2-weighted turbo or fast spin-echo (TSE or FSE) with fat-saturation*: TR, 2000 msec; TE, 100 msec; flip angle, 90°; acquisition time, 2–5 minutes (respiratory-triggered) → traditionally this sequence has been used for the detection of solid liver lesions. Most likely, this sequence will be replaced by newer T2-weighted sequences such as BBEPI.

8) *Magnetic resonance cholangiopancreatography (MRCP)* consists of a 2D heavily T2-weighted sequence with a thick slab of 30–60 mm to provide an overview of the biliary and pancreatic anatomy: TR, 8; TE, 800 msec; flip angle, 90°; acquisition time, 2 sec per slab which are typically acquired as a radial scan of 5–10 slabs around the common bile duct. This thick slab MRCP is often combined with thin slice coronal SSTSE with a TE of about 180 msec and thin sections (< 5 mm).

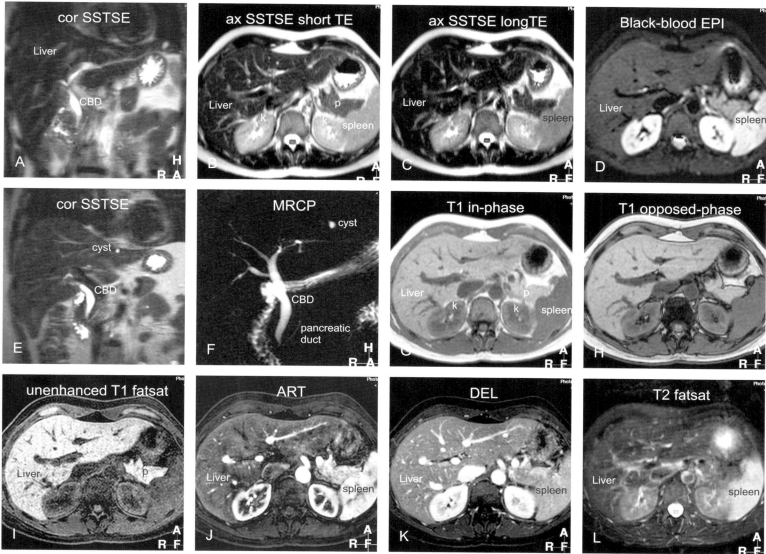

Fig. 113.1. Appendix I: Typical liver MRI protocol. A Coronal single-shot turbo spin-echo (cor SSTSE) image provides an overview of the anatomy (CBD = common bile duct). **B** Axial SSTSE (ax SSTSE) image with a short echo time (TE = 80 ms) shows the liver darker than the spleen (p = pancreas; k = kidneys). **C** Axial SSTSE (ax SSTSE) image with a longer echo time (TE = 120 ms) shows decreased signal in the liver, spleen, pancreas (which indicates the solid nature of the tissues). **D** Axial T2- and diffusion-weighted black-blood echo planar imaging (BBEPI) shows the vessels dark with excellent liver-to-spleen contrast (most liver lesions follow the signal of the spleen). **E, F** Coronal thin-slice (5 mm) and thick-slab (40 mm) SSTSE breath-hold images as part of the MRCP protocol show the relationship of the fluid-filled structures (biliary tree; the pancreatic duct; a cyst) to the solid tissues as well as an overview of the fluid-filled structures, respectively.

G, H Axial T1-weighted in- and opposed-phase gradient-echo (GRE) images show the spleen darker than the liver indicating good T1-weighting; these sequences are sensitive to a small amount of fat. **I** Axial three-dimensional (3D) unenhanced T1-weighted GRE image with fat suppression shows the liver and pancreas (p) with high signal intensity. **J** Axial 3D arterial phase GRE image (ART) shows intense enhancement of the arterial vessels, some enhancement of the portal vein (pv), no enhancement of the hepatic veins (hv), heterogeneous enhancement of the spleen, and intense enhancement of the pancreas. **K** Axial delayed phase image (DEL) shows enhancement of the hepatic veins (hv) and homogeneous enhancement of the organs. **L** Axial respiratory-triggered, fat-suppressed, T2-weighted image (T2 fatsat) with moderate T2-weighting shows spleen with higher signal than the liver; note that – in contrast to the BBEPI – the intrahepatic vessels are bright

114 Appendix II: Liver Segmental and Vascular Anatomy

Segmental Anatomy

Based on external appearance, four lobes of the liver can be distinguished: right, left, quadrate, and caudate. The falciform ligament (fl) divides the liver into the right and left anatomic lobes. The ligament venosum (lv) divides the caudate lobe from the left lobe. In 1957, two classification systems were described. Goldsmith et al. described the right and left lobes and four segments: lateral, medial, anterior and posterior. Each segment consists of two subsegments: superior and inferior. Couinaud described eight segments (Fig. 114.1A–114.1G): one for the caudate lobe (segment I), three on the left (segments II, III and IV) and four on the right (segments V, VI, VII and VIII). The caudate lobe receives vessels both from the left and right branches of the portal vein and hepatic artery: its hepatic veins are independent and drain directly into the inferior vena cava (ivc). Recent studies suggest that the caudate lobe could be divided into a left part or Spiegel's lobe or segment I and the right part or segment IX or paracaval portion.

Hepatic Venous Drainage

The normal hepatic venous anatomy consists of three main venous tributaries that drain into the ivc. The right hepatic vein (rhv) drains liver segments V–VII, the middle hepatic vein (mhv) drains segments IV, V, and VIII, and the left hepatic vein (lhv) drains segments II and III. Accessory veins are a common cause of surgical complications. An accessory rhv occurs in 53 % of patients and two accessory hepatic veins in 12 %, and an accessory vein draining the caudate lobe in 12 %. The most common hepatic venous variant is an accessory inferior rhv (Fig. 114.1I).

Hepatic Arterial Supply

The so-called „normal" hepatic arterial supply occurs only in a small majority of subjects. In 55 % of cases, the common hepatic artery (cha) gives rise to the right hepatic artery (rha), middle hepatic artery (mha), and left hepatic artery (lha) (114.1J); in 11 %, the rha originates from the superior mesenteric artery (sma); in 10 %, a replaced lha is present; in 8 % the rha, mha, and lha arise from the cha with an accessory lha from the left gastric artery (lga); in 7 %, the rha, mha, and lha arise from the cha with an accessory rha from the lga; and in 4.5 %, the entire ha root arises from the sma (Fig. 114.1K). In addition, there are more infrequent variants.

Portal Venous Supply

The normal portal venous anatomy consists of the main portal trunk and its two branching vessels, the right and left portal veins (Fig. 114.1L). Portal venous variants account for about 20 % of all important variants.

Literature

1. Goldsmith NA, Woodburne RT (1957) Surgical anatomy pertaining to liver resection. Surg Gynecol Obstetr 195:310–8
2. Couinaud C (1999) Liver anatomy: portal (and suprahepatic) or biliary segmentation. Digest Surg 16:459–67
3. Abdalla EK, Vauthey JN, Couinaud C (2002) The caudate lobe of the liver. Implications of embryology and anatomy for surgery. Surg Oncol Clin N Am 11:835–48
4. Sahani D, Mehta A, Blake M, et al. (2004) Preoperative hepatic vascular evaluation with CT and MR angiography: implications for surgery. Radiographics 24:1367–1380

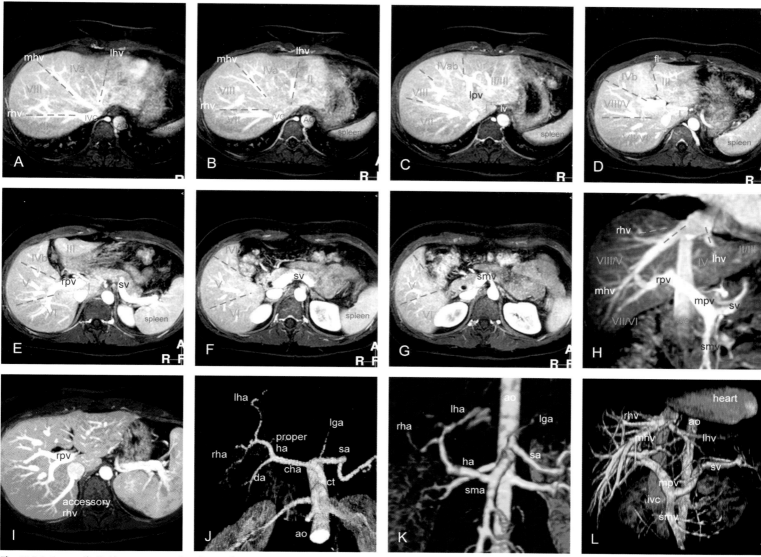

Fig. 114.1. Appendix II: Liver segmental and vascular anatomy. A–G Axial maximum intensity projection (MIP) based on the three-dimensional (3D) gadolinium-enhanced delayed phase gradient echo images at various levels shows the hepatic segments (I–VIII), three hepatic veins, portal vein, and ligaments. **H** Coronal reformat shows the relationship among the hepatic segments, three hepatic veins, portal vein (formed by the splenic and superior mesenteric veins), and inferior vena cava. **I** MIP based on the axial gadolinium-enhanced delayed phase gradient echo image shows an accessory right hepatic vein draining directly into the IVC. **J, K** 3D surface-shaded renderings based on the arterial phase of the gadolinium-enhanced imaging show the normal hepatic arterial vessels (about 55%) and a variant with replaced hepatic artery from the superior mesenteric artery (about 10%). **L** 3D surface-shaded rendering based on the delayed phase of the gadolinium-enhanced imaging rendering shows the normal portal as well as hepatic veins in relation to the aorta and inferior vena cava.

ao = aorta
ct = celiac trunk
da = duodenal artery
fl = falciforme ligament
ha = hepatic artery
ivc = inferior vena cava
lga = left gastric artery
lv = ligament venosum
lha = left hepatic artery
lhv = left hepatic vein
lpv = left portal vein

mhv = middle hepatic vein
mpv = main portal vein
rha = right hepatic artery
rhv = right hepatic vein
rpv = right portal vein
sma = superior mesenteric artery
sa = splenic artery
smv = superior mesenteric vein
sv = splenic vein
I–VIII = indicate the liver segments from 1 to 8

Subject Index